Cardiac Emergencies in the ICU

Editors

SHASHANK S. DESAI
NITIN PURI

CRITICAL CARE CLINICS

www.criticalcare.theclinics.com

Consulting Editor
RICHARD W. CARLSON

July 2014 • Volume 30 • Number 3

ELSEVIER

1600 John F. Kennedy Boulevard • Suite 1800 • Philadelphia, Pennsylvania, 19103-2899

http://www.theclinics.com

CRITICAL CARE CLINICS Volume 30, Number 3
July 2014 ISSN 0749-0704, ISBN-13: 978-0-323-31160-1

Editor: Patrick Manley
Developmental Editor: Casey Jackson

Critical Care Clinics (ISSN: 0749-0704) is published quarterly by Elsevier Inc., 360 Park Avenue South, New York, NY 10010-1710. Months of issue are January, April, July, and October. Business and Editorial Offices: 1600 John F. Kennedy Blvd., Suite 1800, Philadelphia, PA 19103-2899. Customer Service Office: 6277 Sea Harbor Drive, Orlando, FL 32887-4800. Periodicals postage paid at New York, NY and additional mailing offices. Subscription prices are $210.00 per year for US individuals, $503.00 per year for US institution, $100.00 per year for US students and residents, $255.00 per year for Canadian individuals, $630.00 per year for Canadian institutions, $300.00 per year for international individuals, $630.00 per year for international institutions and $150.00 per year for Canadian and foreign students/residents. To receive student/resident rate, orders must be accompanied by name of affiliated institution, date of term, and the signature of program/residency coordinator on institution letterhead. Orders will be billed at individual rate until proof of status is received. Foreign air speed delivery is included in all *Clinics* subscription prices. All prices are subject to change without notice. POSTMASTER: Send address changes to *Critical Care Clinics*, Elsevier Periodicals Customer Service, 11830 Westline Industrial Drive, St. Louis, MO 63146. **Customer Service: 1-800-654-2452 (US). From outside of the US, call 1-314-447-8871. Fax: 1-314-447-8029. E-mail: journalscustomerservice-usa@ elsevier.com (for print support) or journalsonlinesupport-usa@elsevier.com (for online support).**

Reprints. For copies of 100 or more of articles in this publication, please contact the Commercial Reprints Department, Elsevier Inc., 360 Park Avenue South, New York, NY 10010-1710. Tel.: 212-633-3874; Fax: 212-633-3820; E-mail: reprints@elsevier.com.

Critical Care Clinics is also published in Spanish by Editorial Inter-Medica, Junin 917, 1ᵉʳ A, 1113, Buenos Aires, Argentina.

Critical Care Clinics is covered in *MEDLINE/PubMed (Index Medicus)*, *EMBASE/Excerpta Medica*, *Current Concepts/Clinical Medicine*, *ISI/BIOMED*, and *Chemical Abstracts*.

Contributors

CONSULTING EDITOR

RICHARD W. CARLSON, MD, PhD
Chairman Emeritus, Director, Medical Intensive Care Unit, Department of Medicine, Maricopa Medical Center; Professor, University of Arizona College of Medicine; Professor, Department of Medicine, Mayo Graduate School of Medicine, Phoenix, Arizona

EDITORS

SHASHANK S. DESAI, MD
Heart Failure/Transplant Program, Inova Fairfax Hospital, Falls Church, Virginia

NITIN PURI, MD, FCCP
Attending, Pulmonary/Critical Care; Medical Director, Cardiovascular Intensive Care Unit, Inova Fairfax Hospital, Falls Church, Virginia

AUTHORS

LAITH ALTAWEEL, MD
Associate Director, Neuroscience Intensive Care, Department of Medicine, Inova Fairfax Hospital, Falls Church, Virginia

M. KAMRAN ATHAR, MD
Assistant Professor, Division of Critical Care and Neurotrauma, Departments of Neurological Surgery and Medicine, Jefferson College of Medicine, Thomas Jefferson University, Philadelphia, Pennsylvania

EDO Y. BIRATI, MD
Division of Cardiology, Perelman School of Medicine, University of Pennsylvania, Philadelphia, Pennsylvania

LINDA BOGAR, MD
Cardiac Surgeon, Inova Fairfax Hospital; Cardiac Vascular & Thoracic Surgery Associates, Falls Church, Virginia

ALI BOUSHAHRI, MD
Fellow, Cardiovascular Medicine, George Washington University, Medical Faculty Associates, Washington, DC

NELSON BURTON, MD
Cardiac Surgeon, Cardiac Vascular & Thoracic Surgery Associates, Inova Fairfax Hospital, Falls Church, Virginia

LAURENCE W. BUSSE, MD
Section of Critical Care Medicine, Department of Medicine, Inova Fairfax Medical Center, Falls Church, Virginia

JOSEPHINE C. CHOU, MD, MS
Heart and Vascular Institute, University of Pittsburgh Medical Center, Pittsburgh, Pennsylvania

JENNIFER A. COWGER, MD, MS
Heart Failure and Transplant Program, St Vincent Heart Center, Indianapolis, Indiana

CHANDAN M. DEVIREDDY, MD
Associate Professor of Medicine, Division of Cardiology, Department of Medicine, Emory University School of Medicine, Emory University Hospital Midtown, Atlanta, Georgia

PAUL EISENBERG, MD
Assistant Professor, Department of Anesthesiology and Perioperative Medicine, University Hospitals Case Medical Center, Case Western Reserve University School of Medicine, Cleveland, Ohio

MITHIL GAJERA, MD
Department of Internal Medicine, Christiana Care Health System, Newark, Delaware

SASCHA N. GOONEWARDENA, MD
Division of Cardiovascular Medicine, Department of Internal Medicine, University of Michigan Medical Center, Ann Arbor, Michigan

AKRAM W. IBRAHIM, MD
Division of Cardiology, Department of Medicine, Emory University School of Medicine, Emory University Hospital Midtown, Atlanta, Georgia

MOHAMAD KENAAN, MD
Division of Cardiovascular Medicine, Department of Internal Medicine, University of Michigan Medical Center, Ann Arbor, Michigan

CHRISTOPHER KING, MD, FACP, FCCP
Medical Critical Care Service, Inova Fairfax Hospital, Alexandria, Virginia

JOHN C. KLICK, MD
Assistant Professor, Department of Anesthesiology and Perioperative Medicine, University Hospitals Case Medical Center, Case Western Reserve University School of Medicine, Cleveland, Ohio

CHRISTOPHER W. MAY, MD, FACP, FACC
Advanced Heart Failure and Cardiac Transplant Program, Inova Fairfax Hospital, Falls Church, Virginia

JESSICA MITCHELL, MD
Fellow, PGY-5, Department of Critical Care Medicine, Cooper University Hospital, Camden, New Jersey

HOWARD NEARMAN, MD, MBA
Professor, Department of Anesthesiology and Perioperative Medicine; Professor of Surgery, University Hospitals Case Medical Center, Case Western Reserve University School of Medicine, Cleveland, Ohio

LAUREN NG, MD, MPH
Fellow, Division of Critical Care and Neurotrauma and Cerebrovascular Diseases, Departments of Neurology and Neurological Surgery, Thomas Jefferson University, Philadelphia, Pennsylvania

NICHOLAS PESA, MD
Assistant Professor, Department of Anesthesiology and Perioperative Medicine, University Hospitals Case Medical Center, Case Western Reserve University School of Medicine, Cleveland, Ohio

J. EDUARDO RAME, MD, MPhil
Division of Cardiology, Perelman School of Medicine, University of Pennsylvania, Philadelphia, Pennsylvania

THOMAS C. RIDDELL, MD
Division of Cardiology, Department of Medicine, Emory University School of Medicine, Emory University Hospital Midtown, Atlanta, Georgia

PALAK SHAH, MD, MS
Inova Translational Medicine Institute, Inova Fairfax Hospital, Falls Church, Virginia

OKSANA A. SHLOBIN, MD
Assistant Director, Advanced Lung Disease and Transplant Program, Inova Fairfax Hospital, Falls Church, Virginia

JEFFREY J. TEUTEBERG, MD
Assistant Professor of Medicine; Medical Director, Advanced Heart Failure, Heart and Vascular Institute, University of Pittsburgh Medical Center, Pittsburgh, Pennsylvania

CYNTHIA TRACY, MD
Director, Clinical Cardiac Electrophysiology; Professor, Department of Medicine, George Washington University, Washington, DC

JASON S. VOURLEKIS, MD
Section of Critical Care Medicine, Department of Medicine, Inova Fairfax Medical Center, Falls Church, Virginia

JING WANG, PhD
Department of Medicine, Inova Fairfax Hospital, Falls Church, Virginia

JEFFREY WILLIAMS, MD
Medical Critical Care Service, Inova Fairfax Hospital, Falls Church, Virginia

Contents

This article discusses the approach to the management of myocardial infarction (MI) in the intensive care unit setting. It includes an overview of the definition, classification, and underlying pathologic conditions of acute MI and specifically discusses the diagnosis and management of unstable angina, non-ST elevation MI, and ST-segment elevation MI. Diagnosis and treatment of the acute complications of MI are also reviewed.

Patients admitted to the intensive care unit (ICU) are at increased risk for cardiac arrhythmias, the most common of which can be subdivided into tachyarrhythmias and bradyarrhythmias. These arrhythmias may be the primary reason for ICU admission or may occur in the critically ill patient. This article addresses the occurrence of arrhythmias in the critically ill patient, and discusses their pathophysiology, implications, recognition, and management.

Cardiogenic shock is the most common cause of in-hospital mortality for patients who have suffered a myocardial infarction. Mortality exceeds 50% and management is focused on a rapid diagnosis of cardiogenic shock, restoration of coronary blood flow through early revascularization, complication management, and maintenance of end-organ homeostasis. Besides revascularization, inotropes and vasodilators are potent medical therapies to assist the failing heart. Pulmonary arterial catheters are an important adjunctive tool to assess patient hemodynamics, but their use should be limited to select patients in cardiogenic shock.

The assessment of the circulating volume and efficiency of tissue perfusion is necessary in the management of critically ill patients. The controversy surrounding pulmonary artery catheterization has led to a new wave of minimally invasive hemodynamic monitoring technologies, including echocardiographic and Doppler imaging, pulse wave analysis, and bioimpedance. This article reviews the principles, advantages, and limitations of these technologies and the clinical contexts in which they may be clinically useful.

Pulmonary embolism (PE) is a common diagnosis in critical care. Depending on the severity of clot burden, the clinical picture ranges from nearly asymptomatic to cardiovascular collapse. The signs and symptoms of PE are nonspecific. The clinician must have a high index of suspicion to make the diagnosis. PE is risk stratified into 3 categories: low-risk, submassive, and massive. Submassive PE remains the most challenging with regard to initial and long-term management. Little consensus exists as to the appropriate tests for risk stratification and therapy. This article reviews the current literature and a suggested approach to these patients.

Right ventricular failure complicates several commonly encountered conditions in the intensive care unit. Right ventricular dilation and paradoxic movement of the interventricular septum on echocardiography establishes the diagnosis. Right heart catheterization is useful in establishing the specific cause and aids clinicians in management. Principles of treatment focus on reversal of the underlying cause, optimization of right ventricular preload and contractility, and reduction of right ventricular afterload. Mechanical support with right ventricular assist device or veno-arterial extracorporeal membrane oxygenation can be used in select patients who fail to improve with optimal medical therapy.

Patients with cardiothoracic surgical emergencies are frequently admitted to the ICU, either prior to operative intervention or after surgery. Recognition and appropriate timing of operative intervention are key factors in improving outcomes. A collaborative team approach with the cardiothoracic service is imperative in managing this patient population.

The care of the cardiac surgical patient postoperatively is fraught with several complications because of the nature of the surgical procedure itself and the common comorbidities of this patient population. Most complications occurring in the immediate postoperative period are categorized by organ system, and their pathophysiology is presented. Current diagnostic approaches and treatment options are offered. Preventive measures, where appropriate, are also included in the discussion.

CRITICAL CARE CLINICS

Preface

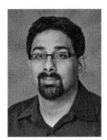 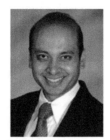

Nitin Puri, MD, FCCP   Shashank S. Desai, MD
Editors

Critical Care and Cardiology have a deeply intertwined history. Modern intensive care units have significant roots in the Coronary Care Units established in the 1960s. The idea of cohorting cardiac patients in a specific location led to a standardization of the management of acute myocardial infarction patients. This was accomplished with continuous ECG monitoring, CPR capabilities, and trained nurses that could start resuscitation. A dramatic reduction in myocardial infarction mortality occurred and the idea spread worldwide. Today, it would be difficult to find an Intensivist who would not know how to treat a myocardial infarction and understand the importance of the "golden hour." A similar revolution is ongoing in the shared space between Critical Care, Cardiology, and Cardiac Surgery with new therapeutic options to treat diseases previously thought intractable.

In this issue of the *Critical Care Clinics*, we seek to explore the common ground between these fields. Although mechanical circulatory support (MCS) devices have been around for more than 50 years, the growing potential for their use in the critically ill is a relatively new phenomenon. The indications, the pitfalls, and the therapeutic potential of different MCS devices are reviewed in this issue. The perplexing disease processes of right heart failure and submassive pulmonary embolisms are similarly delved into. Paradigm-shifting therapies are considered in the Neurologic Complications of Cardiac Emergencies article. "Perioperative Complications of Cardiac Surgery and Postoperative Care" are examined as Intensivists become more involved in the care of cardiac surgery patients. The new pharmaceutical and the MCS options for critically ill cardiac patients are evolving into a new subdivision of critical care that all Intensivists must be familiar with.

Each editor would like to thank his colleagues, who took their time out of their schedules to share their expertise about this rapidly expanding field. We both appreciate those who have guided us in our careers as mentors, colleagues, and trainees. There is much that can be learned from all around us, if we choose to listen carefully. Dr Nitin Puri would like to thank his father, Dr Vinod Puri, and his mother, Dr Kasturi Puri, for his love of medicine, and Dr Richard Carlson, for showing him the path to success as a physician and an educator. Dr Desai would like to express special gratitude for the constant support and encouragement of his loving wife, Nina Phatak, without whom

Crit Care Clin 30 (2014) xi–xii
http://dx.doi.org/10.1016/j.ccc.2014.05.002
0749-0704/14/$ – see front matter © 2014 Elsevier Inc. All rights reserved.

success would not be possible, and children, Dhilan, Annika, and Lara, who make everyday activities worthwhile. Both editors would like to thank their colleagues at the Inova Fairfax Heart Institute and the Heart Failure/Transplant Program at Inova Fairfax Hospital for seemingly daily turning miracles into reality.

Nitin Puri, MD, FCCP
Pulmonary/Critical Care
Cardiovascular Intensive Care Unit
Inova Fairfax Hospital
Falls Church, VA 22042, USA

Shashank S. Desai, MD
Heart Failure/Transplant Program
Inova Fairfax Hospital
Inova Heart and Vascular Institute
3300 Gallows Road
Falls Church, VA 22042, USA

E-mail addresses:
purimon@gmail.com (N. Puri)
shashank.desai@inova.org (S.S. Desai)

Erratum

An error was made in the July 2013 (Volume 29, Issue 3) issue of *Critical Care Clinics*. On page 757 on the title page of the article "Infections in the Elderly" the names of the co-authors have been transposed. The authors' names should read: Hans Jürgen Heppner MD, MHBA, Cornel Sieber MD, Peter Walger MD, Philipp Bahrmann MD, Katrin Singler MD.

Crit Care Clin 30 (2014) xiii
http://dx.doi.org/10.1016/j.ccc.2014.05.001
0749-0704/14/$ – see front matter © 2014 Elsevier Inc. All rights reserved.

Erratum

Acute Myocardial Infarction

Akram W. Ibrahim, MD, Thomas C. Riddell, MD, Chandan M. Devireddy, MD*

KEYWORDS

- Myocardial infarction • Coronary artery disease • Unstable angina
- Fibrinolytic therapy • Primary percutaneous coronary intervention

KEY POINTS

- Cases of acute coronary syndrome demand rapid treatment which varies depending on the underlying type.
- In the intensive care unit setting, chest pain demands immediate evaluation.
- The differential diagnoses to consider with chest pain are many, some of which are benign; but morbid consequences can ensue if high-risk features are not recognized.
- Many causes may be stratified by a focused history alone; but most presentations of chest pain will still require additional testing, such as electrocardiograms, imaging, and laboratory data for a reliable diagnosis.

APPROACH TO PATIENTS WITH ACUTE CHEST PAIN IN THE INTENSIVE CARE UNIT

In the intensive care unit (ICU) setting, chest pain demands immediate evaluation. The differential diagnoses to consider with chest pain are many, some of which are benign; but morbid consequences can ensue if high-risk features are not recognized. Many causes may be stratified by a focused history alone; but most presentations of chest pain will still require additional testing, such as electrocardiograms (ECG), imaging, and laboratory data for a reliable diagnosis.

Acute myocardial infarction (AMI) is the most feared cause of chest pain, but a wide range of cardiac and noncardiac pathophysiology may explain new-onset chest discomfort. It is important to review the common causes of chest pain in the ICU setting not related to AMI.

Common causes of chest pain in ICU setting

- Pericarditis
- Aortic dissection

Disclosure statement: Chandan M. Devireddy, advisory board (2013), Medtronic. The authors have no financial conflicts related to the content of this article.
Division of Cardiology, Department of Medicine, Emory University School of Medicine, Emory University Hospital Midtown, Medical Office Tower, 550 Peachtree Street, Atlanta, GA 30308, USA
* Corresponding author. Emory University School of Medicine, Emory University Hospital Midtown, Medical Office Tower, 6th floor, 550 Peachtree Street, Atlanta, GA 30308.
E-mail address: cdevire@emory.edu

Crit Care Clin 30 (2014) 341–364
http://dx.doi.org/10.1016/j.ccc.2014.03.010
0749-0704/14/$ – see front matter © 2014 Elsevier Inc. All rights reserved.
criticalcare.theclinics.com

- Pulmonary embolism
- Pneumothorax
- Musculoskeletal pain
- Acute myocarditis
- Recommendation for initial assessment
  - A focused history and physical
  - Vital signs (including invasive hemodynamic monitoring if necessary)
  - ECG
  - Chest radiograph or further imaging modality
  - Cardiac biomarkers

Pericarditis

Acute pericarditis refers to inflammation of the pericardial sac, which consists of 2 tissue layers encasing the heart and great vessels in the mediastinum. The potential causes of pericarditis are many and may present as an isolated disorder or part of a systemic process. Although most episodes of pericarditis can be effectively managed with medications, certain high-risk features should be noted in the ICU setting[1]:

High-risk features of acute pericarditis

- Fever and leukocytosis
- Large pericardial effusion or evidence of cardiac tamponade
- Acute trauma
- Recent thoracic surgical procedure or instrumentation
- Anticoagulant therapy
- Immunosuppressed state

Certain specific auscultatory phenomena may occur in acute pericarditis. The pericardial friction rub is the most common finding and is caused by friction between the 2 inflamed pericardial layers.[2] The murmur is generally loudest along the left sternal border and consists of scratching or scraping sounds between S1 and S2.[3]

ECG findings of pericarditis are varied and change with the acuity of the inflammatory process. Typical ECG findings are listed next[4]:

Stage 1 is seen in the first few hours to days and is characterized by diffuse ST elevation (typically concave up) with reciprocal ST depression in leads aVR and V1. There is also an atrial current of injury, reflected by the elevation of the PR segment in lead aVR and depression of the PR segment in other limb leads and in the left chest leads, primarily V5 and V6 (**Fig. 1**).

Stage 2, typically seen in the first week, is characterized by normalization of the ST and PR segments.

Stage 3 is characterized by the development of diffuse T-wave inversions, generally after the ST segments have become isoelectric. However, this stage is not seen in some patients.

Stage 4 is represented by the normalization of the ECG or indefinite persistence of T-wave inversions.

Important distinctions must be made in this setting between ECG features of acute pericarditis and ST-elevation MI (STEMI). The first is that ST elevation in acute pericarditis usually begins at the J point (at the end of the QRS complex and the beginning of the ST segment) and remains concave (see ECG discussed earlier). In STEMI, the ST segments are generally more convex (dome shaped). The ST elevation in pericarditis tends to be widespread, whereas in STEMI the ST-elevation pattern will follow the distribution of a blocked coronary artery. Lastly, the classic PR depression

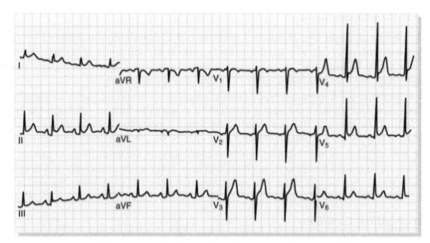

Fig. 1. Acute pericarditis. Note the diffuse ST elevation with concave ST segments. (*From* LeWinter MM, Tischler MD. Pericardial diseases. In: Bonow RO, Mann DL, Zipes DP, et al, editors. Braunwald's heart disease: a textbook of cardiovascular medicine. 9th edition. Philadelphia: Saunders Publishing; 2011; with permission.)

in acute pericarditis is not generally seen in STEMI because of the lack of atrial injury in AMI (**Fig. 2**).

Additional diagnostic modalities to consider in the evaluation of pericarditis include echocardiography to evaluate for effusion, chest radiograph, and laboratory data with comprehensive evaluation of pericardial disease in the proper setting. Although the treatment of pericarditis depends of the cause, the mainstay of therapy is antiinflammatory medications (nonsteroidal antiinflammatory drugs, aspirin, and colchicine). Patients refractory to standard medication or with contraindications may benefit from glucocorticoid therapy. In the case of large pericardial effusion or cardiac tamponade, a timely pericardiocentesis should be considered for diagnosis and therapy (See **Fig. 2**).

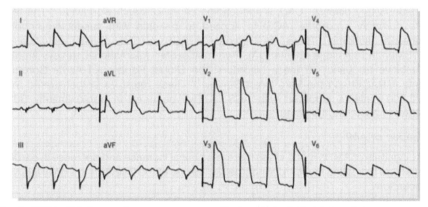

Fig. 2. STEMI. This image demonstrates acute ST elevation of anterior wall MI. You can see the ST changes across the precordium as well as into the lateral leads. Reciprocal changes are also seen in the inferior leads. (*From* Mirvis DM, Goldberger AL. Electrocardiography. In: Bonow RO, Mann DL, Zipes DP, et al, editors. Braunwald's heart disease: a textbook of cardiovascular medicine. 9th edition. Philadelphia: Saunders Publishing; 2011; with permission.)

Venous Thromboembolism

Deep vein thrombosis and pulmonary embolism (PE) constitute the entity of venous thromboembolism (VTE). VTE accounts for hundreds of thousands of hospital admissions annually.[5] Despite advances in medical and catheter-based therapy, mortality remains high for these patients up to 72 hours after admission.[6]

The diagnosis of PE relies heavily on clinical suspicion. The classic triad of tachycardia, hypoxia, and tachypnea may lead a clinician to investigate further. Although the gold standard of diagnosis is the pulmonary angiogram, computed tomography (CT) with contrast is the preferred modality for the diagnosis of PE. The mainstay of treatment of PE is anticoagulation, with heparin or tissue plasminogen activator (tPa). In certain instances, more invasive methods, such as catheter-directed thrombolysis and surgical embolectomy, may be indicated. For more information on PE, please see the article on "Submassive Pulmonary Embolism" by Drs Laurence W. Busse and Jason S. Vourlekis.

Gastrointestinal Conditions

There any many gastrointestinal disorders that may mimic chest pain. Gastroesophageal reflux disease, esophageal spasm, esophageal rupture, or sliding hiatal hernia may all present as acute chest pain in the ICU setting. Although an uncommon complication of transesophageal echocardiogram, esophageal rupture may be catastrophic and lead to complications, such as mediastinitis. In the largest inpatient and surgical setting review, the incidence of esophageal perforation was found to be 0.01%.[7] Chest radiograph is typically abnormal in this group of patients. This complication can be confirmed using water-soluble contrast before the patients' chest radiography.

Musculoskeletal and Other Causes

In the hospital setting, anywhere from 10% to 30% of acute chest pain may be musculoskeletal in origin.[8] Clinical syndromes, such as costochondritis, lower rib pain syndromes, fibromyalgia, or simply muscle spasm, may all be considered and can typically be elicited through physical maneuvers.

AMI
Introduction

Coronary artery disease (CAD) is the leading cause of death worldwide.[9] The term *acute coronary syndrome* (ACS) is applied to patients with suspected ongoing myocardial ischemia. There are 3 types of ACS: STEMI, non–ST-elevation MI (NSTEMI), and unstable angina (UA). Two multicenter, international surveys studied the relative frequency of these disorders: the Global Registry of Acute Coronary Events (GRACE) and the Euro Heart Survey.[10] These registries demonstrated that, in 22,000 patients admitted with ACS, STEMI occurred in approximately 30%, NSTEMI in 25%, and UA in 40%.

Definition of AMI

The diagnosis of AMI is made when there is a typical increase and decrease in cardiac biomarkers indicating myocardial necrosis, plus one of the following to signify injury to myocardium:

- Symptoms of myocardial ischemia
- Ischemic ECG changes (ST segments elevated or depressed)
- Development of pathologic Q waves
- Imaging evidence of new loss of viable myocardium or new regional wall motion abnormalities[1]

The definition was revised in 2012 from the European Society of Cardiology, the American College of Cardiology Foundation, the American Heart Association, and the World Health Federation (ESC/ACCF/AHA/WHF). In addition to the aforementioned definition, any one of the following meets the diagnosis of AMI:

- Cardiac death with symptoms suggestive of myocardial ischemia
- Percutaneous coronary intervention (PCI)–related MI as defined by the elevation of cardiac biomarkers to more than 3 times the upper limit of normal or a 20% increase from baseline with symptoms of ischemia
- Occlusive stent thrombosis when detected by coronary angiogram or autopsy in the setting of acute ischemia
- Coronary artery bypass graft surgery (CABG)–related MI as defined by the elevation of cardiac biomarkers such as cardiac troponin to more than 5 times the upper limit of normal

Classification of MI

The ESC/ACCF/AHA/WHF joint task force further revised the classification of MI according to the cause[11]; this has led to more specific definitions of AMI and addresses different causes of troponin leak commonly seen in the ICU setting.

- Type 1 (spontaneous MI): MI consequent to coronary arterial pathologic conditions (eg, plaque erosion/rupture, fissuring, or dissection), resulting in intraluminal thrombus
- Type 2 (MI secondary to an ischemic imbalance or commonly referred to as *demand ischemia*): MI consequent to increased oxygen demand or decreased supply (eg, coronary endothelial dysfunction, coronary artery spasm, coronary artery embolus, anemia, tachyarrhythmias/bradyarrhythmias, anemia, respiratory failure, hypertension, or hypotension)
- Type 3 (MI resulting in death when biomarker values are unavailable): Sudden unexpected cardiac death before blood samples for biomarkers could be drawn or before their appearance in the blood
- Type 4a (MI related to PCI)
- Type 4b (MI related to stent thrombosis)
- Type 5 (MI related to CABG)

Pathology

Coronary atherosclerosis

Almost all MIs are caused by underlying coronary atherosclerosis, generally superimposed with coronary thrombosis.[2] It has been surmised that chronic, fibrous, atherosclerotic lesions of epicardial arteries are not the cause of AMI. In AMI, it is plaque rupture, often of nonobstructive lesions, that exposes thrombogenic material promoting platelet aggregation and thrombus formation. This acute interruption of blood flow creates an acute supply-demand mismatch of oxygen, leading to myocardial necrosis.[2]

Plaque composition and rupture

Plaques identified at autopsy, from patients with MI, are generally composed of fibrous tissue with superimposed thrombus.[2] Platelet-rich thrombi are commonly found on the surface of these complicated lesions. It is thought that impaired endothelial function may contribute to atherogenesis through the release of certain growth factors.[2] Subsequent luminal narrowing further enhances platelet activation through augmentation of shear forces.

In atherosclerotic plaques that are prone to rupture, there is an increased formation of metalloproteinases that degrade the surrounding extracellular matrix.[12] These proteinases are augmented by activated macrophages and mast cells that are found in increased numbers at sites of plaque formation and rupture.[13] Once plaque rupture has occurred, platelets begin to adhere and are subsequently activated. This process results in a cascade of activation of thrombogenic mediators, including thromboxane A2, serotonin, adenosine diphosphate, platelet-activating factor, thrombin, tissue factor, and oxygen-derived free radicals (**Fig. 3**).

Release of cardiac biomarkers

A variety of cardiac biomarkers are used to evaluate patients with suspected AMI. The most common biomarkers are cardiac troponin I and T as well as the MB isoenzyme of creatine kinase (CK-MB). Although absolute values differ between individual laboratories, reference values greater than the upper level limit should be considered abnormal.

Cardiac troponins (troponin I or troponin T) are the preferred marker for the diagnosis of myocardial injury given the increased specificity and sensitivity compared with CK-MB.[14] Cardiac troponins used in laboratory analysis are regulatory proteins used in the calcium-mediated control of actin and myosin. Cardiac troponin I is unique to adult cardiac myocytes, whereas cardiac troponin T can be found in small amounts in skeletal muscle (**Fig. 4**, graph release biomarkers).[15]

However, it is crucial to examine the context in which elevations of cardiac troponin are interpreted. The new AMI guidelines support the notion that not all elevations in troponin are caused by ACS. Common causes in the hospital setting for elevated troponin not associated with ACS are heart failure, rapid atrial fibrillation, myocarditis, sepsis, and chronic kidney disease.[16] The underlying process elevating troponin in these settings is myocardial strain and necrosis. This process may be caused by direct myocardial injury, such as seen in myocarditis or implantable cardioverter-defibrillator defibrillation, or by elevated pressures in the heart (caused by increased preload or afterload). In the case of elevated troponin levels and sepsis, a small study conducted by Ammann and colleagues[17] demonstrated a significant increase in mortality in patients with systemic inflammatory response syndrome and sepsis. Fifty-five percent

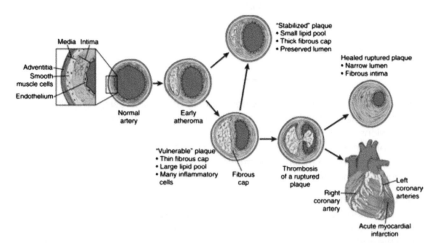

Fig. 3. Atherosclerosis. Progression of arterial plaque. The so-called vulnerable plaque consists of a relatively large lipid core and a thin (<100 mm) fibrous cap. Thrombotic complications can occur as a result of cap rupture, superficial endothelial erosion, intraplaque hemorrhage, or erosion of a calcified nodule in which circulating blood elements come in contact with the thrombogenic lipid core. (*From* Owens CD. Atherosclerosis. In: Cronenwett JL, Johnston KW, editors. Rutherford's vascular surgery. London: Elsevier Saunders; 2014; with permission.)

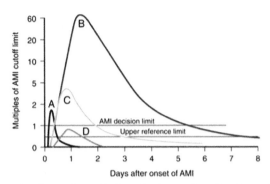

Fig. 4. Release of cardiac biomarkers. Timing of release of cardiac biomarkers following MI. Peak A, early release of myoglobin or CK-MB isoforms after AMI; peak B, cardiac troponin after AMI; peak C, CK-MB after AMI; peak D, cardiac troponin after unstable angina. Data are plotted on a relative scale, whereby 1.0 is set at the AMI cutoff concentration. (*From* Apple FS, Gibler WB. National Academy of Clinical Biochemistry Standards of Laboratory Practice: recommendations for the use of cardiac markers in coronary artery disease. Clin Chem 1999;45:1104; with permission.)

of the patients with sepsis had elevated troponin and had a mortality of 22%, compared with 5% in those without elevated cardiac troponin. Although, there is no specific guideline for determining acceptable troponin elevations in this context, the authors think that the clinical circumstances (eg, patient's medical history and absolute peak level and trend of cardiac biomarkers) should guide whether patients with elevated troponins require further cardiac investigation once stabilized. If a patient's rise in troponin is believed to reflect true cardiac pathology, initiating ASA, unless contraindicated, may prove beneficial because of its low incidence of complications.

Clinical manifestations of myocardial ischemia

An understanding of the cascade of events that occur during ACS will help direct patient care. After acute occlusion of the coronary vessel, myocardial blood flow ceases, leading to initial diastolic and then systolic dysfunction. Myocardial wall motion abnormality and diastolic impairment can be detected with echocardiography. As intracardiac pressures continue to increase, the pulmonary-capillary wedge pressure increases. Electrocardiographic changes will subsequently occur, including ST segment changes; subsequently, patients may present with angina (**Fig. 5**, manifestations).

STEMI
Introduction

STEMI includes a subset of patients with ACS presenting with a typical evolution of ECG changes (described later). The underlying lesions cause transmural infarcts in which myocardial necrosis involves the full thickness of the ventricular wall.[2]

In a retrospective study with hospitalized patients with AMI, the peak time for the onset of symptoms was found to be between 6 AM and 12 PM.[18] This pattern of circadian periodicity corresponds to early morning increases in cortisol, catecholamines, and platelet aggregability.[19]

Recently published observational data describe the mortality of in-hospital STEMI versus outpatient STEMI. Patients who are hospitalized for noncardiac issues and develop STEMI have significantly reduced survival to discharge versus outpatient STEMI (60% vs 96%).[20] This surprising result was primarily driven by a delay to

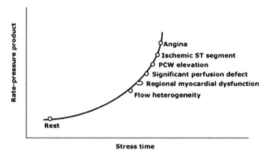

Fig. 5. Manifestations of myocardial ischemia. The relative development of the manifestations of myocardial ischemia as the rate-pressure product is increased. Regional myocardial dysfunction, which can be detected as regional wall motion abnormalities on echocardiography, occurs before ECG changes or anginal chest pain. PCW, pulmonary capillary wedge. (*Adapted from* Beller GA. Myocardial perfusion imaging for detection of silent myocardial ischemia. Am J Cardiol 1988;61:22.)

ECG time, which was 36 minutes longer in the inpatient setting. Although counterintuitive, critical care providers need to be extra vigilant in activating emergency cardiac STEMI protocols for in-hospital patients with STEMI to avoid delays beyond what is experienced for patients presenting in the emergency department or in transfer from another institution. This may be caused by hospitals not having as streamlined a process for STEMI recognition and care activation for in-hospital patients.

Clinical Features

Physical examination
Despite severe symptoms and extensive myocardial damage, physical examination findings during AMI may be unremarkable. Nonspecific findings of cardiac dysfunction may include muffled heart sounds, an S3 or S4, transient systolic murmurs, and pericardial friction rubs.

Electrocardiographic findings
- Although not frequently seen, hyperacute (or peaked) T waves develop initially reflective of localized hyperkalemia.
- Next there is J-point elevation, and the ST segment retains its normal concave configuration.
- Over time, the ST-segment elevation becomes more pronounced, becoming more convex or rounded upward.
- Lastly, the ST segment may become contiguous with the T wave.

Electrocardiographic diagnosis
The joint ESC/ACCF/AHA/WHF developed the following criteria for the diagnosis of STEMI[11]:

- New ST segment elevation at the J point in 2 contiguous leads, with greater than 0.1 mV in all leads other than V2-V3
- For leads V2-V3, greater than 0.2 mV for men older than 40 years or greater than 0.15 mV elevation for women
- New left bundle branch block with consistent changes and only in the setting of a high degree of clinical suspicion

Serum markers of cardiac damage

The diagnosis of AMI necessitates certain clinical findings along with the increase or decrease of cardiac biomarkers. Commonly used biomarkers include the CK isoenzymes (MB) and cardiac-specific troponins. Because of the prevalence of discordant values between cardiac troponins and CK-MB, cardiac troponins are the preferred marker for the diagnosis of AMI.[21]

Recommendations for the evaluation of cardiac biomarkers are constantly changing because of newer technology and availability. It is generally recommended to check Troponin I (TnI) and Troponin T (TnT) at the initial presentation and every 6 to 8 hours if the initial value was negative. It is common in practice, however, to check a second troponin earlier because 80% of patients presenting with AMI have a positive marker within 2 to 3 hours.[22] CK-MB is currently used when cardiac troponin markers are unavailable or to assess for reinfarction as elevated troponins take longer to return to baseline after an initial injury.

Acute Management

Assessment of reperfusion options for STEMI

Rapid reperfusion with early PCI remains the standard of care for patients presenting with STEMI. In a PCI-capable hospital, focus should be made on timely activation of the cardiac catheterization laboratory according to hospital protocols. In non–PCI-capable hospitals, focus should shift to reperfusion therapies with thrombolytics (tPA), emergent transfer to a PCI-capable facility, or both. Guidelines have shifted to pursuing coronary reperfusion within 90 minutes of the first medical contact.

General treatment measures

Aspirin Aspirin is the cornerstone of the initial treatment of ACS. Pharmacologic action relies on blocking the formation of thromboxane A2 in platelets. Aspirin should be chewed in order to facilitate rapid absorption.

β-blockers β-blockers decrease heart rate and systemic arterial pressure, thus, decreasing myocardial oxygen demand. These drugs have been shown to reduce angina and decrease infarct size and should be used in all patients with STEMI unless contraindicated.[23]

Nitrates Nitrates enhance coronary blood flow and decrease ventricular preload. Sublingual nitroglycerin is indicated for almost all patients with STEMI except those in shock or those who have ingested recent phosphodiesterase (type 5) inhibitors, such as sildenafil.

Statins Intensive statin therapy is recommended as early as possible in all patients with STEMI. Clinical trials, such as PROVE IT-TIMI 22 and MIRACL, have demonstrated the efficacy of early statin admisintration.[24]

Anticoagulant and antiplatelet therapy

Antiplatelet therapy $P2Y_{12}$ receptor inhibitors are a central component of antiplatelet therapy in patients with acute coronary syndromes (NSTEMI, STEMI, and UA) (**Fig. 6**). Thienopyridines (clopidogrel, ticagrelor, prasugrel) work by furthering platelet inhibition at the level of the ADP receptor and are indicated in the acute management of ACS. Trials, such as CURE and CLARITY-TIMI 28, have demonstrated improved outcomes in patients with ACS receiving these agents.[25,26]

The latest version of the ACCF/AHA's guidelines on antiplatelet therapies in UA/NSTEMI highlighted the pivotal role of these antiplatelet agents.[27] The use of prasugrel and ticagrelor were approved by the Food and Drug Administration (FDA) following

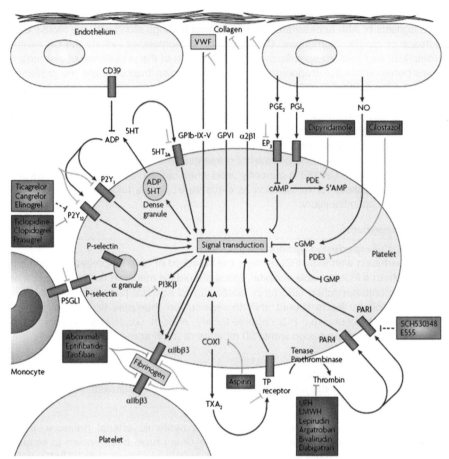

Fig. 6. Anticoagulants and antiplatelets. (*From* Michelson A. Antiplatelet therapies for the treatment of cardiovascular disease. Nat Rev Drug Discov 2010;9:156; with permission.)

head-to-head comparison trials with clopidogrel, in which prasugrel, and ticagrelor were found to be superior to clopidogrel in reducing clinical events at the expense of increased risk of bleeding. The major trial for prasugrel, TRITON-TIMI 38, focused on patients with ACS who were referred for PCI.[28] The loading dose of prasugrel was 60 mg followed by 10 mg daily maintenance dose. There was a significant 2.2% absolute reduction and a 19% relative reduction in the composite event rate of death from cardiovascular causes. However, there was a significant increase in the rate of bleeding, reaching 2.4% of patients taking prasugrel versus 1.8% of patients taking clopidogrel.[28]

The pivotal trial for ticagrelor, Platelet Inhibition and Patient Outcomes (PLATO),[29] was a multicenter randomized controlled trial comparing ticagrelor with clopidogrel. At 12 months, ticagrelor was associated with a 1.9% absolute reduction and 16% relative reduction in the primary composite outcome (time to first occurrence of the composite of vascular death, MI, or stroke). Ticagrelor exhibits a reversible inhibition of the P2Y$_{12}$ receptor and is associated with a more rapid functional recovery of circulating platelets.[29] The FDA approved ticagrelor on July 20, 2011, with a boxed warning indicating that an aspirin daily maintenance dose of greater than 100 mg decreases the effectiveness of ticagrelor.

The ACCF/AHA's guidelines[27] on the choice of P2Y$_{12}$ receptor inhibitors along with aspirin in patients with ACS are based solely on the TRITON-TIMI 38 and PLATO trial, and their clinical use should be determined with this perspective. For instance, prasugrel was administered only in the setting of PCI, whereas ticagrelor was studied in all-comer patients with UA/NSTEMI. Therefore, it is not recommended that prasugrel be administered routinely to patients with UA/NSTEMI before angiography. Additionally, the increased bleeding risks associated with prasugrel and ticagrelor have to be taken into consideration as well as the potential excess risk in the elderly. There is no head-to-head comparison between prasugrel and ticagrelor.

Glycoprotein (GP) IIb/IIIa receptor antagonists' efficacy in patients with ACS has been well established during PCI procedures and in patients with UA/NSTEMI, particularly high-risk patients, such as patients with elevated troponin biomarkers, those with diabetes, and those undergoing revascularization.[27] Most of the evidence on the use of glycoprotein IIb/IIIA receptor antagonists predated the trials that established the benefits of clopidogrel.[27] More recent trials focused on determining the optimal timing of the initiation of GP IIb/IIIa receptor antagonist in patients with UA/NSTEMI. These studies supported the upstream use of a GP IIb/IIIa receptor antagonist as a second agent in combination with aspirin for dual antiplatelet therapy in patients with UA/NSTEMI, especially in high-risk subsets, such as those with elevated cardiac biomarkers, diabetes, and undergoing PCI. The EARLY ACS[30] and ACUITY[31] trials highlighted the potential bleeding risks of the upstream use of GP IIb/IIIa receptor antagonist as part of triple antiplatelet therapy with aspirin and clopidogrel. The trial revealed that the routine use of GP IIb/IIIa receptor antagonists as part of triple antiplatelet therapy is associated with bleeding risks and its use in non–high-risk patients, such as those without diabetes, with normal baseline troponin levels, and patients older than 75 years, should not be adopted.[27]

Timing of discontinuation of P2Y$_{12}$ receptor inhibitor therapy before CABG The ACCF/AHA's 2012 guidelines on the management of patients with UA/NSTEMI suggest discontinuation of clopidogrel therapy for at least 5 days before CABG, a period of at least 7 days in patients receiving prasugrel, and a period of at least 5 days in patients receiving ticagrelor before their planned CABG. In urgent situations demanding more timely operative revascularization, consultation with the cardiothoracic surgeon is warranted.[27]

Anticoagulant therapy Heparin, low-molecular-weight heparin, bivalirudin, and fondaparinux are the major anticoagulants that have been extensively studied in ACS. The current recommendations confer the use of at least one of these anticoagulants regardless of where an invasive or conservative approach is taken. In the group of patients with UA/NSTEMI in whom an initial conservative strategy is selected with no subsequent features that would necessitate diagnostic angiography (recurrent symptoms, heart failure, or serious arrhythmias), it is recommended to start unfractionated heparin (level of evidence [LOE] A) for 48 hours or to administer enoxaparin (LOE A) or fondaparinux (LOE B) over bivalirudin for the duration of hospitalization up to 8 days and then discontinue anticoagulant therapy. For patients with UA/NSTEMI in whom PCI has been selected as a postangiography management strategy, it is recommended to start unfractionated heparin or bivalirudin as opposed to low-molecular-weight heparin and to discontinue anticoagulant therapy after PCI for uncomplicated cases (LOE A).

Fibrinolytic therapy versus invasive strategy
Before the advent of PCI, fibrinolytic therapy was the mainstay of reperfusion therapy in STEMI. Patients receiving fibrinolytics earlier in their course demonstrated the most favorable outcomes, coining the concept that time is muscle.[32] However, thrombolytics

have limitations. Infarct vessel patency was restored in only 60% to 85% of patients. Reocclusion and/or reinfarction occurred in 30% of patients by 3 months, which led to increased mortality. Increased rates of intracranial hemorrhage and other significant bleeding were also demonstrated.

Coronary angiography in a PCI-capable hospital is the current gold standard of treatment in STEMI if this therapy can be delivered within 120 minutes of the first medical contact. Current guidelines support immediate angiography in all patients presenting within 12 hours of symptoms. However, in patients with severe heart failure or cardiogenic shock, PCI should be attempted regardless of the time of presentation. PCI should also be considered early if evidence of failed fibrinolysis is present.[33]

A large 2009 meta-analysis of randomized controlled trials (RCT) and observational studies (OS) was conducted. It compared primary PCI (with balloon angioplasty or stenting) with fibrinolysis. The study found that primary PCI was associated with significant reductions in short-term ($\leq$6 weeks) mortality of 34% in the RCT. It was also associated with significant reductions in long-term (>1 year) mortality of 24% and reinfarction of 51% in the RCT. This finding was not noted in the OS being analyzed.[34]

In summary for most patients, there is a plethora of evidence from clinical trials that demonstrate superiority of primary PCI regardless of whether balloon angioplasty or stenting is performed.

Guidelines for the Management of Patients with STEMI

Stents

The advent of the bare-metal stent (BMS) drastically altered reperfusion strategy since the 1990s (**Fig. 7**). Although dramatically improving procedural success over balloon angioplasty, there still remained a high incidence (10%–20%) of target vessel revascularization. Drug-eluting stents (DES) advanced this mode of interventional therapy and, on the whole, demonstrate a 50% to 70% decrease in repeat revascularization seen with BMS.[35] DES possess antiproliferative drugs that elute from polymers on the metal scaffolding. These drugs decrease the rate of neointimal hyperplasia, the underlying pathophysiologic process behind restenosis.

These antiproliferative coatings delay normal endothelial healing within the stent. During this phase, in the absence of antiplatelet therapy, patients are at increased risk of stent thrombosis. The current guidelines recommend a dual antiplatelet regimen (aspirin plus thienopyridine) for at least 1 month following revascularization with a BMS and 12 months after DES. DES are generally preferred over BMS, given the reduced rates of restenosis, with more pronounced benefit in left main coronary artery PCI, small-caliber vessels, diffuse CAD, diabetes, and saphenous vein grafts. BMS should strongly be considered in patients that have upcoming surgery within 1 year, a history of medical noncompliance, and patients considered to be at high risk for bleeding. Special consideration should be made for patients who will require outpatient systemic anticoagulation with agents such as warfarin.

UA AND NSTEMI

UA is defined as angina pectoris (or an equivalent type of ischemic discomfort) with at least one of 3 features:

- Occurring at rest (or minimal exertion) and usually lasting greater than 20 minutes (if not interrupted by the administration of a nitrate or an analgesic)
- Being severe and usually described as frank pain
- Occurring with a crescendo pattern (ie, pain that awakens patients from sleep or that is more severe, prolonged, or frequent than previously)[36]

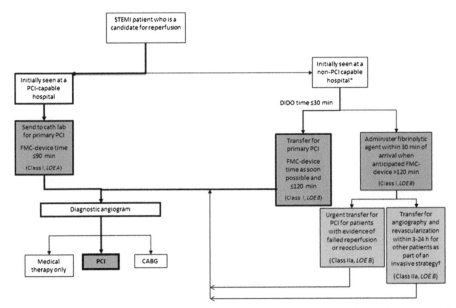

Fig. 7. STEMI algorithm. Reperfusion therapy for patients with STEMI. The *bold arrows* and *boxes* are the preferred strategies. CABG, coronary artery bypass graft; DIDO, door-in–door-out; FMC, first medical contact; LOE, Level of Evidence; MI, myocardial infarction; PCI, percutaneous coronary intervention; STEMI, ST-elevation myocardial infarction. *Patients with cardiogenic shock or severe heart failure initially seen at a non–PCI-capable hospital should be transferred for cardiac catheterization and revascularization as soon as possible, irrespective of time delay from MI onset. †Angiography and revascularization should not be performed within the first 2 to 3 hours after administration of fibrinolytic therapy. (*From* O'Gara, Kushner FG, Ascheim DD, et al. 2013 ACCF/AHA guideline for the management of ST-elevation myocardial infarction: executive summary. Circulation 2013;127:529–55; with permission.)

Approximately two-thirds of patients with UA have evidence of myocardial necrosis from elevated cardiac serum markers, such as cardiac-specific TnT, TnI, and CK-MB, and, thus, have a diagnosis of NSTEMI.[36] With the introduction of more sensitive troponin assays, a higher percentage of patients with UA/NSTEMI will exhibit some release of cardiac biomarkers. This circumstance has led to an increase in the proportion of cases designated as NSTEMI, with a concomitant reduction in the fraction with UA.

Pathophysiology

Five main pathophysiologic processes serve as underlying mechanisms for UA/NSTEMI (**Fig. 8**)[37]:

- Plaque rupture or erosion with superimposed nonocclusive thrombus is the most common.
- Dynamic intracoronary obstruction has a variety of causes, such as epicardial artery spasm or the enhanced action of local platelet-released vasoconstrictors, such as thromboxane A2. Other factors include a disruption in coronary intramural muscular regulatory function; endothelial dysfunction; and adrenergic stimuli, such as cold exposure or cocaine.
- In secondary UA, myocardial oxygen demand outstrips oxygen supply (eg, fever, sepsis, hypotension, anemia).

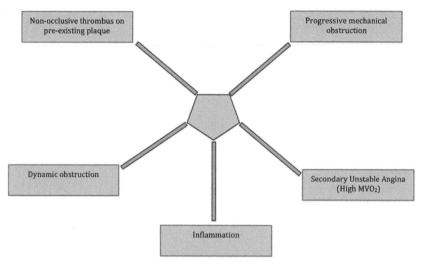

Fig. 8. Pathophysiology of unstable angina: 5 main processes contributing to the development of unstable angina. MVO_2, myocardial oxygen consumption. (*Adapted from* Braunwald EG. Unstable angina: An etiologic approach to management. Circulation 1998;98 2219–22; with permission.)

- Progressive chronic coronary luminal narrowing resulting in downstream myocardial ischemia is also an underlying mechanism.[37]

Electrocardiography and Serum Biomarkers

Electrocardiography

All patients with UA/NSTEMI should be placed on continuous electrocardiographic monitoring to identify ischemia-related arrhythmias and recurrent ST segment changes indicating ongoing ischemia. A repeat ECG should follow the initial ECG obtained in 6 to 12 hours. It has been reported that up to 50% of patients with UA/NSTEMI[38] present with ECG abnormalities, namely, ST depression (transient ST elevation) and T wave changes. Novel ECG changes noted on admission are a reliable measure of ischemia and prognosis. Approximately 10% of patients with UA/NSTEMI exhibit transient (<20 minutes) ST elevation. ST elevation portends a high risk of future cardiac events. It is hypothesized that ST depressions (>0.1 mV) and marked T-wave inversions (>0.3 mV) are sensitive but not specific markers of acute ischemia.

Dynamic ECG changes manifesting as recurrent ST depressions are an independent marker of an adverse outcome.[39]

Serum cardiac biomarkers

It is essential to measure serum cardiac biomarkers in all patients with ACS as these aid in identifying patients with UA or NSTEMI. A cardiac-specific troponin is the preferred marker. In patients with negative cardiac markers within 6 hours of the onset of pain, another sample should be drawn in the 6- to 12-hour time frame. Persistent elevation of troponin after an acute event is associated with worsened outcomes.[40]

Clinical Classification

Patients presenting with UA/NSTEMI compose a heterogeneous population.[41] A clinical classification of patients with UA/NSTEMI provides a useful means to stratify risk. Patients fall into 3 groups depending on the underlying pathophysiology.

- Group A from secondary UA
- Group B suffers from primary UA
- Group C from postinfarction angina[41]

Simultaneously, patients are classified according to the severity of ischemia. This classification (**Table 1**) provides valuable prognostic information. It has the added utility of identifying high-risk patients, mainly those with ongoing or recurrent chest pain and primary/secondary UA (see **Table 1**).[41]

Risk Assessment Scores

Integrating variables from the ECG, serum biomarkers, and clinical variables, multiple risk assessment scores have been derived.

The TIMI risk score assigns one point to each of the following 7 independent risk factors:

- Age greater than 65 years
- Greater than 3 risk factors of CAD
- ST deviation greater than 0.5 mm
- Greater than 2 episodes of angina in the last 24 hours
- Documented CAD at catheterization
- Aspirin use within the prior week
- Elevated cardiac biomarkers

Using the TIMI risk score, patients can be risk stratified across an almost 10-fold gradient of risk of death, urgent revascularization, or MI at 14 days from 4.7% (TIMI 0/1) to 40.9% (TIMI 6/7) (*P*<.001).[36]

It is noted that patients with higher TIMI risk scores have significant reductions in cardiac events when treated with an invasive versus conservative management strategy.[42]

Table 1
Classification of UA

Severity	Clinical circumstances		
	A. Develops in presence of extracardiac condition that intensifies myocardial ischemia (secondary UA)	B. Develops in absence of extracardiac condition (primary UA)	C. Develops within 2 wk after MI (postinfarction UA)
I. New onset of severe angina or accelerated angina, no rest pain	IA	IB	IC
II. Angina at rest within past month but not within preceding 48 h (angina at rest, subacute)	IIA	IIB	IIC
III. Angina at rest within 48 h (angina at rest, acute)	IIIA	IIIB	IIIC

Adapted from Braunwald E. Unstable angina: a classification. Circulation 1989;80:410; with permission.

Another helpful risk assessment score is the GRACE score. This score has also identified factors associated independently with increased mortality:

- Age
- Killip classification (**Table 2**)
- Increased heart rate
- ST-segment depression
- Signs of heart failure
- Lower systolic blood pressure
- Cardiac arrest at presentation
- Elevated serum creatinine or cardiac biomarkers[43]

Treatment strategies and interventions
There are 2 main approaches to the management of patients with UA/NSTEMI:

- The early invasive approach (**Fig. 9**) is a strategy that involves early cardiac catheterization followed by PCI, CABG, or more intensive medical therapy.[36]
- The conservative approach (**Fig. 10**) is a treatment arm that focuses on medical management with cardiac catheterization reserved for patients with recurrent ischemia either at rest or on a noninvasive stress test with subsequent revascularization if deemed appropriate.[36]

To date, the aforementioned approaches were studied in 10 large randomized trials, 6 of which demonstrated a significant benefit of an early invasive strategy.[44–46] A recent meta-analysis of the more recent trials has concluded that managing NSTEMI by an early invasive strategy results in an overall significant reduction in death, MI, or rehospitalization and of mortality during a mean follow-up of 2 years whereby the incidence of all-cause mortality was 4.9% in the early invasive group compared with 6.5% in the conservative group (risk ratio = 0.75, 95% confidence interval 0.63 to 0.90, P = .001). It also demonstrated a benefit of an early invasive strategy in all men and high-risk women but not in low-risk women.[46]

Indications for Invasive Versus Conservative Management Strategies

Based on the results of several recent randomized trials and meta-analyses, an early invasive strategy is the recommended strategy in patients with UA/NSTEMI with the following:

- ECG changes, namely, ST depressions
- Positive troponins
- Other high-risk features, including recurrent ischemia and evidence of congestive heart failure[36]

Table 2 Killip classification		
Killip Subgroup	**Clinical Characteristics**	**Hospital Mortality (%)**
I	No congestion signs	<6
II	S3, basal rales	<17
III	Acute pulmonary edema	38
IV	Cardiogenic shock	81

Data from Killip T, Kimball J. Treatment of myocardial infarction in a coronary care unit: a two year experience with 250 patients. Am J Cardiol 1967;20:457–65.

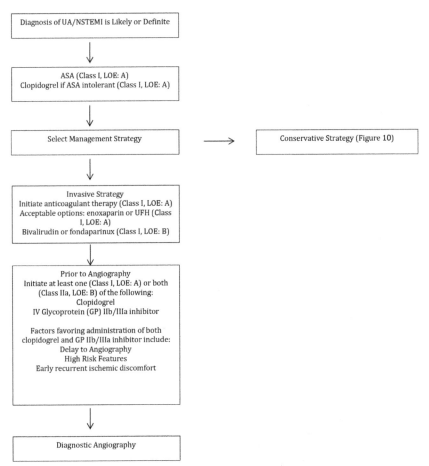

Fig. 9. Algorithm for patients with UA/NSTEMI managed by an initial invasive strategy. ASA, aspirin; IV, intravenous; UFH, unfractionated heparin. (*From* Anderson JL, Adams CD, Antman EM, et al, 2011 Writing Group Members, ACCF/AHA Task Force Members. 2011 ACCF/AHA focused update incorporated into the ACC/AHA 2007 guidelines for the management of patients with unstable angina/non-ST-elevation myocardial infarction: a report of the American College of Cardiology Foundation/American Heart Association Task Force on Practice Guidelines. Circulation 2011;123(18):e426–579. http://dx.doi.org/10.1161/CIR.0b013e318212bb8b; with permission.)

The following two trials have provided evidence to a very early invasive strategy, especially in high-risk patients:

- In the Intracoronary Stenting with Antithrombotic Regimen Cooling-Off (ISAR-COOL) trial,[47] immediate invasive strategies were beneficial with an average time from randomization to catheterization of 2 hours compared with 4 days with a delayed invasive strategy.
- In the TIMACS trial,[48] the primary end point was death, stroke, and MI. It compared early (median = 14 hours after randomization) with later (median = 50 hours) angiography. A trend in reduction of the primary end point (death, MI, and stroke) was noted in the overall group but a significant reduction in the primary end point was achieved in patients with a high GRACE risk score. There was also a significant 28% reduction of the secondary end point of death, MI, and refractory ischemia with earlier angiography.

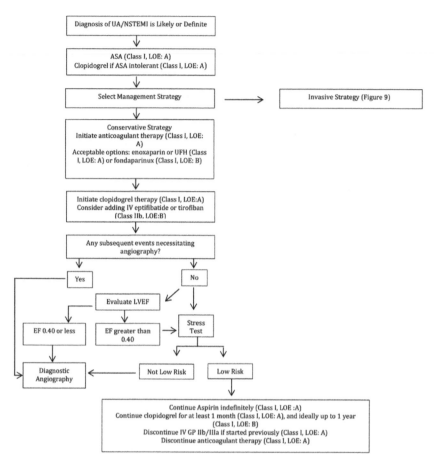

Fig. 10. Algorithm for patients with UA/NSTEMI managed by an initial conservative strategy. ASA, aspirin; EF, ejection fraction; IV, intravenous; LVEF, left ventricular ejection fraction; UFH, unfractionated heparin. (*From* Anderson JL, Adams CD, Antman EM, et al, 2011 Writing Group Members, ACCF/AHA Task Force Members. 2011 ACCF/AHA focused update incorporated into the ACC/AHA 2007 guidelines for the management of patients with unstable angina/non-ST-elevation myocardial infarction: a report of the American College of Cardiology Foundation/American Heart Association Task Force on Practice Guidelines. Circulation 2011;123(18):e426–579. http://dx.doi.org/10.1161/CIR.0b013e318212bb8b; with permission.)

ACUTE COMPLICATIONS OF MI

- Free wall rupture

  The incidence of this complication seems to be decreasing with significant improvement in time to reperfusion. It is noted that rupture of the free wall of the infarcted ventricle occurs in up to 10% of patients dying in the hospital of STEMI.[36]

  This condition occurs more commonly in the elderly, women, and usually involves the anterior or lateral walls of the left ventricle in the area of terminal distribution of the left anterior descending artery. It also occurs more frequently in patients with STEMI who were subjected to fibrinolytic therapy as opposed to PCI.[49] Rupture of the free wall is commonly associated with hemopericardium and death from cardiac tamponade. Incomplete rupture may occur when organizing thrombus and hematoma seal a left ventricular rupture and prevent the development of hemopericardium. The tenous patch of thrombus results in the formation of pseudoaneurysm that communicates with the left ventricular cavity.

- Rupture of the interventricular septum

    The risk of a rupture causing ventricular septal defect increases with increasing age, the lack of development of a collateral network, and anterior infarction.[50] Clinically, this condition appears by the presence of a new harsh, loud holosystolic murmur that is heard best at the lower left sternal border and accompanied by a thrill.[51] Diagnosis is usually made by echocardiography with color flow.

- Rupture of a papillary muscle

    This complication is a rare yet fatal complication of a transmural MI. Anterolateral wall MI can lead to the rupture of the anterolateral papillary muscle, yet inferior wall infarction can lead to the rupture of the posteromedial papillary muscle, which occurs more commonly. The sudden onset of severe mitral regurgitation is a catastrophic result of a complete transection of a papillary muscle and is not compatible with life. The rupture of a partial portion of the papillary muscle will present less dramatically.[36] Patients with this condition develop a new holosystolic murmur that may attenuate as the systemic arterial pressure decreases. The diagnosis of this condition can be promptly made by echocardiography. Color flow Doppler can differentiate acute mitral regurgitation from a ventricular septal defect.

Surgical treatment remains the most definitive treatment modality for patients with a mechanical complication caused by MI. Often, however, surgery is not an option either because of hemodynamic instability or from a lack of suitable tissue in which to operate on. Percutaneous options for closure of post-MI ventricular septal defects exist but are made difficult by the friability of infarct scar and the serpiginous track of infarcted tissue. Any post-MI mechanical complication demands urgent cardiovascular consultation to determine if any treatment options exist and to evaluate the potential benefits of ventricular assist options in the setting of clinical instability.

POST-MI CARE

The following is according to the 2013 guidelines from the ACCF/AHA and the ESC for the management of AMI in patients presenting with STEMI[52,53]:

All hospitals participating in the care of patients with STEMI should have a coronary care unit (CCU) equipped to provide all aspects of care for patients with STEMI, including treatment of ischemia, severe heart failure, arrhythmias, and common comorbidities (class I, LOE C).[53]

All patients should have an echocardiography for the assessment of infarct size and resting left ventricular function (class I, LOE C[52]; class I, LOE B[53]). Patients undergoing uncomplicated successful reperfusion therapy should be kept in the CCU for a minimum of 24 hours, after which they may be moved to a step-down monitored bed for another 24 to 48 hours (class I, LOE C).[53] The Primary Angioplasty in Myocardial Infarction II (PAMI-II) trial showed that low-risk patients with successful primary PCI could be safely discharged from the hospital at day 3 without noninvasive testing.[54]

To identify these low-risk patients, schemes such as the PAMI-II criteria designate low-risk patients as

1. Less than 70 years of age

2. Left ventricular ejection fraction greater than 45%
3. One- or 2-vessel disease, successful PCI, and no persistent arrhythmias

In general, the decision to transfer patients out of the CCU involves the physician and nursing staff and is usually favored in the following:

1. Absence of recurrent chest pain
2. Presence of hemodynamic stability
3. Down trending cardiac biomarkers
4. Successful uncomplicated revascularization
5. The absence of unstable arrhythmias or dynamic ECG changes

Long-term antithrombotic and antiplatelet therapy at hospital discharge should be continued depending on the adopted ACS management strategy (conservative vs invasive in UA/NSTEMI) and depending on whether a bare-metal or drug-eluting intra-coronary stent was deployed (**Fig. 11**).

Secondary prevention and long-term management strategies should also be initiated, with benefits that are seen even with early initiation in the ICU setting. These strategies include counseling on smoking cessation, a target blood pressure goal less than 140/90 mm Hg (or <130/90 if diabetes or chronic kidney disease is present), and intensive lipid management therapy with high-intensity statins.[55] The goal of treatment with statin therapy is to achieve a low-density-lipoprotein cholesterol (LDL-C) of 100 mg/dL. For very-high-risk patients, namely, those with established CAD plus (1)

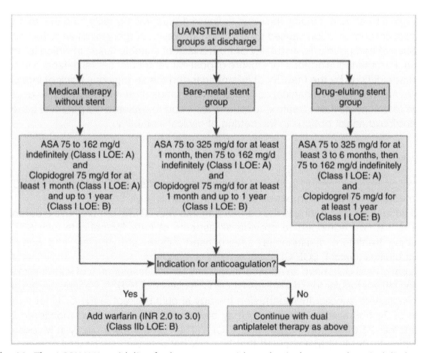

Fig. 11. The ACC/AHA's guideline for long-term antithrombotic therapy at hospital discharge after UA/NSTEMI. INR, international normalized ratio. (*From* Cannon CP, Braunwald EG, editors. Unstable angina and non–ST elevation myocardial infarction. In: Bonow RO, Mann DL, Zipes DP, et al, editors. Braunwald's heart disease: a textbook of cardiovascular medicine. 9th edition. Saunders Publishing; 2011; with permission.)

multiple major risk factors (especially diabetes), (2) severe and poorly controlled risk factors (especially continued cigarette smoking), (3) multiple risk factors of the metabolic syndrome (especially high triglycerides >200 mg/dL plus non–high-density-lipoprotein cholesterol [HDL-C] >130 mg/dL with low HDL-C <40 mg/dL), and (4) patients with acute coronary syndrome, an LDL-C target of 70 mg/dL is reasonable.[55] In addition, cardiac rehabilitation and secondary prevention programs are recommended for patients with STEMI.[54] Finally, patients should be on optimal medical therapy, including antiplatelet therapy, as per the ACC/AHA's guidelines listed in **Fig. 11**.

REFERENCES

1. Imazio M, Cecchi E, Demichelis B, et al. Indications for poor prognosis in setting of acute pericarditis. Circulation 2007;115(21):27–39.
2. Braunwald E. Heart disease, a textbook of cardiovascular medicine. 6th edition. New York: Saunders; 2001. p. 1115, 1828.
3. Spokick DH. Pericardial rub. A prospective multiple observer investigation of pericardial friction in 100 patients. Am J Cardiol 1975;35(3):357.
4. Spodick DH. The pericardium: a comprehensive textbook. New York: Marcel Dekker; 1997.
5. Yusuf HR. Venothromboembolism in adult hospitalizations. JAMA 2012;308(6): 559–61.
6. Soloff LA. Acute pulmonary embolism: II. Am Heart J 1967;74(6):829.
7. Hilberath JN, Oakes DA, Shernan SK, et al. Safety of transesophageal echocardiolgraphy. J Am Soc Echocardiogr 2010;23(11):1115–27.
8. Cilia C, Malatino LS, Puccia G, et al. The prevalence of the cardiac origin of chest pain: the experience of a rural area of southeast Italy. Intern Emerg Med 2010;5(5):427.
9. Roger VL, Go AS, Lloyd-Jones DM, et al. Executive summary: heart disease and stroke statistics-2012 update: a report from the American Heart Association. Circulation 2012;125:188–97.
10. Hasdai D, Behar S, Wallentin L, et al. A prospective survey of the characteristics, treatments and outcomes of patients with acute coronary syndromes in Europe and the Mediterranean basin; the Euro Heart Survey of Acute Coronary Syndromes (Euro Heart Survey ACS). Eur Heart J 2002;23(15):1190–201.
11. Thygesen K, Alpert JS, Jaffe AS, et al. Third universal definition of myocardial infarction. Circulation 2012;126(16):2020–35.
12. Ross R. Atherosclerosis- an inflammatory disease. N Engl J Med 1999;340:115–26.
13. Ardissino D, Merlini PA, Ariens R, et al. Tissue-factor antigen and activity in in human coronary atherosclerotic plaques. Lancet 1997;349(9054):769–71.
14. Alpert JS. Myocardial infarction redefined–a consensus document of the Joint European Society of Cardiology/American College of Cardiology Committee for the redefinition of myocardial infarction. J Am Coll Cardiol 2000;36(3):959–69.
15. Jaffe AS, Vasile VC, Milone M, et al. Diseased skeletal muscle: a noncardiac source of increased circulating concentrations of cardiac troponin T. J Am Coll Cardiol 2011;58(17):1819.
16. Babuin L, Vasile VC, Rio Perez JA, et al. Elevated cardiac troponin is an independent risk factor for short- and long-term mortality in medical intensive care unit patients. Crit Care Med 2008;36(3):759–65.
17. Ammann P, Maggiorini M, Bertel O, et al. Troponin as a risk factor for mortality in critically ill patients without acute coronary syndromes. J Am Coll Cardiol 2003; 41(11):2004.

18. Kloner RA, Leor J. Natural disaster plus wake up time: a deadly combination of triggers. Am Heart J 1999;137(5):779–81.
19. Muller JE, Abela GS, Nesto RW, et al. Triggers, acute risk factors and vulnerable plaques. J Am Coll Cardiol 1994;23(3):809–13.
20. Dai X, Bumgarner J, Spangler A, et al. Acute ST elevation myocardial infarction in patients hospitalized for noncardiac conditions. J Am Heart Assoc 2013;2(2): e000004.
21. Goodman SG, Steg PG, Eagle KA, et al. The diagnostic and prognostic impact of the redefinition of acute myocardial infarction: lessons from the GRACE registry. Am Heart J 2006;151(3):654–60.
22. Macrae AR, Kavsak PA, Lustig V, et al. Assessing the requirement for the 6-hour interval between specimens in the American Heart Association Classification of Myocardial Infarction in Epidemiology and Clinical Research Studies. Clin Chem 2006;5(52):812–8.
23. Chamberlain D. Beta-blockers and calcium antagonists. Management of acute myocardial infarction. London: WB Saunders; 1994. p. 193–221.
24. Schwartz GG, Olsson AG, Ezekowitz MD, et al. Effects of atorvastatin on early recurrent ischemic events in acute coronary syndromes: the MIRACL study. JAMA 2001;285(13):1711–8.
25. Sabatine MS, Cannon CP, Gibson CM, et al. Addition of clopidogrel to aspirin and fibrinolytic therapy for myocardial infarction with ST-segment elevation. N Engl J Med 2005;352(12):1179–89.
26. Gibson CM, Murphy SA, Pride YB, et al. Effects of pretreatment with clopidogrel on nonemergent percutaneous coronary intervention after fibrinolytic administration for ST-segment elevation myocardial infarction: a Clopidogrel as Adjunctive Reperfusion Therapy-Thrombolysis in Myocardial Infarction (CLARITY-TIMI) 28 study. Am Heart J 2008;155(1):133–9.
27. Jneid H, Anderson JL, Wright RS, et al. 2012 ACCF/AHA focused update of the guideline for the management of patients with unstable angina/non–ST-elevation myocardial infarction (updating the 2007 guideline and replacing the 2011 focused update). J Am Coll Cardiol 2012;60(7):645–81.
28. Wiviott SD, Braunwald E, McCabe CH, et al. Prasugrel versus clopidogrel in patients with acute coronary syndromes. N Engl J Med 2007;357:2001–15.
29. Mahaffey KW, Wojdyla DM, Carroll K, et al. Ticagrelor compared with clopidogrel by geographic region in the Platelet Inhibition and Patient Outcomes (PLATO) trial. Circulation 2011;124:544–54.
30. PRISM-PLUS Study Investigators. Inhibition of the platelet glycoprotein IIb/IIIa receptor with tirofiban in unstable angina and non-Q-wave myocardial infarction: Platelet Receptor Inhibition in Ischemic Syndrome Management in Patients Limited by Unstable Signs and Symptoms (PRISM-PLUS) Study Investigators. N Engl J Med 1998;338:1488–97.
31. PURSUIT Trial Investigators. Inhibition of platelet glycoprotein IIb/IIIa with eptifibatide in patients with acute coronary syndromes: the PURSUIT Trial Investigators: platelet glycoprotein IIb/IIIa in unstable angina: receptor suppression using Integrilin therapy. N Engl J Med 1998;339:436–43.
32. Boersma E, Maas AC, Deckers JW, et al. Impact of time to thrombolysis. Lancet 1996;348(9030):771–5.
33. Bates ER, Blankenship JC, Bailey SR, et al. 2011 ACCF/AHA/SCAI guideline for percutaneous intervention: executive summary. Circulation 2011;124(23):2574–609.
34. Huynh T, Perron S, O'Loughlin J, et al. Comparison of primary percutaneous coronary intervention and fibrinolytic therapy in ST-segment-elevation-myocardial

infarction: bayesian hierarchical meta-analyses of randomized controlled trials and observational studies. Circulation 2009;119(24):3101–9.

35. Moses JW, Leon MB, Popma JJ, et al. Sirolimus-eluting stents versus standard stents in patients with stenosis in a native coronary artery. N Engl J Med 2003; 349(14):1315.

36. Cannon C, Braunwald E. Braunwald's heart disease. Philadelphia: Elsevier Saunders; 2012. p. 1178–209.

37. Braunwald E. Unstable angina: an etiologic approach to management. Circulation 1998;98(21):2219–22.

38. Cannon CP, McCabe CH, Stone PH, et al. The electrocardiogram predicts one-year outcome of patients with unstable angina and non–Q wave myocardial infarction: results of the TIMI III Registry ECG Ancillary Study. J Am Coll Cardiol 1997;30(1):133–40.

39. Scirica BM, Morrow DA, Budaj A, et al. Ischemia detected on continuous electrocardiography following acute coronary syndrome: observations from the MERLIN-TIMI 36 trial. J Am Coll Cardiol 2009;53(16):1411–21.

40. Morrow DA, Cannon CP, Rifai N, et al. Ability of minor elevations of troponin I and T to predict benefit from an early invasive strategy in patients with unstable angina and non–ST elevation myocardial infarction: results from a randomized trial. JAMA 2001;286(19):2405–12.

41. Braunwald E. Unstable angina: a classification. Circulation 1989;80(2):410–4.

42. Cannon CP, Weintraub WS, Demopoulos LA, et al. Comparison of early invasive and conservative strategies in patients with unstable coronary syndromes treated with the glycoprotein IIb/IIIa inhibitor tirofiban. N Engl J Med 2001; 344(25):1879–87.

43. Granger CB, Goldberg RJ, Dabbous O, et al. Predictors of hospital mortality in the global registry of acute coronary events. Arch Intern Med 2003;163(19):2345–53.

44. Morrow DA, Scirica BM, Fox KA, et al. Evaluation of a novel antiplatelet agent for secondary prevention in patients with a history of atherosclerotic disease: design and rationale for the Thrombin-Receptor Antagonist in Secondary Prevention of Atherothrombotic Ischemic Events (TRA 2 P)–TIMI 50 trial. Am Heart J 2009;158(3):335–41.

45. O'Donoghue M, Boden WE, Braunwald E, et al. Early invasive vs. conservative treatment strategies in women and men with unstable angina and non–ST-segment elevation myocardial infarction. A meta-analysis. JAMA 2008;300(1):71–80.

46. Bavry AA, Kumbhani DJ, Rassi AN, et al. Benefit of early invasive therapy in acute coronary syndromes: a meta-analysis of contemporary randomized clinical trials. J Am Coll Cardiol 2006;48(7):1319–25.

47. Neumann FJ, Kastrati A, Pogatsa-Murray G, et al. Evaluation of prolonged antithrombotic pretreatment ("cooling-off" strategy) before intervention in patients with unstable coronary syndromes: a randomized controlled trial. JAMA 2003; 290(12):1593–9.

48. Mehta SR, Granger CB, Boden WE, et al. Early versus delayed invasive intervention in acute coronary syndromes. N Engl J Med 2009;360(21):2165–75.

49. Lloyd-Jones D, Adams R, Carnethon M, et al. Heart disease and stroke statistics 2009 update: a report from the American Heart Association Statistics Committee and Stroke Statistics Subcommittee. Circulation 2009;119(3):480–6.

50. Birnbaum Y, Fishbein MC, Blanche C, et al. Ventricular septal rupture after acute myocardial infarction. N Engl J Med 2002;347(18):1426–32.

51. Antman EM, Anbe DT, Armstrong PW, et al. ACC/AHA guidelines for the management of patients with ST-elevation myocardial infarction: a report of the

American College of Cardiology/American Heart Association Task Force on Practice Guidelines (Committee to Revise the 1999 Guidelines for the Management of Patients with Acute Myocardial Infarction). Circulation 2004;110(9): e82–292.

52. O'Gara PT, Kushner FG, Ascheim DD, et al. 2013 ACCF/AHA guideline for the management of ST elevation myocardial infarction: executive summary. Circulation 2013;127(4):529–55.

53. Steg PG, James SK, Atar DM, et al. ESC Guidelines for the management of acute myocardial infarction in patients presenting with ST-segment elevation. Eur Heart J 2012;33(20):2569–619.

54. Grines CL, Marsalese DL, Brodie B, et al. Safety and cost-effectiveness of early discharge after primary angioplasty in low risk patients with acute myocardial infarction. PAMI-II Investigators. Primary angioplasty in myocardial infarction. J Am Coll Cardiol 1998;31(5):967–72.

55. Smith SC, Benjamin EJ, Bonow RO, et al. AHA/ACCF secondary prevention and risk reduction therapy for patients with coronary and other atherosclerotic vascular disease: 2011 update: a guideline from the American Heart Association and American College of Cardiology Foundation. Circulation 2011; 124(22):2458–73.

Managing Arrhythmias in the Intensive Care Unit

Cynthia Tracy, MD[a],*, Ali Boushahri, MD[b]

KEYWORDS

- Cardiac arrhythmia • Intensive care unit • Tachyarrhythmia • Bradyarrhythmia

KEY POINTS

- Patients admitted to the intensive care unit (ICU) are at increased risk for cardiac arrhythmias.
- Cardiac arrhythmias are common in the ICU, and can be either the initial reason for admission to the ICU or a consequence of the medical condition.
- Exacerbating and contributing factors are multiple, and management of the patient requires a careful determination of these factors and correction where possible.

INTRODUCTION

Patients admitted to the intensive care unit (ICU) are at increased risk for cardiac arrhythmias, which may be either the primary reason for ICU admission or a contingency in the critically ill patient. This article addresses the occurrence of arrhythmias in the critically ill patient, and their pathophysiology, implications, recognition, and management.

PATHOPHYSIOLOGY

Although patients can be admitted to the ICU with a variety of conditions, the critical nature of their underlying processes and the supportive measures used to treat them can contribute to an elevated catecholamine state. Coupled with fluctuations in intravascular volume, electrolyte disturbances, and other metabolic derangements, this places patients at risk for cardiac arrhythmias. The incidence of arrhythmia in the ICU patient can approach 40%, most typically associated with conditions such as septic shock and respiratory failure.[1] The most common arrhythmias in the ICU setting can be divided into 2 basic categories: (1) tachyarrhythmias (eg, atrial fibrillation [AF] and atrial flutter, ventricular arrhythmias, and other supraventricular tachycardias [SVTs]) and (2) bradyarrhythmias (eg, junctional rhythm, sinus bradycardia, and atrioventricular [AV] conduction block).

[a] Department of Medicine, George Washington University, 2150 Pennsylvania Avenue, Northwest, Washington, DC 20037, USA; [b] Cardiovascular Medicine, George Washington University, Medical Faculty Associates, 2150 Pennsylvania Avenue, Northwest, Washington, DC 20037, USA
* Corresponding author.
E-mail address: ctracy@mfa.gwu.edu

Crit Care Clin 30 (2014) 365–390
http://dx.doi.org/10.1016/j.ccc.2014.03.009   criticalcare.theclinics.com
0749-0704/14/$ – see front matter © 2014 Elsevier Inc. All rights reserved.

Predictors of tachyarrhythmia occurrence in ICU patients include the use of stimulant drugs such as norepinephrine, and a high APACHE II score ($\geq$25) (see the article on Cardiogenic Shock by Shah and colleagues elsewhere in this issue). For those with bradyarrhythmias, identified predictors include the use of norepinephrine (which is a predictor of both tachyarrhythmia and bradycardia), arterial pH less than 7.3, and HCO_3 level of 18 mEq/L or higher (see **Box 1** for common risk factors).[1]

CONSEQUENCES OF ARRHYTHMIAS IN THE INTENSIVE CARE UNIT

The presence of arrhythmia, especially ventricular fibrillation (VF), symptomatic sinus bradycardia, and junctional bradycardia, in the medical ICU has been associated with higher in-hospital mortality. Tongyoo and colleagues[1] reported on a single-center population of 247 ICU patients (mean age 58.5 years; mean APACHE II score 20.1). In this group of critically ill patients, arrhythmias were seen in 39.7%. The mortality among patients who developed arrhythmias was significantly higher than among those who did not. Among those who developed significant bradyarrhythmias (sinus or junctional) the mortality was 88.7%, and in those with tachyarrhythmias (particularly VF) the mortality was 66.7%, compared with 18.1% mortality ($P<.001$) in patients free of arrhythmias.

Similar results were seen by Annane and colleagues[2] among 1341 medical ICU patients, sustained arrhythmias being seen in 12% of patients. In this population, in-hospital death rates were 17% in patients without arrhythmia; 29% in patients with supraventricular arrhythmia (SVA); 73% in patients with ventricular arrhythmia (VA); and 60% in patients with conduction abnormalities.

The occurrence of arrhythmias in the ICU population can be associated with a prolonged stay in hospital.[3] Polanczyk and colleagues[3] reported on 4181 patients aged 50 years or older who presented in sinus rhythm and underwent nonemergency, noncardiac procedures. In this group of patients, perioperative SVAs were seen in in 317 patients (7.6%). Independent preoperative correlates for the occurrence of these arrhythmias included male sex, age 70 years or older, history of valvular heart disease or heart failure, and prior history of SVA or asthma. The occurrence of SVA was associated with a 33% increase in length of stay after adjustment for other clinical data ($P<.001$).

Goodman and colleagues[4] reported on both short-term and long-term consequences of arrhythmias in the ICU population. This study included 611 patients

---

Box 1
Risk factors for arrhythmia in the intensive care unit

- Male gender
- Age greater than 70 years
- Cardiac disease (coronary artery disease, heart failure, valvular disease)
- Pulmonary disease (asthma)
- Thyroid disease
- Critically ill (APACHE score $\geq$25)
- Volume fluctuations
- Electrolyte disturbances
- Metabolic derangements
- Vasopressors

admitted to the general ICU who were evaluated for the development of SVA. Patients were followed through hospital discharge, and 48-month mortality was evaluated. New-onset SVA was found in 9% of patients, and preexisting history of SVA in 12%. In-hospital mortalities were 18% in those with no SVA, 56% in the new-onset SVA group, and 32% in those with prior histories of SVA ($P<.05$ for any SVA vs no SVA; $P<.05$ for history SVA vs new-onset SVA). Similarly to other studies, mortality was associated with high APACHE II scores, sepsis, acute renal failure, and myocardial ischemia. For those with new-onset SVA the APACHE II score was 23.8 ± 8 versus 16 ± 8 for those without SVA ($P<.05$).[4] Of note, for those surviving to discharge the postdischarge mortality rates were 20% in the no-SVA group, 36% in the new-onset SVA group, and 45% in the history of SVA group ($P<.05$ for any SVA vs no SVA; $P<.05$ for history SVA vs new-onset SVA). Most deaths in the new-onset SVA group occurred during the acute hospital stay and were typically associated with multiorgan system failure as reflected in the APACHE II scores.[4] Moreover, in this study new-onset SVAs were not found to be associated with a preadmission history of cardiac disease, being more closely associated with a history of underlying pulmonary disease and hypothyroidism.

DIAGNOSTIC APPROACH
Determine Urgency

As in any other patient population, the management of arrhythmias in the ICU patient is determined by the acuity of the problem (**Box 2**). An initial critical step is determining whether an arrhythmia truly exists, or if an artifact is recorded as a result of electrical interference created by devices in the patient environment, or is created by motion (**Fig. 1**). If an arrhythmia is confirmed, the urgency of treatment will depend on a determination of whether the rhythm itself is causing compromise to the patient. Management will be more urgent in the setting of an acute arrhythmia that is resulting in symptomatic hypotension and/or hypoperfusion to vital organs.

Identify Causes

Regardless of whether urgent steps are required, identification of correctable underlying causes should be undertaken when the patient is sufficiently stabilized (**Box 3**). Multiple electrolytes and acid-base abnormalities are common in the ICU patient population, and in one study were reported in around 67% of patients.[5] Hypokalemia is a well-recognized contributor to cardiac arrhythmia, and in the population with ischemic heart disease the likelihood of VF as almost twice as high among patients with potassium levels of less than 3.6 mEq/L as in those with higher levels (odds ratio 1.97).[6,7] In up to 40% of patients with hypokalemia there is concomitant hypomagnesemia, and unless this is corrected it may not be possible to correct the potassium level.[8]

Box 2
Determinants of urgency

- Hypotension
- Ischemia
- Heart failure
- Altered mentation
- Other signs of hypoperfusion: hypoxia, decreased urine output

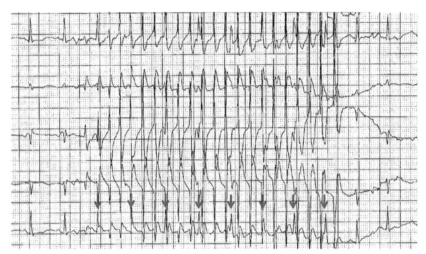

Fig. 1. Telemetry strip demonstrating artifact initially thought to be ventricular tachycardia. Close examination reveals underlying sinus rhythm with motion artifact (*arrows* indicate QRS complexes).

The relation between potentially life-threatening arrhythmias and inappropriate ventilation, hypoxemia, hypo- or hyperventilation, and metabolic acidosis has long been appreciated.[9] Patients in the ICU are at risk for these potentially reversible causes of arrhythmias. Critically ill patients are with volume overload can be arrhythmogenic because of atrial stretch.[10] In patients with an indwelling catheter such as a peripherally inserted central catheter or other central line, mechanical stimulation may lead to arrhythmias.

Advanced Cardiac Life Support (ACLS) guidelines emphasize the "5 H" and "5 T" reversible causes of arrhythmias applicable in all clinical scenarios: Thrombosis, pulmonary/cardiac; Tension pneumothorax; Tamponade, cardiac; Trauma; Toxins; and Hypoxia; Hydrogen ions (acidosis); Hypothermia; Hypovolemia; Hypo-/Hyperkalemia.[11] Care should be taken in the ICU patient to prevent or correct these potential

---

Box 3
Causes of arrhythmia

- Hypoxia/hypoventilation
- Hypovolemia/hypervolemia
- Electrolyte imbalances (potassium, magnesium)
- Metabolic acidosis
- Hypothermia
- Coronary ischemia
- Cardiac tamponade
- Acute pulmonary process (pulmonary embolism, pneumothorax)
- Trauma
- Intoxication
- Mechanical stimulation (central line)

causes and contributors to arrhythmias. Without correction, management of the arrhythmia may not be possible.

UNDERSTANDING MECHANISMS OF ARRHYTHMIAS

An understanding of the basic mechanisms of cardiac arrhythmias is helpful in determining correct therapeutic approaches.

Bradyarrhythmias

Bradyarrhythmias (**Table 1**) arise from problems in impulse generation (automaticity) and/or impulse conduction (heart block). Diminished automaticity in the sinus node results in sinus bradycardia, and in more extreme cases sinus pauses. Heart block is usually due to disease (more commonly fibrosis, less commonly ischemia) in the AV node or His-Purkinje system, the latter being associated with higher grades of AV block. The degree of heart block is determined by the extent of impulse conduction from the atria to the ventricles: in first-degree heart block all impulses are conducted, albeit at a slower rate (prolonged PR interval); in second-degree heart block they are intermittently conducted; and in third-degree heart block none of the atrial impulses are conducted. Bradyarrhythmias can be seen in a variety of settings in the ICU, such as with elevated intracranial pressure, exaggerated vagal activity (coughing, vomiting), carotid sinus pressure (tight collar), hypothyroidism, hypothermia, ischemia, metabolic abnormalities (hyperkalemia), and various drugs (β-blockers, calcium-channel blockers, antiarrhythmics, digoxin, clonidine, opioids, lithium, dexmedetomidine).[12]

Tachyarrhythmias

Tachyarrhythmias (**Table 2**) have 3 general mechanisms: increased automaticity, reentry, and triggered activity. Enhanced automaticity can occur in the atrium, AV node, or within the ventricle. These automatic foci in the atria, AV junction, or ventricles can accelerate and drive an ectopic tachyarrhythmia, such as paroxysmal atrial tachycardia. Automatic tachyarrhythmias (both atrial and ventricular) are commonly encountered in the ICU, as they are triggered by metabolic disturbances such as electrolyte abnormalities (namely potassium and magnesium disturbances), acid-base disturbances, hypoxemia, and ischemia. Use of vasopressors and inotropes can also contribute, given their sympathomimetic properties.

Reentry

Reentry is the most common mechanism for tachyarrhythmias. For reentry to occur, 2 pathways (or tissue) with different conduction properties must exist and be anatomically oriented in such a way as to form an electrical circuit. These circuits may be congenital (eg, dual AV node) or acquired (surrounding or within scar tissue of uneven electrical properties). As such, reentry can occur around anatomic barriers such as scar, or by utilizing anatomically distinct pathways such as the slow and fast pathways of the AV node. Reentrant arrhythmias are often provoked by premature complexes arising in either the atrium or the ventricle. A well-timed electrical impulse takes

Table 1 Bradyarrhythmias	
Mechanism of Bradyarrhythmia	**Examples**
Decreased automaticity	Sinus bradycardia Sinus pause/arrest
Impaired conduction	Heart block (first, second, and third degree)

Table 2 Tachyarrhythmias	
Mechanism of Tachyarrhythmia	**Examples**
Increased automaticity	Paroxysmal atrial tachycardia Multifocal atrial tachycardia
Reentry	Atrial flutter Atrioventricular (AV) nodal reentrant tachycardia AV reentrant tachycardia Ventricular tachycardia
Triggered activity	Digoxin toxicity Torsades de pointes

advantage of the discrepancies in conduction properties, penetrating one limb of the circuit while the second is refractory owing to the prematurity of the stimulus. The impulse travels forward on the anterograde limb, and can then proceed retrograde up the second pathway of the reentrant loop, which will now have recovered its ability to conduct. The impulse can create an endless loop of reentry while simultaneously activating adjacent myocardium. Perpetuation of the circuit depends on the ability of both limbs to maintain the tachycardia (**Fig. 2**). Common reentrant arrhythmias encountered in the ICU, as well as other clinical settings, include AV nodal reentrant tachycardia (AVNRT), atrial flutter, and ventricular tachycardia (VT). AV reentrant tachycardia (AVRT) is less frequently seen, and depends on the substrate (accessory pathway, as in Wolff-Parkinson-White [WPW] syndrome) being present. Reentry is favored when there is differential conduction in the two limbs or the circuit and this is favored by changes in heart rate and autonomic tone,[13] ischemia, and pH and electrolyte abnormalities.

Triggered activity

Triggered activity involves the premature activation of the cardiac cell during the repolarization (recovery) period, which is referred to as an afterdepolarization. These

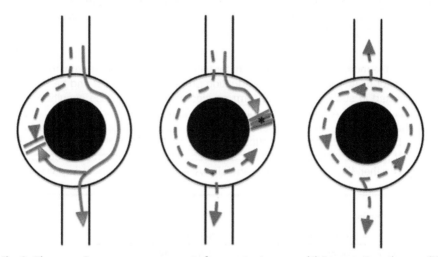

Fig. 2. There are 3 necessary components for reentry to occur: (1) 2 separate pathways, (2) unidirectional block in 1 pathway (*asterisk*), and (3) slow conduction along the other pathway. To persist, both pathways must be capable of maintaining conduction.

afterdepolarizations are capable of sustaining a tachyarrhythmia and are the likely underlying mechanism in certain rhythms. Digoxin has been implicated in the occurrence of delayed afterdepolarizations, which likely are at least partly responsible for the various tachyarrhythmias seen in the setting of digoxin toxicity (such as paroxysmal atrial tachycardia with block).[14] Triggered activity has also been implicated in the pathogenesis of torsades de pointes, whereby early afterdepolarizations in the setting of a prolonged QT interval can precipitate polymorphic VT (PMVT). The prolonged QT interval can be congenital or acquired, as in the setting of numerous drugs (including antiarrhythmics, antimicrobials, antihistamines, and psychotropics),[15,16] metabolic abnormalities (hypokalemia, hypomagnesemia, hypocalcemia), ischemia, and hypothermia. PMVT in the setting of acquired long QT is usually pause dependent, and is precipitated by long-short RR intervals.[17]

DIAGNOSIS AND MANAGEMENT OF SPECIFIC ARRHYTHMIAS ENCOUNTERED IN THE ICU
Atrial Fibrillation

AF is the most common sustained arrhythmia in the general population, and occurs in up to 31% of ICU patients (**Fig. 3**).[18] Risk factors for AF include: advancing age (≥33% of patients with AF are ≥80 years); presence of structural heart disease; and chronic conditions: cardiac (eg, hypertension) and noncardiac (eg, renal failure, chronic obstructive pulmonary disease).[19,20] Risk factors for AF in the ICU setting include hypotension, use of vasopressors or inotropes, septic shock, fluid overload, electrolyte imbalance, heart failure, and postoperative status, among others (**Box 4**).[21] Mechanisms causing and sustaining AF are multifactorial, and AF can be complex and difficult for clinicians to manage. In the structurally normal heart variations in autonomic tone have been implicated in the initiation of AF, as surges in vagal and sympathetic tone have been detected in the minutes that precede initiation of the arrhythmia.[22,23] AF is associated with a 5-fold increased risk of stroke,[24] 3-fold increased risk of heart failure,[25–27] and 2-fold increased risk of mortality.[24] In the United States, AF alone contributes to nearly 10,000 deaths per year.

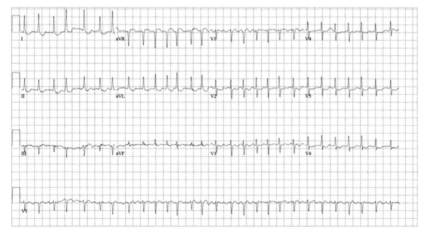

Fig. 3. Typical appearance of atrial fibrillation with rapid ventricular response. ST-segment changes are noted, which were not previously seen during sinus rhythm, and likely reflect demand ischemia.

Box 4
Predisposing factors for atrial fibrillation in the intensive care unit

- Advanced age
- Structural heart disease
- Chronic cardiovascular conditions (hypertension)
- Chronic noncardiac conditions (renal failure, chronic obstructive pulmonary disease)
- Hypotension and shock
- Fluid overload
- Electrolyte imbalances
- Vasopressors and inotropes
- Postoperative state

In AF there is loss of (or diminished) atrial contribution to ventricular preload, which accounts for 25% of ventricular end-diastolic volume in the normal heart.[28] Though of little consequence in the normal heart, this may become hemodynamically significant with systolic dysfunction, diastolic dysfunction (noncompliant ventricle), and rapid heart rates (decreased ventricular filling).

The acute management of AF involves 3 strategies: rhythm control (cardioversion), rate control, and anticoagulation. Cardioversion can be accomplished electrically or pharmacologically. Immediate electrical direct current (DC) cardioversion is indicated in patients with AF who have severe hemodynamic compromise (eg, hypotension, decompensated heart failure) thought to be related to the arrhythmia. If tolerated, premedication with a benzodiazepine or opiate is preferable. Shocks should be synchronized with the QRS complex. In general, pads placed anterior to posterior provide greater efficacy than do anterior and lateral positioning, and a biphasic waveform typically requires less energy than a monophasic waveform. If a single shock fails to result in conversion to sinus rhythm, repositioning pads, applying pressure over the anterior pad (to reduce impedance), and using a bipolar waveform may facilitate cardioversion.[29,30] DC cardioversion should not be attempted in the setting of digoxin toxicity or uncorrected hypokalemia.

Pharmacologic cardioversion may be appropriate in patients who are not immediately hemodynamically compromised and not experiencing cardiac ischemia as a result if the arrhythmia. Several antiarrhythmic agents are available, and the choice of drug will depend on the underlying myocardial function, but ibutilide and amiodarone are most commonly chosen in the ICU (**Table 3**). Intravenous ibutilide has a reported success rate of up to 50%, but has not been specifically tested in the ICU population.[31] Given its effects on repolarization, ibutilide can significantly prolong

---

Table 3
Dosing for atrial fibrillation pharmacologic cardioversion

Medication	Dose
Ibutilide	<60 kg: 0.01 mg/kg intravenously (IV) over 10 min ≥60 kg: 1 mg IV over 10 min May repeat once if arrhythmia does not terminate
Amiodarone	150 mg IV over 10 min, then IV drip 1 mg/min for 6 h followed by 0.5 mg/min for 18 h (total 1.05 g over 24 h)

the QT interval and provoke torsades de pointes, which has been reported in up to 3.9% of cases.[32,33] The risk of torsades de pointes is higher (and should therefore be avoided) in patients with heart failure, prolonged QT interval at baseline, or hypokalemia.[34] Ibutilide can facilitate electrical cardioversion, but this has not been specifically tested in the ICU setting.[35] Amiodarone is often the preferred agent in the ICU setting, particularly in patients with depressed ejection fractions given its better safety profile in this population. In the acute setting, amiodarone may provide rate control and can be used for longer-term rhythm control, as it has been shown to decrease AF recurrence.[36,37]

More than 50% of episodes of AF convert spontaneously without specific antiarrhythmic intervention within the first 72 hours,[38] and cardioversion may not be necessary unless symptoms are distressing. Management of AF in the hemodynamically stable patient focuses on adequate control of ventricular rate, and management of the underlying cardiac substrate and any coexisting conditions that could be contributing to the arrhythmia. In the ICU setting where ongoing illnesses may dominate the clinical picture, maintenance of sinus rhythm after cardioversion may be impossible even with antiarrhythmic medications, and a strategy of rate control may be needed.[39,40]

Acute rate control can be achieved with numerous drugs (**Table 4**). β-Blockers are particularly effective when adrenergic/sympathetic tone is elevated, such as in the postoperative period. Metoprolol may be initiated as intravenous boluses (up to 15 mg total within a 15-minute period) and followed by oral doses when rate control is achieved. The short half-life of intravenous esmolol makes it a good option in patients at risk for hemodynamic instability. In patients who cannot tolerate β-blockers or do not achieve adequate ventricular rate control, nondihydropyridine calcium-channel blockers such as diltiazem or verapamil may be used. However, calcium-channel blockers should be avoided in patients with heart failure and reduced ejection fraction, given their negative inotropic effects and potential to worsen hemodynamics. Alternatively, digoxin may be considered for use in patients with heart failure and marginal blood pressures. It should be used cautiously in patients with renal insufficiency, and has a relatively delayed onset of action (at least 1 hour), which is why it is not usually a first-line agent for rate control. Amiodarone may also cause slowing of the ventricular rate via its β-blocking and calcium-channel–blocking effects, and may provide better rate control than other agents.[41]

Magnesium has been shown to prevent the development of AF in some instances, and may have a synergistic effect when used with amiodarone for the suppression of AF.[42] A combination of the aforementioned drugs may be used if a single class is

Table 4	
Drugs for rate control in atrial fibrillation	
Medication	**Dose**
β-Blockers	
Metoprolol	2.5–5 mg IV over 2–5 min (up to 15 mg in 15 min)
Esmolol	0.5 mg/kg IV over 1 min, then IV drip 50–200 μg/kg/min
Calcium-Channel Blockers	
Diltiazem	0.25 mg/kg IV over 2 min, then IV drip 5–15 mg/h
Verapamil	0.075–0.15 mg/kg IV over 2 min
Digoxin	0.25 mg IV every 2 h (up to 1.5 mg in 24 h)
Amiodarone	150 mg IV over 10 min, then IV drip 1 mg/min for 6 h followed by 0.5 mg/min for 18 h (total 1.05 g over 24 h)

unable to adequately control the ventricular rate, but these patients must be very closely monitored because they are at increased risk for cumulative adverse effects, namely bradycardia and heart block.

In patients with WPW syndrome and AF, β-blockers should be used with caution, as they may facilitate anterograde conduction down the accessory pathway.[43] In AF with preexcitation, intravenous procainamide or ibutilide may be used to restore sinus rhythm.[44] However, intravenous amiodarone, adenosine, digoxin, or nondihydropyridine calcium-channel antagonists may accelerate the ventricular rate, and these drugs should be avoided.[45]

Postoperative AF is reported in 30% to 40% of patients undergoing coronary artery bypass surgery and in 60% of patients undergoing valve surgery, and usually appears in the first 4 postoperative days.[46] Risk factors include valvular surgery, advanced age, and failure to resume β-blocker therapy after surgery. β-Blockers are preferred for rate control of AF in this setting.[47] This arrhythmia is usually self-limited, and more than 90% of patients will convert to sinus rhythm within 6 to 8 weeks.[48]

Strategies for anticoagulation in general are based on the risk of embolization in the individual patient. This risk is generally calculated according to known risk factors for systemic embolization as described in the CHA_2DS_2-VASc score classification of risk (**Table 5**).[49] The annual risk for stroke is based on the total score calculated based on identified risk factors (**Table 6**).[50] In general, for patients with prior stroke, TIA, or CHA_2DS_2-VASc score of 2 or higher, oral anticoagulants are recommended. Oral anticoagulant options include warfarin, dabigitran, apixiban, and rivaroxiban.[51–54] The decision to anticoagulate any patient must be weighed against the risk of bleeding. In the general population, the HAS-Bled score can be calculated, with 1 point ascribed to risk factors for bleeding including hypertension, abnormal liver or renal function, history of stroke or bleeding, labile international normalized ratios, elderly age (>65 years), use of drugs that promote bleeding, or excess alcohol. Patients with a HAS-Bled score of 3 or greater are considered to be at high risk for bleeding while anticoagulated.[55] Patients in the ICU may be at particular risk for bleeding because of their underlying medical conditions, polypharmacy, and altered metabolism; in general, if anticoagulation is deemed necessary based on the CHA_2DS_2-VASc score, extreme caution should be used.

Atrial Flutter

Although the two are often seen in the same patient, atrial flutter is an arrhythmia distinct from AF. The incidence of atrial flutter is lower than that of AF in the ICU

Table 5	
CHA_2DS_2-VASc score classification of risk	
CHA_2DS_2-VASc Clinical Predictor	**Score**
Congestive heart failure, decreased ejection fraction	1
Hypertension	1
Age ≥75 y	2
Diabetes mellitus	1
Vascular disease (prior myocardial infarction, peripheral arterial disease)	1
Stroke/transient ischemic attack	2
Age 65–74 y	1
Sex: female	1
Maximum potential score	9

Table 6
Stroke risk stratification associated with CHA$_2$DS$_2$-VASc score

CHA$_2$DS$_2$-VASc Score	Adjusted Stroke Rate (%/y)
0	0
1	1.3
2	2.2
3	3.2
4	4.0
5	6.7
6	9.8
7	9.6
8	6.7
9	15.2

population, and in the study by Reinelt and colleagues[18] atrial flutter accounted for 3.6% of arrhythmia episodes. Management concerns and anticoagulation for atrial flutter are similar to those for AF. It can be more difficult to achieve rate control in atrial flutter than in AF, because fewer wavefronts penetrate the AV node in flutter in comparison with fibrillation, resulting in less suppression of AV-node conduction in flutter.[56] However, drug management is similar to that already described.

Atrial flutter is a macro-reentrant arrhythmia that registers a sawtooth pattern on the electrocardiogram (ECG) (**Fig. 4**). Typical flutter involves a macro-reentrant loop in the right atrium traversing from inferior to superior, resulting in negative waves in the inferior leads and positive flutter waves in V1. Atrial rates in typical flutter range from 240 to 300 beats per minute.[57] The degree of AV block varies, and with rapid A to V conduction the rhythm may be more difficult to determine until AV block is achieved with medication. In the ICU setting where sympathetic tone can be high or where sympathomimetic drugs are in use, ventricular rates may be rapid, as these situations favor enhanced AV conduction. Adenosine can facilitate unmasking of the underlying flutter waves. Adenosine results in transient block in the AV node but does not affect the flutter circuit itself. As with AF, adenosine should not be used in any case where there

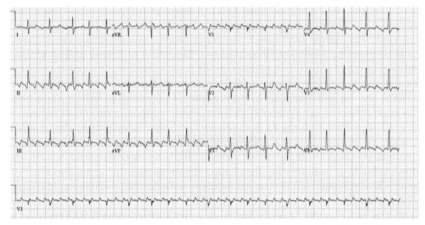

Fig. 4. Typical counterclockwise atrial flutter with characteristic sawtooth pattern of flutter waves.

is a question of anomalous AV conduction such as in WPW syndrome. The blockade of the AV node may permit conduction of electrical impulses unopposed down a rapidly anterograde conducting accessory pathway, which can result in VF.[45]

In some instances, the flutter wave can be reversed and result in a clockwise circuit in the right atrium, which gives rise to positive flutter waves in the inferior leads (II, III, and aVf) and a negative flutter in V1. It can be difficult to determine the circuitry in some instances of flutter, and perhaps a better descriptive term for these rhythms is noncavotricuspid isthmus dependent macro-reentrant atrial tachycardia. These rhythms can arise in the left atrium and may be quite complex, and can occur in the setting of prior ablation procedures or following cardiac surgery.[57] Management in the acute setting remains the same. Acute cardioversion of atrial flutter can require lower energies than are used for AF, and ibutilide can result in conversion to sinus rhythm in 38% to 76% of patients.[58]

Supraventricular Tachycardias

Among the SVTs there are essentially 3 types based on their anatomic origins: sinus node dependent (eg, sinus tachycardia, sinus node reentry, inappropriate sinus tachycardia); atrial dependent (eg, atrial flutter/fibrillation [see earlier discussion], atrial tachycardia); AV-node dependent (eg, AVNRT, AVRT [accessory pathway involved in circuit], junctional tachycardia).

For the patient presenting with a narrow complex tachycardia, the administration of an AV nodal blocking agent such as adenosine can prove useful both therapeutically and diagnostically. Adenosine would be expected to terminate (at least temporarily) SVTs that are AV-node dependent. Rarely will an automatic atrial tachycardia terminate with adenosine, and other non–AV-node dependent SVTs will be unmasked as the AV node is blocked, permitting visualization of the underlying atrial activity (**Fig. 5**).[59] Certain conditions may exist in the ICU patient that would interfere with adenosine usage. For example, methylxanthines have adenosine receptor antagonist activity and may render the patient less sensitive to adenosine. Adenosine must be used with caution in patients with reactive airway disease, as it can provoke bronchospasm. Dipyridamole can block adenosine transport back into the cell and can enhance the response to adenosine (**Fig. 6**).

AV-node dependent arrhythmias

AVNRT is much more common than AVRT. If these arrhythmias prove refractory to adenosine or if they recur after adenosine administration, further suppression may be needed. For either termination or suppression, nondihydropyridine calcium-channel blockers or β-blockers may be used. Digoxin is of limited utility because of its delayed onset of action. Use of these drugs is with caution in the patient with overt preexcitation. Nondihydropyridine calcium-channel blockers and β-blockers may destabilize the patient because of their potential hypotensive effects, and should not be used for acute conversion in the hemodynamically compromised patient. Primary antiarrhythmics can cause hypotension and may have proarrhythmic effects, and should be avoided unless AV nodal blocking agents are ineffective and cardioversion cannot be done. Potential antiarrhythmics that can be considered include amiodarone, sotalol, procainamide, flecainide, disopyramide, or propafenone.[60] For patients with depressed left ventricular function, amiodarone, β-blockers, and digoxin may be preferred.

Junctional tachycardia typically arises as a result of enhanced automaticity, and may occur in the ICU setting as a result of digitalis toxicity or excessive use of exogenous catecholamines. These inciting/exacerbating agents should be withdrawn.

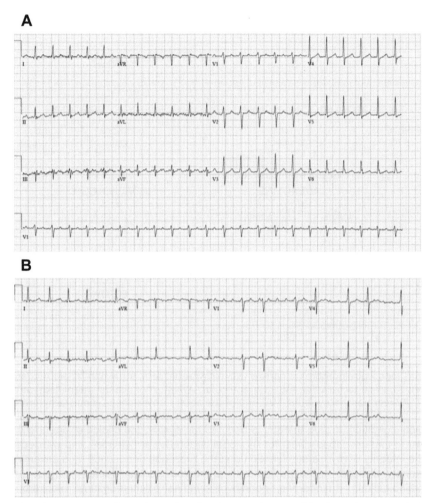

Fig. 5. (*A*) Narrow complex tachycardia of unclear mechanism. (*B*) After adenosine administration, underlying atrial tachycardia is unmasked.

Cardioversion is ineffective in converting junctional tachycardia related to increased automaticity, and may be harmful if the junctional tachycardia is caused by digitalis toxicity. If the arrhythmia persists despite removal of the inciting agents(s), the choice of medical therapy will depend on the underlying cardiac function. For patients with preserved ejection fraction, choices may include amiodarone, β-blockers, or nondihydropyridine calcium-channel blockers. For those with depressed function, amiodarone is preferred.

Atrial-dependent arrhythmia

A regular atrial tachycardia can occur from an ectopic atrial focus as a result of enhanced automaticity, and in the ICU setting this may be related to stimulant drugs used (eg, catecholamines) or to pulmonary disease. These arrhythmias are best treated by correcting the underlying cause, as cardioversion has no role. Before initiating specific treatment, it is important to determine whether there is any hemodynamic compromise related to the rhythm itself rather than the patient's underlying

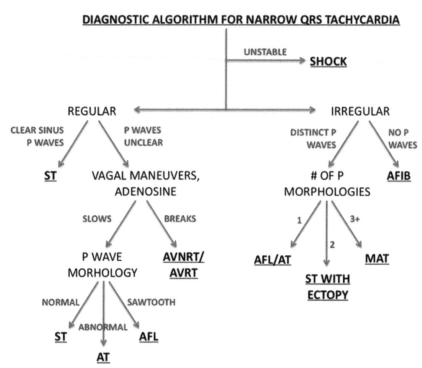

Fig. 6. Diagnostic algorithm for narrow QRS tachycardia. AFIB, atrial fibrillation; AFL, atrial flutter; AT, atrial tachycardia; AV, atrioventricular; AVNRT, AV nodal reentrant tachycardia; AVRT, AV reentrant tachycardia; MAT, multifocal atrial tachycardia; ST, sinus tachycardia.

medical condition. If drug therapy is deemed necessary, the choice of agent will be similar to that described earlier for AV nodal dependent arrhythmias, and will depend on the integrity of myocardial function and the presence or absence (and severity) of pulmonary disease. In the patient with preserved ejection fraction without other contraindications, amiodarone, nondihydropyridine calcium-channel blockers, or β-blockers may be used. In the patient with preserved ejection fraction, no absolute contraindications, and multifocal atrial tachycardia (MAT) (**Fig. 7**), the therapeutic options are the same.[61] MAT is typically associated with underlying pulmonary disease and is characterized by the identification of 3 or more separate P-wave morphologies in a rapid irregular rhythm. Medications may achieve clinical benefit as a result of their suppression of AV-node conduction and slowing of heart rate, rather than arrhythmia suppression. In patients with depressed ejection fraction, medication choices include amiodarone, β-blockers, and digoxin.

Sinus node–dependent arrhythmia
Sinus tachycardia occurs typically in response to the underlying medical problem, and correction depends on identifying and correcting possible causes (eg, fever, sepsis, pulmonary embolism, blood loss). Sinoatrial nodal reentrant tachycardia (SANRT) is a difficult diagnosis to make clinically. Technically this rhythm falls into the category of a macro-reentrant atrial arrhythmia involving the sinus node. Typical rates are in the range of 100 to 150 beats/min, and the P-wave is identical to that seen in sinus rhythm, often with underlying structural heart disease.[62,63] Like other reentrant arrhythmias, onset and offset are often abrupt, and episodes may last for hours.

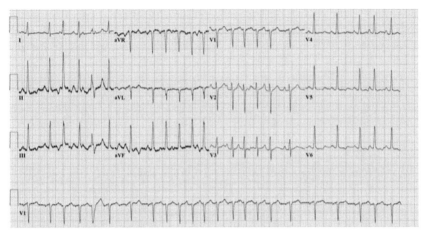

Fig. 7. Multifocal atrial tachycardia characterized by multiple (≥3) P-wave morphologies.

Adenosine can terminate SANRT, and suppression can sometimes be achieved with verapamil or amiodarone.[64,65]

Wide Complex Tachycardias

Wide complex tachycardias can be of either supraventricular or ventricular origin. There are several well-published guidelines for electrocardiographic distinction that can be helpful (**Box 5**). When possible, it is extremely useful to obtain the baseline ECG to determine whether there is a preexistent conduction abnormality. In general, aberration of an SVT in a patient without an underlying conduction abnormality will electrocardiographically appear more like a typical bundle branch block morphology. In patients with an underlying conduction abnormality, the QRS complex will appear similar to the baseline morphology, but may be wider owing to rate-related conduction delays. Virtually any SVT with intact AV nodal conduction can result in a wide complex tachycardia. The presence of AV dissociation is a strong indicator that the rhythm is of ventricular origin.

In patients with WPW syndrome, the most common tachycardia is orthodromic AV reentry (electrical impulse traveling anterograde down the AV node and retrograde up the accessory pathway). In some patients with WPW syndrome, an antidromic AV reentrant arrhythmia can occur (down the accessory pathway and up the AV node) (**Fig. 8**). The ECG will appear wide and the morphology will not appear as a typical

---

Box 5
Wide complex tachycardia is more likely ventricular tachycardia if…

- Atrioventricular dissociation
- Very wide QRS (>160 milliseconds if left bundle branch block, >140 milliseconds if right bundle branch block)
- Bizarre QRS morphology
- Abnormal axis ("NW axis")
- Concordance across precordial leads
- Capture beats
- Fusion beats

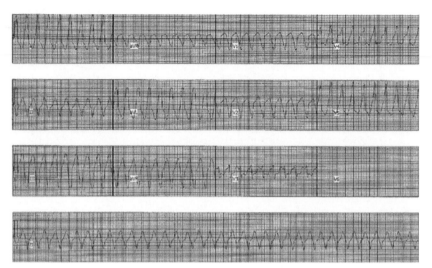

Fig. 8. Antidromic atrioventricular (AV) reentrant tachycardia with anterograde conduction via a posteroseptal accessory pathway and retrograde conduction via the AV node.

bundle branch block, and may be difficult to distinguish from VT. AF in the patient with WPW may appear wide and bizarre if anterograde conduction is present. A hallmark of preexcited AF is the capacity to (in some cases where the properties of the pathway permit) conduct at very rapid rates and to have varying morphologies as more, or less of the impulse travels anterograde to the ventricle down the accessory pathway.

In a patient with a cardiac implanted electrical device (pacemaker or defibrillator), a wide complex tachycardia can occur under a variety of situations, including (1) true superseding arrhythmia unrelated to the device or (2) device involvement in the rhythm. Examples of device-related tachycardias can include ventricular tracking of a rapid atrial rate (eg, AF, atrial flutter, or sinus tachycardia) or pacemaker-mediated tachycardia. The latter usually results when there is loss of atrial capture but intact ventricular capture, followed by retrograde atrial activation through an intact AV node and subsequent ventricular pacing based on the sensed atrial event. Most devices can be programmed to avoid or terminate these rapid rhythms, and application of a magnet will terminate pacemaker-mediated tachycardia. Device interrogation is critical to determining the nature of the rhythm and taking corrective steps.

The other major cause of wide complex tachycardia is, of course, VT which accounts for 80% of wide complex tachycardias.[66] Although there may be clinical clues as to whether the rhythm is of supraventricular, or ventricular origin, it is not wise to rely on the apparent stability of the patient to make the distinction. VT should be suspected in the patient with underlying heart disease, such as cardiomyopathy, prior myocardial infarction, or valvular heart disease. In the postinfarct patient, 90% of cases of wide complex tachycardia will be VT, and this should be considered the diagnosis of exclusion.[67] Despite several algorithms available for distinguishing VT from SVT, it is often difficult in the acute setting to determine the origin of wide complex tachycardias **(Fig. 9)**.[68]

The acute management of the patient with wide complex tachycardia will depend on the clinical stability of the patient. Unless it is known with certainty that the patient has a preexisting conduction defect, and that the rapid rhythm is morphologically the same as the sinus ECG, adenosine should only be used with extreme caution. In

DIAGNOSTIC ALGORITHM FOR WIDE QRS TACHYCARDIA

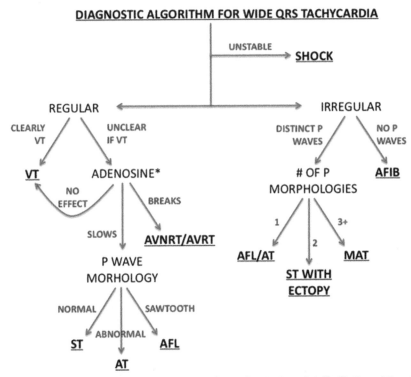

Fig. 9. Diagnostic algorithm for wide QRS tachycardia. AFIB, atrial fibrillation; AFL, atrial flutter; AT, atrial tachycardia; AV, atrioventricular; AVNRT, AV nodal reentrant tachycardia; AVRT, AV reentrant tachycardia; MAT, multifocal atrial tachycardia; ST, sinus tachycardia; VT, ventricular tachycardia. * Use caution with adenosine if there is possible VT.

preexcited arrhythmias (antidromic AVRT or preexcited AF), adenosine will not block the accessory pathway (and may even enhance its conduction) but may block the AV node, leaving anterograde conduction down the accessory pathway unopposed, and placing the patient at risk for degeneration to VF.[69] Patients with a wide complex tachycardia may appear hemodynamically stable, but the acute vasodilatory effect of adenosine may destabilize the patient in VT, and not terminate the abnormal rhythm.[70]

   If the patient presents with hemodynamically stable wide complex tachycardia, use of an antiarrhythmic may be considered, recognizing that an apparently stable patient may decompensate rapidly either owing to the duration of the rhythm or to the hemodynamic effects of drugs. As with adenosine, drugs that are appropriate for SVT both diagnostically and for therapy such as β-blockers or nondihydropyridine calcium-channel blockers may cause rapid clinical deterioration in the patient with VT.[68] Acute administration of these drugs should be avoided in wide complex tachycardia of uncertain mechanism. If the patient is stable enough, steps should be taken to best determine the mechanism of the arrhythmia to better target the most appropriate treatment. Useful steps include evaluation of the baseline ECG, determining the likelihood of VT versus SVT with aberration based on the clinical history (assume VT in the postinfarct patient), determining prior episodes of arrhythmia, reviewing telemetry strips if available for prior nonsustained arrhythmias, and determining family history for potentially hereditary conditions such as WPW syndrome or channelopathies.

If the patient has hemodynamically unstable wide complex tachycardia, immediate steps should be taken toward cardioversion. Depending on patient stability, administration of analgesics or sedatives may be prudent. Extreme care must be taken to avoid clinical deterioration related to these drugs. Intravenous access, continuous monitoring, and supplemental oxygen should be in place before synchronous cardioversion. Although lower energies may convert atrial arrhythmias, it is the authors' practice to use higher energy levels immediately, rather than titrating upwards.

After initial stabilization, a thorough evaluation for underlying causes such as electrolyte imbalance, drug toxicity, ischemia, or catecholamine excess should be undertaken and remediable causes treated. In the event of recurrent VT or wide complex tachycardia of uncertain mechanism, antiarrhythmic therapy will likely be needed (**Table 7**). Amiodarone is typically the drug of choice (other than in cases of WPW) because of its superior efficacy. If WPW is suspected, procainamide may be an appropriate agent, as it can block the accessory pathway. Procainamide can be useful for SVT and VT, but its utility is limited by its tendency to induce hypotension. Lidocaine is also an appropriate agent but will not benefit most patients in whom the mechanism is SVT, owing to its lack of effect on atrial and AV nodal tissue. Lidocaine can slow or block accessory pathway conduction and can affect distal conduction.

Monomorphic VT

Most cases of monomorphic VT occur in the presence of underlying heart disease; the mechanism is typically reentry, as described earlier, and depends on discrepancies in conduction and refractoriness within the ventricular myocardium, usually in border zones of damaged and normal tissue. The characteristic appearance of this VT is of uniform QRS morphology. As with all arrhythmias, identification of underlying or exacerbating conditions is required. Similarly to the strategy described earlier, management is based on the stability or instability of the patient at the time of the arrhythmia. When drug therapy is needed, amiodarone and β-blockers are the preferred agents.[71,72] Lidocaine may also be used.[73] In general, agents that can compromise hemodynamics such as sotalol or intravenous procainamide should be avoided in the ICU patient unless the patient is completely hemodynamically stable. Long-term suppression depends on definitive correction, where possible, of reversible causes, and removal of inciting agents such as pressors.

Polymorphic VT

The hallmark electrocardiographically of PMVT is beat-to-beat variation in the QRS morphology. The mechanism of PMVT is different from monomorphic VT and is often hemodynamically unstable, and sustained episodes require urgent cardioversion.

Table 7 Drugs for wide complex tachycardia	
Medication	**Dose**
Amiodarone	150 mg IV over 10 min, may repeat every 10 min as needed; then IV drip 1 mg/min for 6 h followed by 0.5 mg/min for 18 h (max. cumulative dose 2.2 g over 24 h)
Procainamide	15–18 mg/kg over 25–30 min or 100 mg given no faster than 50 mg/min, may repeat every 5 min (max. cumulative dose 1 g); then IV drip 1–4 mg/min
Lidocaine	1–1.5 mg/kg IV, may repeat 0.5–0.75 mg/kg every 5–10 min (max. cumulative dose 3 mg/kg); then IV drip 1–4 mg/min

PMVT may occur in the setting of either normal or long QT, and the baseline ECG should be evaluated to determine the QTc interval.

When seen in the setting of long QT, PMVT is termed torsades de pointes, and the approach is directed at correction of the QT (**Fig. 10**). Long QT can be hereditary or associated with several drug toxicities. In the setting of a congenital channelopathy associated long QT, torsades de pointes in more often associated with accelerated sinus rates with lengthening or inappropriate shortening of the QT interval. In acquired long QT torsades de pointes is often pause dependent, with further prolongation of the QT interval after the pause. In these instances, overdrive pacing and isoproterenol may be effective at arrhythmia suppression. Intravenous magnesium can also be effective at improving rhythm control in the patient with PMVT either with or without long QT, and correction of hypokalemia is critical.[74,75]

PMVT with normal QT is often associated with myocardial ischemia, which needs to be rapidly identified and corrected. This approach may require urgent cardiac catheterization and revascularization. Amiodarone and β-blockers may be effective for arrhythmia suppression.

Electrical Storm Recurrent VT/VF or ICD Discharges

Extreme electrical instability with recurrent episodes of VT or VF is infrequent and is typically seen in settings such as patients with acute myocardial ischemia or drug

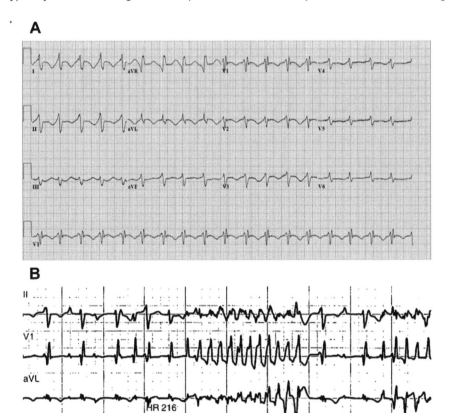

Fig. 10. (A) Sinus tachycardia with marked QT prolongation in a patient with Takotsubo cardiomyopathy. (B) Onset of torsades de pointes.

toxicity (including alcohol), and acute or worsened heart failure in patients with cardiomyopathy.[75,76] Less frequently, the patient will have an underlying primary electrical cause such as Brugada syndrome or long-QT syndrome. By definition, electrical storm exists when there are 3 or more episodes of VT or VF or appropriate discharges from an implanted cardioverter-defibrillator (ICD) in a 24-hour period.[75] As always, device interrogation is mandatory to ensure that the shocks are clinically appropriate and that the device is functioning normally. Among patients with implanted ICDs, the incidence of electrical storm may be 10% to 20%.[77] Gaining control of the arrhythmia is paramount given the potentially life-threatening nature of the arrhythmia itself, in addition to the potential long-term deleterious effects of multiple ICD therapies in the ICD patient population.[78]

The initial therapy is directed at identifying and correcting any potential underlying mechanism such as hypokalemia, other electrolyte imbalances, ischemia, worsening heart failure, or other remediable factors.[75] The pharmacologic agents that are most useful in electrical storm are amiodarone and β-blockers.[75,79] During cardiac arrest or electrical storms, the sympathetic nervous system is activated, and β-blockers are often very effective at suppressing recurrent VT/VF.[80] For the patient with an ICD, reprogramming the device to maximize attempts at pace termination rather than shocks, prolonging the time before ICD discharge, and other changes may be helpful acutely. For the ICD recipient who has repeated shocks despite optimization of medical therapy and device reprogramming, radiofrequency ablation may be considered, recognizing that the procedure is not without risk.[81]

In some cases, particularly where arrhythmia is pause dependent or in the setting of long QT, overdrive pacing with a temporary pacemaker may suppress the arrhythmia. The utility of isoproterenol for VT/VF suppression is limited to those patients with primary electrical abnormalities such as Brugada syndrome or long-QT syndrome.[82] Long-term management of the patient with electrical storm is directed toward maximizing therapy for heart failure, definitive ischemia correction through revascularization where feasible, and reducing risk for future events through optimization of electrolytes and other metabolic parameters.

Bradyarrhythmias

In the ICU setting, bradyarrhythmias are often the result of medical conditions, medications, or respiratory status (see earlier discussion on mechanisms). As such, many causes of bradycardia or heart block are anticipated to be reversible in the ICU setting. However, in situations where recurrent bradycardia is compromising the patient or impeding care, temporary pacing may be required. For very rare episodes of symptomatic pauses or if a definite need for transvenous pacing has not been established, external transcutaneous pacing is available. Another indication for transcutaneous pacing might be during right heart manipulation (eg, placement of right heart catheter) in a patient with an underlying left bundle branch block. Long-term or continuous transcutaneous pacing is not appropriate, as this form of pacing can be unreliable and painful.

Temporary transvenous right ventricular pacing can usually be accomplished at the bedside in the ICU without the use of fluoroscopy. If dual-chamber pacing is required (eg, patient does not tolerate right ventricular pacing, for overdrive suppression of atrial arrhythmias), placement of a right atrial lead is facilitated with the use of fluoroscopy.

Many postoperative cardiac patients will have epicardial leads placed at the time of surgery. A variety of temporary pacing electrodes are available for transvenous insertion, including a balloon-tipped catheter that is easiest for bedside insertion, but is more likely to become dislodged and not optimal in the setting of cardiac arrest whereby forward flow is absent. Temporary screw-in leads are fairly reliable but require fluoroscopy for placement. Transvenous access from the right subclavian or internal jugular vein is preferred for ease of lead placement, patient comfort, and sterility. Careful site management is required to avoid contamination, and leads may be left in for 7to 10 days.

In the setting of acute myocardial infarction, temporary pacing is indicated for symptomatic bradyarrhythmias unresponsive to medical treatment.[83]

Special Circumstances: Patient with Ventricular Assist Device

The use of ventricular assist devices is becoming more common in patients with advanced heart failure, either as destination therapy or as a bridge to transplant. By definition, these patients are inherently at risk for arrhythmias related to their underlying cardiac disease, and the implantation of the assist device can create arrhythmic foci in the ventricle. Even though the presence of the assist device may mitigate the immediate compromise of a VA, left ventricular assist device flow may be decreased and contribute can contribute to mortality.[84] These patients may require advanced techniques for arrhythmia management, such as cryoablation or radiofrequency ablation.

SUMMARY

Cardiac arrhythmias are common in the ICU, and can be either the initial reason for admission to the ICU or a consequence of the medical condition. Exacerbating and contributing factors are multiple, and management of the patient requires a careful determination of these factors and correction where possible. Arrhythmias in the ICU are associated with short-term and long-term consequences. Such arrhythmias may occur in patients with underlying cardiac and pulmonary disease, but can occur in the medically ill or postoperative patient regardless of underlying pathology. A stepwise approach facilitates care.

1. Determine whether the patient is compromised by the arrhythmia as opposed to the underlying condition.
2. Aggressively manage life-threatening arrhythmias as per ACLS guidelines.
3. Determine the nature of the arrhythmia: what am I treating?
4. Determine underlying causes and identify correctable causes.
5. Determine appropriate drug therapy based on clinical condition.

REFERENCES

1. Tongyoo S, Permpikul C, Haemin R, et al. Predicting factors, incidence and prognosis of cardiac arrhythmia in medical, non-acute coronary syndrome, critically ill patients. J Med Assoc Thai 2013;96(Suppl 2):S238–45.
2. Annane D, Sébille V, Duboc D, et al. Incidence and prognosis of sustained arrhythmias in critically ill patients. Am J Respir Crit Care Med 2008;178(1):20–5.
3. Polanczyk CA, Goldman L, Marcantonio ER, et al. Supraventricular arrhythmia in patients having noncardiac surgery: clinical correlates and effect on length of stay. Ann Intern Med 1998;129(4):279–85.
4. Goodman S, Shirov T, Weismann C. Supraventricular arrhythmias in intensive care unit patients: short and long-term consequences. Anesth Analg 2007; 104:880–6.

5. Adekola OO, Soriyan OO, Meka I, et al. The incidence of electrolyte and acid-base abnormalities in critically ill patients using point of care testing (i-STAT portable analyser). Nig Q J Hosp Med 2012;22(2):103–8.
6. Volpi A, Cavalli A, Santoro L, et al. Incidence and prognosis of early primary ventricular fibrillation in acute myocardial infarction—results of the Gruppo Italiano per lo Studio della Sopravvivenza nell'Infarto Miocardico (GISSI-2) database. Am J Cardiol 1998;82(3):265.
7. Macdonald JE, Struthers AD. What is the optimal serum potassium level in cardiovascular patients? J Am Coll Cardiol 2004;43:155–61.
8. Whang R, Whang DD, Ryan MP. Refractory potassium repletion. A consequence of magnesium deficiency. Arch Intern Med 1992;152(1):40.
9. Ayres SM, Grace WJ. Inappropriate ventilation and hypoxemia as causes of cardiac arrhythmias: the control of arrhythmias without antiarrhythmic drugs. Am J Med 1969;46(4):495–505.
10. Jhanjee R, Templeton GA, Sattiraju S, et al. Relationship of paroxysmal atrial tachyarrhythmias to volume overload: assessment by implanted transpulmonary impedance monitoring. Circ Arrhythm Electrophysiol 2009;2:488–94.
11. Nuemar RW, Otto CW, Link MS, et al. Part 8: adult advanced cardiovascular life support. 2010 American Heart Association guidelines for cardiopulmonary resuscitation and emergency cardiovascular care. Circulation 2010;122:S729–67.
12. Ebert TJ, Hall JE, Barney JA, et al. The effects of increasing plasma concentrations of dexmedetomidine in humans. Anesthesiology 2000;93:382–94.
13. Hirose M, Carlson MD, Laurita KR. Cellular mechanisms of vagally mediated atrial tachyarrhythmia in isolated arterially perfused canine right atria. J Cardiovasc Electrophysiol 2002;13(9):918–26.
14. Gorgels AP, Vos MA, Smeets JL, et al. Delayed afterdepolarizations and atrial and ventricular arrhythmias. In: Rosen MR, Janse MJ, Wit AL, editors. Cardiac electrophysiology: a textbook. Mount Kisco (NY): Futura Publishing; 1990. p. 341.
15. Yap YG, Camm AJ. Drug induced prolongation and torsades de pointes. Heart 2003;89(11):1363.
16. De Ponti F, Poluzzi E, Cavalli A, et al. Safety of non-antiarrhythmic drugs that prolong the QT interval or induce torsades de pointes: an overview. Drug Saf 2002;25(4):263.
17. Jackman WM, Friday KJ, Anderson JL, et al. The long QT syndromes: a critical review, new clinical observations and a unifying hypothesis. Prog Cardiovasc Dis 1988;31(2):115.
18. Reinelt P, Karth GD, Geppert A, et al. Incidence and type of cardiac arrhythmias in critically ill patients: a single center experience in a medical-cardiological ICU. Intensive Care Med 2001;27(9):1466–73.
19. Camm AJ, Kirchhof P, Lip GY, et al. Guidelines for the management of atrial fibrillation: the Task Force for the Management of Atrial Fibrillation of the European Society of Cardiology (ESC). Eur Heart J 2010;31:2369–429.
20. Go AS, Hylek EM, Phillips KA, et al. Prevalence of diagnosed atrial fibrillation in adults: national implications for rhythm management and stroke prevention: the AnTicoagulation and Risk Factors in Atrial Fibrillation (ATRIA) Study. JAMA 2001;285:2370–5.
21. Kanji S, Williamson DR, Yaghchi BM, et al. Epidemiology and management of atrial fibrillation in medical and noncardiac surgical adult intensive care unit patients. J Crit Care 2012;27:326.e1–8.

22. Fioranelli M, Piccoli M, Mileto GM, et al. Analysis of heart rate variability five minutes before the onset of paroxysmal atrial fibrillation. Pacing Clin Electrophysiol 1999;22(5):743–9.
23. Herweg B, Dalal P, Nagy B, et al. Power spectral analysis of heart period variability of preceding sinus rhythm before initiation of paroxysmal atrial fibrillation. Am J Cardiol 1998;82(7):869–74.
24. Kannel WB, Wolf PA, Benjamin EJ, et al. Prevalence, incidence, prognosis, and predisposing conditions for atrial fibrillation: population-based estimates. Am J Cardiol 1998;82:2N–9N.
25. Wang TJ, Larson MG, Levy D, et al. Temporal relations of atrial fibrillation and congestive heart failure and their joint influence on mortality: the Framingham Heart Study. Circulation 2003;107:2920–5.
26. Krahn AD, Manfreda J, Tate RB, et al. The natural history of atrial fibrillation: incidence, risk factors, and prognosis in the Manitoba Follow-Up Study. Am J Med 1995;98:476–84.
27. Stewart S, Hart CL, Hole DJ, et al. A population-1 based study of the long-term risks associated with atrial fibrillation: 20-year follow-up of the Renfrew/Paisley study. Am J Med 2002;113:359–64.
28. Guyton AC. The relationship of cardiac output and arterial pressure control. Circulation 1981;64:1079–88.
29. Agency for Healthcare Research and Quality. Treatment of atrial fibrillation. Available at: http://effectivehealthcare.ahrq.gov/index.cfm/search-for-guides-reviews-and-reports/?productid=946&pageaction=displayproduct. Accessed May 9, 2014.
30. Kirchhof P, Andresen D, Bosch R, et al. Short-term versus long-term antiarrhythmic drug treatment after cardioversion of atrial fibrillation (Flec-SL): a prospective, randomised, open-label, blinded endpoint assessment trial. Lancet 2012;380:238–46.
31. Dunn AB, White CM, Reddy P, et al. Efficacy and cost analysis of ibutilide. Ann Pharmacother 2000;34(11):1233–7.
32. VerNooy RA, Mounsey P. Antiarrhythmic drug therapy in atrial fibrillation. Cardiol Clin 2004;22:21–34.
33. Gowda RM, Khan IA, Punukollu G, et al. Female preponderance in ibutilide-induced torsade de pointes. Int J Cardiol 2004;95(2–3):219.
34. Stambler BS, Wood MA, Ellenbogen KA, et al. Efficacy and safety of repeated intravenous doses of ibutilide for rapid conversion of atrial flutter or fibrillation. Ibutilide Repeat Dose Study Investigators. Circulation 1996;94(7):1613.
35. Li H, Natale A, Tomassoni G, et al. Usefulness of ibutilide in facilitating successful external cardioversion of refractory atrial fibrillation. Am J Cardiol 1999;84(9): 1096–8, A10.
36. Clemo HF, Wood MA, Gilligan DM, et al. Intravenous amiodarone for acute heart rate control in the critically ill patient with atrial tachyarrhythmias. Am J Cardiol 1998;81(5):594.
37. Roy D, Talajic M, Dorian P, et al. Amiodarone to prevent recurrence of atrial fibrillation. Canadian Trial of Atrial Fibrillation Investigators. N Engl J Med 2000; 342(13):913.
38. Danias PG, Caulfield TA, Weigner MJ, et al. Likelihood of spontaneous cardioversion of atrial fibrillation to sinus rhythm. J Am Coll Cardiol 1998;31:588–92.
39. Sleeswijk ME, Van Noord T, Tulleken JE, et al. Clinical review: treatment of new-onset atrial fibrillation in medical intensive care patients- a clinical framework. Crit Care 2007;11:233.

40. Miller S, Crystal E, Garfinkle M, et al. Effects of magnesium on atrial fibrillation after cardiac surgery: a meta-analysis. Heart 2005;91:618–23.

41. Delle KG, Geppert A, Neunteufl T, et al. Amiodarone versus diltiazem for rate control in critically ill patients with atrial tachyarrhythmias. Crit Care Med 2001;29:1149–53.

42. Cagli K, Ozeke O, Ergun K, et al. Effect of low-dose amiodarone and magnesium combination onatrial fibrillation after coronary artery surgery. J Card Surg 2006;21:458–64.

43. Kim RJ, Gerling BR, Kono AT, et al. Precipitation of ventricular fibrillation by intravenous diltiazem and metoprolol in a young patient with occult Wolff-Parkinson-White syndrome. Pacing Clin Electrophysiol 2008;31:776–9.

44. Blomstrom-Lundqvist C, Scheinman MM, Aliot EM, et al. ACC/AHA/ESC guidelines for the management of patients with supraventricular arrhythmias—executive summary. a report of the American College of Cardiology/American Heart Association Task Force on Practice Guidelines and the European Society of Cardiology Committee for Practice Guidelines (writing committee to develop guidelines for the management of patients with supraventricular arrhythmias) developed in collaboration with NASPE-Heart Rhythm Society. J Am Coll Cardiol 2003;42:1493–531.

45. Boriani G, Biffi M, Frabetti L, et al. Ventricular fibrillation after intravenous amiodarone in Wolff-Parkinson-White syndrome with atrial fibrillation. Am Heart J 1996;131:1214–6.

46. Hogue CW, Creswell LL, Gutterman DD, et al. American College of Chest Physicians guidelines for the prevention and management of postoperative atrial fibrillation after cardiac surgery: epidemiology, mechanisms, and risks. Chest 2005;128(Suppl 2):9S–16S.

47. Martinez EA, Epstein AE, Bass EB. American College of Chest Physicians guidelines for the prevention and management of postoperative atrial fibrillation after cardiac surgery. Pharmacological control of ventricular rate. Chest 2005; 128(Suppl 2):56S–60S.

48. Fuster V, Rtyden LE, Asinger RW, et al. ACC/AHA/ESC guidelines for the management of patients with atrial fibrillation: a report of the American College of Cardiology/American Heart Association Task Force on Practice Guidelines and the European Society of Cardiology Committee on Practice Guidelines and Policy Conferences. J Am Coll Cardiol 2001;38:1266i–1xx.

49. Camm AJ, Lip GY, De CR, et al. 2012 focused update of the ESC Guidelines for the management of atrial fibrillation: an update of the 2010 ESC Guidelines for the management of atrial fibrillation. Developed with the special contribution of the European Heart Rhythm Association. Eur Heart J 2010;31:2369–429.

50. Lip GY, Tse HF, Lane DA. Atrial fibrillation. Lancet 2012;379:648–61.

51. Mason PK, Lake DE, DiMarco JP, et al. Impact of the CHA2DS2-VASc score on anticoagulation recommendations for atrial fibrillation. Am J Med 2012;125:603–6.

52. Connolly SJ, Ezekowitz MD, Yusuf S, et al. Dabigatran versus warfarin in patients with atrial fibrillation. N Engl J Med 2009;361:1139–51.

53. Granger CB, Alexander JH, McMurray JJ, et al. Apixaban versus warfarin in patients with atrial fibrillation. N Engl J Med 2011;365:981–92.

54. Patel MR, Mahaffey KW, Garg J, et al. Rivaroxaban versus warfarin in nonvalvular atrial fibrillation. N Engl J Med 2011;365:883–91.

55. Pisters R, Lane DA, Nieuwlaat R, et al. A novel user-friendly score (HAS-BLED) to assess 1-year risk of major bleeding in patients with atrial fibrillation: the Euro Heart Survey. Chest 2010;138:1093–100.

56. Gelzer AR, Moise NS, Vaidya D, et al. Temporal organization of atrial activity and irregular ventricular rhythm during spontaneous atrial fibrillation: an in vivo study in the horse. J Cardiovasc Electrophysiol 2000;11:773–84.
57. Saoudi N, Cosio F, Waldo A, et al. Classification of atrial flutter and regular atrial tachycardia according to electrophysiologic mechanism and anatomic bases: a statement from a joint expert group from the Working Group of Arrhythmias of the European Society of Cardiology and the North American Society of Pacing and Electrophysiology. J Cardiovasc Electrophysiol 2001;12:852–66.
58. Trappe H-J, Brandts B, Weismueller P. Arrhythmias in the intensive care patient. Curr Opin Crit Care 2003;9(5):345–55.
59. Camm AJ, Garratt CJ. Adenosine and supraventricular tachycardia. N Engl J Med 1991;325(23):1621.
60. Jordaens L, Gorgels A, Stroobandt R, et al. Efficacy and safety of intravenous sotalol for termination of paroxysmal supraventricular tachycardia. The Sotalol Versus Placebo Multicenter Study Group. Am J Cardiol 1991;68(1):35.
61. Kouvaras G, Cokkinos DV, Halal G, et al. The effective treatment of multifocal atrial tachycardia with amiodarone. Jpn Heart J 1989;30(3):301.
62. Gomes JA, Mehta D, Langan MN. Sinus node reentrant tachycardia. Pacing Clin Electrophysiol 1995;18(5 Pt 1):1045.
63. Garson A Jr, Gillette PC. Electrophysiologic studies of supraventricular tachycardia in children. I. Clinical-electrophysiologic correlations. Am Heart J 1981; 102(2):233.
64. Engelstein ED, Lippman N, Stein KM, et al. Mechanism-specific effects of adenosine on atrial tachycardia. Circulation 1994;89(6):2645.
65. Gomes JA, Hariman RJ, Kang PS, et al. Sustained symptomatic sinus node reentrant tachycardia: incidence, clinical significance, electrophysiologic observations and the effects of antiarrhythmic agents. J Am Coll Cardiol 1985;5(1):45.
66. Akhtar M, Shenasa M, Jazayeri M, et al. Wide QRS complex tachycardia. Reappraisal of a common clinical problem. Ann Intern Med 1988;109(11):905.
67. Tchou P, Young P, Mahmud R, et al. Useful clinical criteria for the diagnosis of ventricular tachycardia. Am J Med 1988;84(1):53.
68. Stewart RB, Bardy GH, Greene HL. Wide complex tachycardia: misdiagnosis and outcome after emergent therapy. Ann Intern Med 1986;104(6):766.
69. Garratt CJ, Griffith MJ, O'Nunain S, et al. Effects of intravenous adenosine on antegrade refractoriness of accessory atrioventricular connections. Circulation 1991;84(5):1962.
70. Sharma AD, Klein GJ, Yee R. Intravenous adenosine triphosphate during wide QRS complex tachycardia: safety, therapeutic efficacy, and diagnostic utility. Am J Med 1990;88(4):337.
71. Eifling M, Razavi M, Massumi A. The evaluation and management of electrical storm. Tex Heart Inst J 2011;38(2):111–21.
72. Naccarelli GV, Jalal S. Intravenous amiodarone. Another option in the acute management of sustained ventricular tachyarrhythmias. Circulation 1995; 92(11):3154.
73. Griffith MJ, Linker NJ, Garratt CJ, et al. Relative efficacy and safety of intravenous drugs for termination of sustained ventricular tachycardia. Lancet 1990; 336(8716):670.
74. Tzivoni D, Banai S, Schuger C, et al. Treatment of torsade de pointes with magnesium sulfate. Circulation 1988;77(2):392.
75. Zipes DP, Camm AJ, Borggrefe M, et al, American College of Cardiology/American Heart Association Task Force, European Society of Cardiology Committee

for Practice Guidelines, European Heart Rhythm Association, Heart Rhythm Society. ACC/AHA/ESC 2006 guidelines for management of patients with ventricular arrhythmias and the prevention of sudden cardiac death: a report of the American College of Cardiology/American Heart Association Task Force and the European Society of Cardiology Committee for Practice Guidelines (writing committee to develop guidelines for management of patients with ventricular arrhythmias and the prevention of sudden cardiac death): developed in collaboration with the European Heart Rhythm Association and the Heart Rhythm Society. Circulation 2006;114(10):e385.

76. Greene M, Newman D, Geist M, et al. Is electrical storm in ICD patients the sign of a dying heart? Outcome of patients with clusters of ventricular tachyarrhythmias. Europace 2000;2(3):263.

77. Emkanjoo Z, Alihasani N, Alizadeh A, et al. Electrical storm in patients with implantable cardioverter-defibrillators: can it be forecast? Tex Heart Inst J 2009;36(6):563–7.

78. Gatzoulis KA, Andrikopoulos GK, Apostolopoulos T, et al. Electrical storm is an independent predictor of adverse long-term outcome in the era of implantable defibrillator therapy. Europace 2005;7(2):184–92.

79. Kudenchuk PJ, Cobb LA, Copass MK, et al. Amiodarone for resuscitation after out-of-hospital cardiac arrest due to ventricular fibrillation. N Engl J Med 1999; 341(12):871–8.

80. Nademanee K, Taylor R, Bailey WE, et al. Treating electrical storm: sympathetic blockade versus advanced cardiac life support-guided therapy. Circulation 2000;102(7):742–7.

81. Aliot EM, Stevenson WG, Almendral-Garrote JM, et al. EHRA/HRS expert consensus on catheter ablation of ventricular arrhythmias: developed in a partnership with the European Heart Rhythm Association (EHRA), a Registered Branch of the European Society of Cardiology (ESC), and the Heart Rhythm Society (HRS); in collaboration with the American College of Cardiology (ACC) and the American Heart Association (AHA). Heart Rhythm 2009;6(6):886–933.

82. Ohgo T, Okamura H, Noda T, et al. Acute and chronic management in patients with Brugada syndrome associated with electrical storm of ventricular fibrillation. Heart Rhythm 2007;4(6):695–700.

83. O'Gara PT, Kushner FG, Ascheim DD, et al. 2013 ACCF/AHA guideline for the management of ST-elevation myocardial infarction: executive summary: a report of the American College of Cardiology Foundation/American Heart Association Task Force on Practice Guidelines. Circulation 2013;127:529–55.

84. Bedi M, Kormos R, Winowich S, et al. Ventricular arrhythmias during left ventricular assist device support. Am J Cardiol 2007;99(8):1151–3.

Cardiogenic Shock

Palak Shah, MD, MS[a],*, Jennifer A. Cowger, MD, MS[b]

KEYWORDS

- Cardiogenic shock • Intra-aortic balloon pump
- Percutaneous ventricular assist device • Inotropes • Revascularization

KEY POINTS

- Cardiogenic shock is the leading cause of death for patients hospitalized with an acute myocardial infarction.
- Early revascularization is the therapy of choice for patients with cardiogenic shock complicating an acute myocardial infarction.
- Intra-aortic balloon pumps have not been shown to improve survival for patients who are suffering from an acute myocardial infarction in the modern era of early revascularization.
- Percutaneous ventricular assist devices are a promising therapy for temporary support of patients in cardiogenic shock, but rigorous clinical data demonstrating improved outcomes are lacking.
- Routine utilization of a pulmonary artery catheter in managing patients with cardiogenic shock is unnecessary, but may be vital to determining a care plan in select patients being considered for mechanical support or transplant.

Shock is characterized by a state of end-organ hypoperfusion resulting in abnormal organ homeostasis, leading to high patient morbidity and mortality. Cardiogenic shock (CS) is a clinical syndrome characterized by systemic hypotension and hypoperfusion secondary to insufficient cardiac output. In states of pure CS, cardiac filling pressures are elevated and cardiac output is low.[1] CS can lead to multisystem organ failure, manifested by oliguria, lactic acidosis, altered mentation, and cool extremities. Most commonly, CS is the direct sequelae of an acute myocardial infarction (MI), and acute ischemic CS carries an in-hospital mortality of greater than 50%.[2,3] However, CS can also arise as an acute presentation of a cardiomyopathy of nonischemic cause or as a severe decompensation of chronic (ischemic or nonischemic) cardiomyopathy. The latter presentations are less common and account for only 1% of acute heart failure syndromes.[4]

Disclosures: None relevant.
[a] Inova Translational Medicine Institute, Inova Fairfax Hospital, 3300 Gallows Road, Falls Church, VA 22042, USA; [b] Heart Failure and Transplant Program, St Vincent Heart Center, 8333 Naab Road, Suite 400, Indianapolis, IN 46260, USA
* Corresponding author. Transplant Program, Inova Fairfax Hospital, 3300 Gallows Road, Falls Church, VA 22042.
E-mail address: palak.shah@inova.org

Critical care management is centered on an efficient, rapid, and organized approach to the shock patient using a multidisciplinary care approach between intensivists, heart failure specialists, cardiac surgery, and interventional cardiology. The tenets of therapy include restoring cardiac output and identifying and treating one or multiple potential causative factors: hypoxia, hypervolemia, acidosis, arrhythmias, coronary ischemia, and mechanical complications of an MI. In certain clinical situations (eg, requirement for multiple inotropes or vasopressors, worsening hemodynamics despite inotrope support), it may be prudent to refer the patient to the nearest left ventricular assist device (LVAD)/transplant program for further management.

PHYSICAL FINDINGS

The importance of a focused physical examination in the management of a patient with CS should be emphasized. It is at this critical juncture in the clinical evaluation process that obtaining the correct information can direct the caregiver down the right diagnostic and therapeutic pathway. A thorough assessment allows for evaluation of intravascular volume status and adequacy of end-organ function (**Box 1**).

Jugular Venous Pressure and S_3 Gallop

The internal jugular vein forms a direct fluid column with the right atrium and provides a noninvasive measure of right atrial pressure. The correct method for determining jugular venous pressure (JVP) is depicted in **Fig. 1**. The patient should be placed in bed at a 45° angle, which can be confirmed by use of the ball found commonly on the side of a

---

Box 1
Components of the heart failure physical examination

JVP

Rales

Displaced and sustained point of maximal impulse

Gallops—third or fourth heart sounds

Heart murmurs

Cool extremities

Peripheral, scrotal, or presacral edema

Right ventricular heave/parasternal lift

Hypotension

Tachycardia

Tachypnea

Abdominal ascites

Hepatomegaly

Pulsatile liver

Pulsus alternans

Orthopnea

Dullness to percussion in lung bases

Restlessness

Temporal wasting

Elevated jugular venous pressure

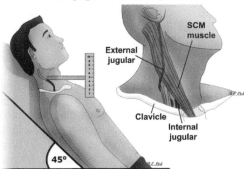

Fig. 1. Assessment of JVP. The appropriate assessment of JVP relies on an estimation of the distance of the meniscus of the jugular venous pulsation above the sternal angle and is correctly performed by having the patient in a semi-recumbent position with the body angled at 45°. The distance of the meniscus of the jugular venous pulsation over the angle of Louis is then added to 5 cm to estimate the JVP or the right atrial pressure. SCM, sterno-cleidomastoid muscle. (*From* Clinical examination of the cardiovascular system DVD-3, Bloomsbury Educational Ltd, 97 Judd Street, London WC1H 9JB; with permission.)

hospital bed. Careful observation of internal jugular vein with the head and neck as aligned in **Fig. 1** allows one to appreciate the JVP. It is important to avoid having the patient extend their neck because this can cause the internal jugular vein to flatten. Once the meniscus of the JVP has been located, an estimate of the right atrial pressure can be made by adding 5 cm to the distance of the JVP meniscus above the angle of Louis. The constant of 5 cm is added because it represents the distance from the sternum to the right atrium. The normal JVP is 6 to 8 cm of water, and 1 cm of water is equivalent to 0.74 mm Hg. In patients who have a very low or high JVP, it is often necessary to lay the patient flat or elevate the head of the bed at 90°, respectively, to appreciate the meniscus of the JVP.[5,6]

The ventricular gallop, S_3, or third heart sound is a relatively specific finding of heart failure in the adult population. In the setting of heart failure, an S_3 gallop occurs because of early and rapid ventricular filling often in a dilated ventricle. The sound can originate from either the right or the left ventricle and leads to a right-sided or left-sided third, early diastolic heart sound (S_3). The quality and intensity of the S_3 gallop are related to the atrial pressure, ventricular compliance, and diastolic filling rate. An S_3 tends to be louder in states of volume overload and can be heard with significant mitral regurgitation (MR) even in those with normal left ventricular function.[7] In pregnant women and children, an S_3 may also be a benign finding.

The JVP and S_3 gallop are not only useful tools for diagnosing heart failure, but are also predictive of patient outcome. The prognostic importance of these physical examination findings was studied within the large multicenter Studies of Left Ventricular Dysfunction trial, which evaluated the efficacy of enalapril in the treatment of systolic heart failure.[8,9] In a multivariable analysis that included ejection fraction, age, as well as other demographic and clinical variables, the only predictors of death or hospitalization for heart failure were JVP and an S_3 gallop.[9] The presence of elevated JVP in heart failure patients was associated with an increased risk of death (relative risk = 1.52) compared with patients without an elevation of JVP.[9] A similar increased risk of death was seen in patients with an S_3 gallop (relative risk = 1.35) compared with those patients with heart failure and no ventricular gallop.[9]

Determining the Cardiac Output on Examination

JVP, dependent edema, and rales are all physical examination findings associated with fluid overload, but give little information as to the adequacy of end-organ perfusion by the myopathic heart. A variety of physical examination findings can be used to assist in determining whether the cardiac output is normal or low. These findings include, but are not limited to, the presence of cool or mottled extremities with a reduced capillary refill, the presence of a pulsus alternans, a narrow pulse pressure, hypotension, and impaired mentation.[10] Patients can be grouped into 4 profiles based on the presence of elevated filling pressures and the adequacy of cardiac output as outlined in **Fig. 2**.[11] These profiles guide the usage and timing of diuretics, vasodilators, and vasoactive and inotropic medications. These hemodynamic profiles not only guide therapy but also have prognostic implications similar to those obtained by invasive measurements of cardiac output and pulmonary capillary wedge pressure.[12,13]

Physical Examination Pitfalls

A common pitfall in the evaluation of heart failure patients is the overreliance on certain physical examination findings to determine a volume overloaded state. Although wet

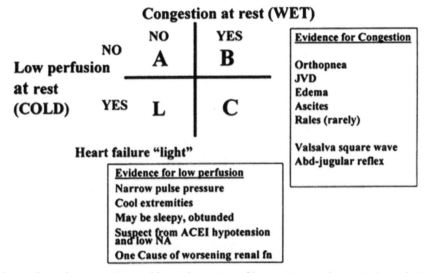

Fig. 2. Physical examination and hemodynamic profiles. Patients with systolic heart failure can be assigned to 1 of 4 profiles, based on a clinical assessment of congestion and perfusion as proposed by Stevenson.[11] Congestion is assessed based on the presence of elevated JVP, dependent edema, rales, orthopnea, ascites, or hepatojugular reflux. Perfusion can be determined based on cool extremities, altered mentation, worsening renal function, hypotension, pulsus alternans, and narrow pulse pressure. The hemodynamic profile then dictates the appropriate course of therapy. Profile A patients are stable and require no escalation of therapy. Profile B ("wet and warm") patients benefit from diuretics to reduce congestion. Profile L ("dry and cold") patients are adequately compensated at rest, but usually have severe functional intolerance. Finally, profile C ("wet and cold") patients are in CS and require vasodilators or inotropic support to augment cardiac output and then diuretics to help reduce symptoms of congestion. Abd, abdominal; ACEI, angiotensin converting enzyme inhibitor; fn, function; JVD, jugular venous distention; NA, sodium. (*From* Stevenson LW. Tailored therapy to hemodynamic goals for advanced heart failure. Eur J Heart Fail 1999;1(3):251–7; with permission.)

crackles (ie, rales) may be appreciated in patients with acute heart failure, they may be absent on examination of CS patients with a past history of chronic heart failure.[14] Patients with chronic heart failure tend to exhibit rales only in very severe states of volume overload because their pulmonary lymphatics accommodate higher pulmonary venous pressures over time. Rales may not be heard in some individuals with chronic heart failure presenting with acute shock until left ventricular filling pressures are very high. Peripheral edema is neither sensitive nor specific for CS. Although lower extremity edema can be a marker of elevated right-sided filling pressures, edema can also occur in the setting of protein calorie malnutrition or venous incompetence.

HEMODYNAMIC ASSESSMENT

The first pulmonary arterial catheterization (PAC) was performed by Lewis Dexter in 1945 and was performed to diagnose congenital heart disease.[15] It was not until 1970 when Swan and and colleagues[16] developed the balloon-tipped catheter that widespread use of the device became popular. Initial excitement for the device has contemporaneously been tempered by a growing body of evidence that its routine use in managing a variety of patient groups may be unwarranted and potentially harmful.[17–20] Over the past decade, the utilization of PACs has fallen dramatically and some would argue that many clinicians now lack adequate training in how to place, interpret, or manage a PAC.[21,22]

The routine use of PACs in patients with an acute exacerbation of heart failure was studied in the multicenter Evaluation Study of Congestive Heart Failure and Pulmonary Artery Catheterization Effectiveness (ESCAPE) trial.[23] Patients who had their heart failure managed in conjunction with a PAC failed to demonstrate an improvement in hospital length of stay or mortality compared with those managed without a PAC. The PAC group had an increased incidence of adverse events largely driven by catheter-related complications including line infection.[23] It is important to note, however, that these patients were not necessarily in CS: the mean cardiac index was 1.9 L/min/m^2 and the trial explicitly excluded those patients receiving an intravenous inotrope.[23]

Studies specifically looking at PAC use in patients after an MI showed similar results to that of the ESCAPE trial. In an analysis of greater than 26,000 patients presenting with an acute coronary syndrome who were enrolled in to the Global Utilization of Streptokinase and TPA for Occluded Coronary Arteries (GUSTO) IIb and III trials, only 735 patients received a PAC.[24] Pulmonary arterial catheters were more commonly used in the post-MI setting when patients had higher resource utilization (eg, coronary artery bypass grafting, percutaneous coronary intervention) and/or a more unstable clinical presentation (eg, need for mechanical ventilation, intra-aortic balloon pumps [IABP]).[24] PAC use was associated with an increased risk of adverse events including an adjusted 6-fold increase in 30-day mortality. However, when looking at the subgroup of patients with CS, the use of a PAC had a neutral effect on mortality. The nonrandomized nature of this study makes the findings about the utility of PAC placement questionable.[24]

The PAC measurements also provide prognostic information in the setting of acute MI. The Forrester criteria assess pulmonary congestion (pulmonary capillary wedge pressure greater than 18 mm Hg) and systemic hypoperfusion (cardiac index less than 2.2 L/min/m^2) by using PAC data to categorize patients in quartiles.[25] Patients who exhibit both pulmonary congestion and systemic hypoperfusion have a 60% in-hospital mortality. It is important to note that the study was performed in the 1970s and management of acute coronary syndromes and CS has changed dramatically since then. Nevertheless, an appreciation for the severity of the hemodynamic derangement allows for an objective assessment of myocardial dysfunction and may prompt evaluation for advanced therapies including mechanical circulatory support.

Although routine invasive hemodynamic monitoring in patients with an acute heart failure exacerbation seems unwarranted, use in CS may still be clinically indicated. Potential indications for a PAC are listed in **Box 2**; these indications lack quality evidence from rigorously conducted randomized trials but continue to be supported in professional society guidelines, largely because of expert opinion.[26,27] Further details on PACs and hemodynamic monitoring are presented in the article in this issue by Kenaan and colleagues.

ILLNESS SEVERITY CLASSIFICATION SYSTEMS
Killip Class

The most widely recognized illness classification system to characterize patients with heart failure after an MI was developed by Killip and Kimball in 1967.[28] These physicians are credited with not only developing the Killip Classification system for heart failure severity (**Table 1**) but also creating the modern day coronary care unit. In the global registry of acute coronary events risk score, a higher Killip classification at time of hospital presentation was associated with a 2-fold increased risk of death per increase in Killip class.[29,30] Similar prognostication potential is also seen when the Killip classification system is applied to patients with non–ST-elevation acute coronary syndromes.[31]

APACHE II and SOFA Score

Although no well-validated tools have been developed for the explicit purpose of prognosticating outcome in patients presenting with CS, various risk scores derived for predicting outcome in a wide breadth of patients admitted to an intensive care unit (ICU) have been extrapolated to those in CS. The Acute Physiology and Chronic Health

---

Box 2
Recommendations for the use of pulmonary artery catheter

The routine use of invasive hemodynamic monitoring in patients with decompensated heart failure is not recommended.

Invasive hemodynamic monitoring should be considered in patients

a. When volume status and cardiac filling pressures are unclear

b. When refractory to initial therapy

c. Who have clinically significant hypotension or persistent symptoms

d. With worsening renal function during therapy

e. Being considered for cardiac transplant or mechanical circulatory support

f. To assess the response to vasoactive medications

g. When chronic outpatient infusion is being considered and documentation of an adequate hemodynamic response to the inotropic agent is necessary.

Data from Yancy CW, Jessup M, Bozkurt B, et al. 2013 ACCF/AHA guideline for the management of heart failure: a report of the American College of Cardiology Foundation/American Heart Association task force on practice guidelines. J Am Coll Cardiol 2013;62:e147–239; and Lindenfeld J, Albert NM, Boehmer JP, et al. HFSA 2010 comprehensive heart failure practice guideline. J Card Fail 2010;16(6):e1–194.

Table 1 Killip classification	
Class A	No heart failure. No clinical signs of cardiac decompensation.
Class B	Heart failure. Diagnostic criteria include rales, S_3 gallop, and venous hypertension.
Class C	Severe heart failure. Frank pulmonary edema.
Class D	CS. Signs include hypotension (systolic pressure of 90 mm Hg or less) and evidence of peripheral vasoconstriction, such as oliguria, cyanosis, and diaphoresis. Heart failure, often with pulmonary edema, has also been present in most of these patients.

Data from Killip T 3rd, Kimball JT. Treatment of myocardial infarction in a coronary care unit. A two year experience with 250 patients. Am J Cardiol 1967;20(4):457–64.

Evaluation II (APACHE II) was developed to prognosticate outcomes in patients presenting to the ICU with various unstable medical maladies.[32] The 12-item model calculates a risk score ranging from 0 to 71, taking into account patient age, chronic illnesses/comorbidities, physiologic measurements, end-organ function, the Glasgow coma scale, and postoperative state. Generally lower scores are assigned to patients in the postoperative state and higher overall scores predict a higher in-hospital mortality.[32] For those patients with a score greater than 25, in-hospital mortality exceeds 50%. Although the initial APACHE II validation cohort comprised a limited number of patients with cardiovascular disease, subsequent studies applying the APACHE II score to patients presenting in CS have demonstrated good predictive power.[33–35] In a study of more than 6000 patients presenting with an acute MI in Spain, each unit increase in APACHE II score was associated with a 16% increase in mortality.[34]

The Sequential Organ Failure Assessment (SOFA) score,[36] originally devised for describing complications in those with multisystem dysfunction due to sepsis, has also been used to predict mortality in patients with multisystem organ failure due to cardiac causes. The SOFA score comprises markers of renal function (serum creatinine or urine output), hepatic function (serum bilirubin), hemodynamic stability (mean arterial pressure or use of vasopressors), neurologic function (Glasgow coma scale), hematologic derangement (platelet count), and respiratory stability (the ratio of PaO_2/FiO_2). In a retrospective analysis of 726 acute MI patients, each unit increase in SOFA score was associated with a 1.3-fold increase in mortality.[37] The score offered reasonable risk discrimination with an area under the receiver operating characteristic curve of 0.79.

Although both the APACHE II and the SOFA models were not derived from a CS cohort, the leading cause of death in these patients is multisystem organ failure, which accounts for the prognostication of both models. The models do not predict long-term outcome after hospital discharge or death due to arrhythmias. Large studies comparing the APACHE II, SOFA, and the (updated) APACHE III scoring systems in the patients in CS are lacking.

INTERMACS Profiles

As durable ventricular assist devices become increasingly common in the management of patients with refractory end-stage heart failure, a unique patient registry that tracks clinical outcomes in LVAD recipients has been devised: the Interagency Registry for Mechanically Assisted Circulatory Support (INTERMACS).[38] The registry is supported by the National Institutes of Health, Food and Drug Administration,

Centers for Medicaid and Medicare Services, industry, and the individual institutions that participate. From the group who developed the registry, there has also been a parallel development of a heart failure classification scheme termed INTERMACS profiles. INTERMACS profiles (**Table 2**) are more appropriate than the New York Heart Association (NYHA) classification scheme or the American College of Cardiology Foundation/American Heart Association (ACC/AHA) heart failure stages (A–D) for categorizing disease severity and predicting outcome in patients who have end-stage heart failure (ie, NYHA class IIIB–IV symptoms and stage D status).[39,40] The profiles implicate a certain clinical course that provides prognostic information to the health team that can assist in clinical decision-making.[41] Patients in profile 1 are termed "Crash and Burn" and are in a state of severe end-organ malperfusion caused by CS. Patients in profile 2 (also known as "sliding on inotropes") have evidence of cardiac insufficiency (eg, worsening renal function) despite inotrope dependence, and patients in profile 3 are clinically stable, but are dependent on inotrope therapy. Although profile 3 patients are the most "stable" of the described scenarios, inotrope dependence is associated with a greater than 50% mortality at 1 year.[42] Even those who receive intravenous inotropes for heart failure support who are not deemed inotrope dependent at hospital discharge have higher morbidity and mortality than those with heart failure who have never received inotropes.[43]

MECHANICAL COMPLICATIONS

Patients with any type of mechanical complication post-MI carry a higher mortality when compared with patients with CS due to left ventricular dysfunction alone.[44] Previously, it was thought that these complications occurred at a predictable time course after an MI and was largely driven by the extent of tissue necrosis and timing of myocardial fibrosis.[45] As revascularization strategies have improved for MI, the modern day incidence of mechanical complications has dropped to less than 1% and most events occur within the first 24 hours of presentation.[46] Detection of a mechanical complication necessitates careful clinical attention to patient's signs and symptoms coupled with prompt echocardiographic evaluation to confirm the diagnosis.

Right Ventricular Infarction

One of the most widely recognized, but difficult to diagnose, complications of an inferior MI is a right ventricular infarction (RVI). The marginal branches that supply the right

Table 2
INTERMACS profiles

INTERMACS Profile	Profile Description	Clinical Example
1	Critical CS	Crash and burn
2	Progressive decline	Sliding on inotropes
3	Stable, but inotrope dependent	Dependent stability
4	Resting symptoms	Dyspnea at rest
5	Exertion intolerant	Dyspnea with activities of daily living
6	Exertion limited	Dyspnea with independent activities of daily living
7	NYHA class IIIB	Limited to mild physical activity

INTERMACS, Interagency Registry for Mechanically Assisted Circulatory Support.[40]

ventricle with blood typically originate from the right coronary artery, the culprit vessel in most inferior MIs. RVI complicating an inferior MI occurs at a rate of approximately 30% to 50% and accurate diagnosis is often difficult.[47] A right-sided V_4 electrocardiogram lead has a sensitivity and specificity of 88% and 78%, respectively, for the diagnosis.[47] Overall RVI is responsible for the development of CS in only 5% of CS cases, but carries a high mortality.[48] Patients with RVI also have a 3-fold higher risk of ventricular arrhythmias and atrioventricular node block compared with inferior MI patients without right ventricular involvement.[49]

The mainstay of therapy in RVI has been to maintain right ventricular preload by avoidance of nitrates and diuretics. Other strategies for management include adequate saline hydration such that the central venous pressure (ie, right atrial pressure) is above 10 mm Hg. In those patients with significant hypotension and bradycardia, insertion of a temporary pacemaker and/or initiation of inotrope support may be indicated to maintain a higher heart rate. This strategy of promoting relative tachycardia seems counterintuitive in an acute MI but is often necessary to maintain adequate left ventricular filling. Of note, the right ventricle is extremely resilient and often shows dramatic recovery on both clinical and echocardiographic follow-up, indicating the underlying pathophysiology of right ventricular dysfunction may represent stunning more so than myocardial necrosis.[50]

Acute MR

Acute MR after MI is associated with a poor survival.[51] Risk factors for the development of MR after MI include older age, female sex, and inferior or posterior infarction.[52] In a study of 773 patients presenting with an acute MI, mild MR occurred in 38% of subjects and an additional 12% had moderate or severe MR.[51] Event-free survival at 5 years was 84%, 74%, and 35% for those with no, mild, and moderate or severe MR, respectively. The Should We Emergently Revascularize Occluded Coronaries for Cardiogenic Shock (SHOCK) trial studied 1190 patients presenting in CS due to an acute MI and found that severe MR complicated 8% of patient courses.[52] Despite a mean left ventricular ejection fraction of 38%, in-hospital mortality was 55% in those with severe MR.

Mild or moderate MR during acute ischemia is often transient and resolves after restoration of blood flow, unlike acute papillary muscle rupture, which is life-threatening. Acute papillary muscle rupture occurs in about 7% of CS patients and affords about 5% of the mortality in patients presenting with an acute MI.[2,53] The occurrence of papillary muscle rupture has to do with the location of coronary occlusion and the time to reperfusion. There are 2 papillary muscles that attach to the mitral valve leaflets via chordae tendineae: the anterolateral and posteromedial papillary muscles. The anterolateral papillary muscle receives dual blood supply from the left anterior descending artery and marginal branches from the left circumflex artery, whereas the posteromedial papillary muscle has a singular blood supply from the posterior descending artery alone. Because of the blood supply pattern, the posteromedial papillary muscle is much more likely to rupture and this complication can be seen in the setting of an inferior infarction.[54,55] Rupture of the muscle can be either partial or complete with the clinical severity corresponding directly to the degree of muscle rupture (**Fig. 3**).[56] Older literature cited an onset of rupture of 3 to 7 days post-MI, but in the contemporary era of rapid reperfusion, the time clock for rupture has moved earlier (median time of 13 hours in the SHOCK trial)[52] and is likely caused by reperfusion injury (inflammation) in the territory of the injured papillary muscle.

Clinically, the presentation of acute MR secondary to papillary muscle rupture is often sudden with patients developing flash pulmonary edema (**Fig. 4**) and rapid

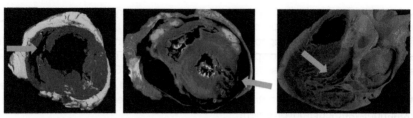

Fig. 3. Mechanical complications of an MI. Mechanical complications of a MI are depicted, from left to right, as: ventricular septal defect, free wall rupture, and papillary muscle rupture. (*From* Antman EM, Anbe DT, Kushner FG, et al. ACC/AHA guidelines for the management of patients with ST-elevation myocardial infarction. Circulation 2004;110:e82–292; with permission.)

hemodynamic instability. Because of rapid equalization of pressures between the left atrium and ventricle, a murmur may be absent. Therapy is focused on prompt clinical recognition, urgent echocardiographic visualization, afterload reduction with vasoactive medications, and/or an IABP followed by emergent surgical correction.[57–59]

Ventricular Septal Defects

Unlike papillary muscle rupture, ventricular septal defects typically occur in the setting of an anterior MI.[60] The incidence is quite uncommon, occurring in only 0.2% of patients in the current reperfusion era.[61] The mortality with medical management of acute septal defect is greater than 50%, and survival at 30 days is 71% to 100% in those with rapidly recognized and surgically corrected defects.[61,62] As percutaneous treatment of structural heart disease continues to develop, use of a septal occlusion device has shown some promise as a potential therapy for MI-associated ventricular

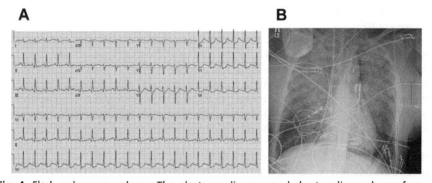

Fig. 4. Flash pulmonary edema. The electrocardiogram and chest radiograph are from a 60-year-old woman who presented to the emergency department with stuttering chest pain for 2 days. On presentation, her electrocardiogram showed inferior ST-segment elevation (*A*). She was promptly taken to the cardiac catheterization laboratory, where she was found to have total occlusion of her right coronary artery (*B*). The patient underwent percutaneous coronary intervention and stent placement. Four days later in the ICU, she was noted to develop acute-onset hypoxia and found to be in flash pulmonary edema. The patient was diagnosed with posteromedial papillary muscle partial rupture and underwent mitral valve replacement with preservation of the mitral valve apparatus as well as single-vessel coronary artery bypass surgery. She survived to discharge and was doing well on follow-up 1-year after surgery.

septal defects.[63,64] Use of a septal occlusion device may be particularly attractive in those patients who are deemed nonoperative candidates due to other medical comorbidities. Until a head-to-head study or large retrospective analysis comparing septal occlusion to surgery is completed, surgery continues to be the "gold standard" for treatment of ventricular septal defects in the setting of an MI (see **Fig. 3**).

Free Wall Rupture

Ventricular rupture of the free wall presents dramatically with electromechanical dissociation and pericardial tamponade (see **Fig. 3**). Free wall rupture occurs in less than 3% of patients with an acute MI, but accounts for more than 10% of the mortality; it is a common finding at autopsy in both out-of-hospital and in-hospital acute MI deaths.[65] Acute free wall rupture only occurs in patients with a transmural MI with a median time to onset of 5 days post-MI. The complication is more likely to occur in patients who are older, who are female gender, who have had anterior ST-elevation myocardial infarctions (STEMI), and for those in whom there is a delay in coronary revascularization.[66] Management is focused on hemodynamic support with fluids and vasoactive medications, bedside pericardiocentesis, followed by prompt surgical correction.

REVASCULARIZATION

The beneficial effects of revascularization of MI patients presenting in CS were established with the landmark SHOCK trial.[67] In patients presenting with CS as a complication of their MI, early revascularization with primary angioplasty and/or coronary artery bypass grafting was associated with a nonsignificant reduction in the primary endpoint of mortality at 30 days when compared with medical therapy alone. There was, however, a significant reduction in the prespecified secondary endpoints of 6-month and 1-year mortality, with an absolute reduction of mortality by 13%.[67,68] In the parallel SHOCK registry, the benefits of early revascularization were similarly noted.[2] At the time of the SHOCK trial in the late 1990s, early revascularization time was defined as occurring within 6 hours of presentation and only 36% of the revascularization patients received coronary stenting. In the current "door-to-balloon" era of revascularization, where most MI patients receive prompt revascularization with primary percutaneous coronary intervention, stent placement, and aggressive adjunctive medical therapy (ie, dual antiplatelet therapy, statins, anticoagulants, β-blockers, angiotensin converting enzyme inhibitors (ACE-I) and angiotensin II receptor blockers (ARBs), and aldosterone blockade), the rates of CS have dropped to approximately 5% for patients presenting with an STEMI.[69] Furthermore, general trends have shown a decreased incidence in the overall rate of STEMI over time, dropping from 47% in 1999 to 23% by 2008, which has also contributed to the reduced rate of CS over time.[70] The mortality from CS has also dropped from 60% in 1995 to 48% in 2004.[71]

One controversial finding in the original SHOCK trial was the patient group aged 75 years or older had no additional mortality benefit with revascularization when compared with their younger counterparts.[68] However, conclusions from this subgroup analysis should be interpreted with caution because only one-sixth of the overall randomized trial population was aged 75 or older. Results of subsequent clinical registries have shown that the benefit of revascularization extends to those over the age of 75 and even the oldest old, aged 85 years or older.[2,72] Reflecting this clinical data, the most recent ACC/AHA guidelines no longer use age to differentiate which patients will benefit from revascularization.[73] If primary angioplasty is not available, thrombolytic therapy should be initiated, although the results are generally less favorable.[74]

MEDICAL MANAGEMENT

Medical management of patients in CS should focus on improving cardiac output and addressing complications of CS (eg, electrolyte disturbances, hypoxia) that may amplify the effects of shock. Options for medical management include intravenous inotrope and vasopressor support, and patients in severe CS often need both to maintain organ perfusion. Patients with low-grade CS/insufficiency who are not requiring vasopressor support may (paradoxically) gain benefit from the cautious addition of vasodilators.

Inotrope Support

The routine use of inotrope support in heart failure for short-term or long-term support is clearly linked to an increased mortality.[43,75] The routine use of these agents in management of most heart failure syndromes is inappropriate and should be discouraged,[43] but they have an important role in maintaining systemic perfusion and restoring end-organ function for patients in CS.[26] Both dobutamine and milrinone increase the inotropy of the failing heart to improve cardiac output. Dobutamine stimulates both β_1 receptors and β_2 receptors, triggering the G-protein adenylate cyclase cascade that leads to increased cyclic AMP production. Although dobutamine is mainly a β_1 agonist, stimulation of peripheral β_2 receptors can lead to a drop in blood pressure noted on medication initiation. Typical doses of dobutamine range from 2.5 to 20 μg/kg/min. In rare cases, patients may develop an allergic reaction to dobutamine, which is manifested as acute, unexplained, renal failure and eosinophilia in both urine and blood smears and (often) evidence of eosinophilic infiltration on myocardial biopsy. Discontinuation of the agent is required and a reintroduction of the medication in the future should be done with caution as recurrence is known to occur.

Milrinone is a selective phosphodiesterase-3 inhibitor that increases intramyocyte cyclic AMP levels leading to increased intracellular calcium for myofilament binding. The net result is a vasodilatory effect in the pulmonary and systemic circulations and increased inotropy within the heart without significant chronotropic alterations.[76] Typical milrinone doses are 0.125 to 0.75 μg/kg/min. Because of a long half-life (2.5 hours), the agent takes about 7 hours before peak effects can be seen. The long time to drug onset may be offset with an intravenous bolus load (50 μg/kg/min), but this practice is strongly discouraged (especially in unstable patients) due to the increased risk for acute hypotension. Active and inactive metabolites of milrinone are renally cleared and dose adjustments should be made in patients with low glomerular filtration rates.

Both dobutamine and milrinone are associated with an increased risk of atrial and ventricular arrhythmias and systemic hypotension. Dobutamine has a shorter half-life, which is associated with an earlier onset of action and elimination from the body should ectopy or hypotension develop. Because of milrinone's long half-live, it is the preferred agent for outpatient parenteral therapy and is a more potent pulmonary arterial vasodilator.[77] Clinical outcomes are similar and the choice of agent is generally determined by clinician preference, institutional availability, and potential need to transition to outpatient parenteral therapy.[78]

One other intravenous inotropic agent is Levosimendan. This drug binds to troponin C and sensitizes the myofilament to calcium.[79] When compared head-to-head with dobutamine, there was no beneficial effect on clinical outcomes at 180 days and this drug remains unapproved for clinical use within the United States.[80]

Vasodilators

Although the use of a vasodilator in patients with critical CS is contraindicated, they can be initiated with caution in patients with low-grade shock. Intravenous vasodilators include nitroglycerin, nitroprusside, and nesiritide. Nitroglycerin is a strong venodilator that is effective in reducing preload and in vasodilating the coronary vasculature.[81] Unfortunately, tachyphylaxis requiring dose escalation is common, limiting its clinical application to mainly those patients with refractory angina. Nitroprusside vasodilates the arterial and venous vasculature by means of the guanyl cyclase pathway. This agent is commonly used in acute heart failure syndromes in patients without evidence of severe shock to reduce systemic and pulmonary afterload. In selected patient with lower grades of CS stabilized with inotropes, the addition of nitroprusside may lead to a reduction in left and right ventricular afterloads, leading to improved left-sided and right-sided stroke volumes. Paradoxically, because of the benefits in cardiac output, blood pressures can even increase with nitroprusside therapy. In head-to-head comparisons with inotropic agents, nitroprusside has been shown to reduce the systemic and pulmonary vascular resistance, pulmonary capillary wedge pressure and improve cardiac output as effectively as an inotrope.[82] The very short half-life of nitroprusside compared with other intravenous vasodilators makes it particularly attractive for ICU management of those with cardiac insufficiency. Nitroprusside should be started at low doses (0.5 µg/kg/min) with an arterial line in place. The dose may be titrated by 0.5 µg/kg/min increments while maintaining a goal blood pressure. It is important to monitor patients for signs and symptoms of cyanide toxicity. Patients with cyanide toxicity may present with confusion, nausea, vomiting, or hyperreflexia and laboratory test results may demonstrate new or worsening lactic acidosis. Monitoring of serum thiocyanate levels is useful if provided by an in-hospital laboratory in a timely fashion. Toxicity is more common in patients with renal dysfunction and with prolonged administration.

The last class of intravenous vasodilators used for patients in CS includes nesiritide. Nesiritide is a recombinant B-type natriuretic peptide that is an arterial and venous vasodilator and has natriuretic peptide properties. Initial studies of this drug showed not only a favorable hemodynamic profile but also improved short-term mortality.[83] Later pooled analyses showed worsening renal function and higher short-term mortality in patients receiving nesiritide, curbing a high initial enthusiasm for the medication.[84,85] Nevertheless, the drug remains a useful adjunctive agent for managing patients with CS.

Vasopressors

For those patients with profound hypotension, use of vasopressors is often required to maintain adequate blood pressure and organ homeostasis. Dopamine has classically been used in the management of heart failure patients who are suffering from acute hypotension because this medication has been shown to vasodilate the renal vasculature.[86] Despite these assumed beneficial effects in heart failure patients, dopamine appears to offer a less favorable short-term mortality when compared with norepinephrine.[87] In 280 patients with CS managed with vasopressor support, dopamine was associated with increased tachyarrhythmias and mortality compared with norepinephrine.[87] Given the high mortality for any patient receiving vasopressor therapy, the focus of treatment should not be on the specific agent, but rather on the restoration of normal cardiac output and resumption of normal organ homeostasis. In appropriate patients, use of temporary mechanical support should supersede addition or further titration of vasopressors.

MECHANICAL CIRCULATORY SUPPORT

Temporary circulatory support is a promising option for management of patients in CS.

Intra-Aortic Balloon Pump

In the landmark SHOCK trial, more than 86% of patients with CS received IABP support.[67] In the subsequent SHOCK registry, the use of an IABP with or without thrombolytics was associated with a significant reduction in in-hospital mortality from 72% to 50%.[88] Despite the widespread use of IABP counterpulsation to manage patients with CS, the data supporting favorable outcomes are quite limited, particularly in the setting of early revascularization. A recent meta-analysis that evaluated both randomized clinical trials and observational cohort studies of STEMI patients with CS showed an increased mortality for those patients receiving an IABP at the time of primary percutaneous coronary intervention.[89] In CS patients treated with fibrinolytics, mortality was reduced with IABP support.[89]

Two recent randomized clinical trials have been undertaken to evaluate the efficacy of IABPs for patients in CS: the IABP-SHOCK I and II trials. The initial IABP-SHOCK trial was a small, single-center study that randomized 45 patients with MI and CS.[90] The primary endpoint was a reduction in the APACHE II score at 4 days. There was a reduction in APACHE II scores for both patient groups, suggesting no added benefit of IABP therapy.[90] To confirm these results, the IABP-SHOCK II trial was conducted in 600 patients with CS complicating an acute MI.[91] Across all analyzed outcomes — including adverse events — there was no difference found between groups.[91] In the most recent revision of the ACC/AHA STEMI guidelines, the use of an IABP for patients with CS has been downgraded from a class I to a class IIa recommendation.[73,92]

Percutaneous Ventricular Assist Devices

As mechanical circulatory support continues to grow with improvements in LVAD technology, a parallel growth is occurring within percutaneous ventricular assist devices. As the technology continues to evolve, a durable entirely percutaneous implantable ventricular assist device is not unfathomable. Some of the more commonly used percutaneous devices include the TandemHeart (Cardiac Assist Inc, Pittsburgh, PA, USA), Impella 2.5, Impella CP (Abiomed Inc, Danvers, MA, USA), and peripheral extracorporeal membrane oxygenation (ECMO) (**Fig. 5**). The Impella 2.5 and CP are placed across the aortic valve using a transcatheter approach. Both devices have an axial-flow rotor that withdraws blood from the left ventricle via a pigtail and ejects blood into the ascending aorta directly above the coronary ostia. The Impella 2.5 provides up to 2.5 L of flow, whereas the CP can provide 3.5 L of flow. Hemolysis and pigtail migration are not infrequent complications. The TandemHeart device withdraws oxygenated blood from an inflow cannula that is placed via the femoral vein in the left atrium through a transseptal puncture. Oxygenated blood returns to a pump, which sits outside the patient and is then returned via a cannula placed within the femoral artery. The TandemHeart device is capable of providing 4 to 5 L of flow depending on the size of the return cannula used. Complications with this device include catheter dislodgment, hemolysis, bleeding, and limb ischemia, with limb ischemia being alleviated with the use of antegrade perfusion catheter.

Well-powered, randomized studies of percutaneous support devices in CS are lacking. Two small randomized studies have been conducted comparing the use of the

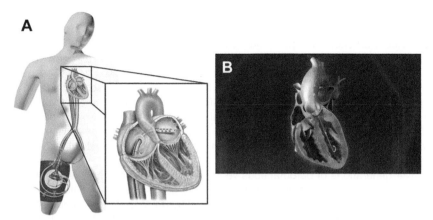

Fig. 5. Percutaneous ventricular assist devices. Demonstration of 2 percutaneous ventricular assist devices. (*A*) The TandemHeart device, where oxygenated blood is removed from the left atrium via a 21-F inflow cannula, which originates in the femoral vein and is placed in the left atrium via a transeptal puncture using intracardiac or transesophageal echocardiographic guidance. The oxygenated blood then flows through the pump and is returned to the body via a 15-F or 17-F cannula placed in the femoral artery. (*B*) The Impella devices are placed in the femoral artery using either a 13-F (Impella 2.5) or a 14-F (Impella CP) sheath. The device has a pigtail that sits across the aortic valve where blood is removed, rotated through the axial-flow rotor, which sits across the aortic valve. Blood is then ejected from the pump above the ostia of the coronary arteries. (*Courtesy of* CardiacAssist, Inc, Pittsburg, PA; with permission.)

TandemHeart versus IABP in CS patients.[93,94] Both studies showed an improvement in hemodynamic parameters, such as cardiac index or pulmonary capillary wedge pressure, but showed no significant difference in mortality.[93,94] Each study only included approximately 40 patients and were underpowered to assess mortality. Another randomized study compared the Impella 2.5 device with an IABP in 25 CS patients and found similar improvement in hemodynamics, but again no improvement in clinical outcomes.[95] A recent meta-analysis of all 3 trials showed no improvement in short-term mortality when these devices are used in patients with CS.[96] Importantly, these studies have failed to look at the efficacy of the percutaneous ventricular assist device when used as a bridge-to-bridge strategy for patients who go on to receive a durable LVAD. There is some data that suggest these devices may be effective in improving outcomes after a durable LVAD is implanted (eg, right ventricular failure, renal failure, and operative mortality).[97]

The artificial heart-lung machine was developed in 1937 by John Heysham Gibbon Jr, MD to allow performance of open heart surgery.[98,99] The initial experience was complicated by hemolysis, thrombocytopenia, and hemorrhage due to direct contact of the blood and gases used for oxygenation. The technology was improved through the use of a membrane to separate the gas from blood,[100] and after years of work, the use of extracorporeal membrane oxygenation to support adults and children with respiratory failure successfully became reported.[101,102] Because of decades of experience and a relatively inexpensive cost compared with newer percutaneous devices, ECMO continues to be the device of choice for many institutions in patients with critical CS. It has been used successfully as a bridge-to-bridge device to mitigate the risks of putting in a durable LVAD.[103,104] There are, however, some potential advantages of a percutaneous ventricular assist device over ECMO: (1) the ability to decompress the cardiac chambers; (2) a reduction in wall stress and oxygen consumption should myocardial recovery be an intent; (3) normalization of hemodynamics (central venous and pulmonary capillary wedge pressures); and (4) physiologically mimicking a durable ventricular assist device by allowing one a "guess-estimate" of the expected response to a more durable LVAD. Because of the perceived beneficial effects of ventricular decompression, some centers have begun to use the Impella 2.5 device with ECMO and others decompress the LV using the TandemHeart.[105] As reviewed later in this issue, mortality following initiation of ECMO in patients with cardiac arrest and CS remains high. Survival with the use of any percutaneous support is best when instituted before a patient is "crashing and burning."

Newer generations of percutaneous ventricular assist devices promise to increase the cardiac output without the requirement for a larger French-size access sheath or the need for a surgical cut down. Some upcoming devices in order of potential clinical availability include the following: the Reitan Catheter Pump (Kiwimed, London, UK), iVAC 3L PVAD (PulseCath BV, Amsterdam, the Netherlands), and the Percutaneous Heart Pump (Thoratec Corp, Pleasanton, CA, USA).

PERSPECTIVE FOR THE FUTURE

The improvements in clinical outcomes following the onset of CS have largely been driven by early revascularization. Adjunctive therapies such as inotropes, IABPs, and PACs have not been shown to improve outcomes systematically. Clinically, we exist at a plateau, where despite continued improvements in adjunctive pharmacology and revascularization techniques, CS mortality remains high. With newer percutaneous support devices, the ability to rest or recover the heart until the stunned myocardium recruits or until a durable LVAD can be placed is a hope. The field will only move forward, however, with increased randomized clinical trials such as the SHOCK trial—which is now more than a decade old—seemingly the only influential trial of CS patients.

REFERENCES

1. Califf RM, Bengtson JR. Cardiogenic shock. N Engl J Med 1994;330(24): 1724–30.
2. Hochman JS, Buller CE, Sleeper LA, et al. Cardiogenic shock complicating acute myocardial infarction–etiologies, management and outcome: a report from the SHOCK trial registry. Should we emergently revascularize occluded coronaries for cardiogenic shock? J Am Coll Cardiol 2000;36(3 Suppl A):1063–70.
3. Goldberg RJ, Spencer FA, Gore JM, et al. Thirty-year trends (1975 to 2005) in the magnitude of, management of, and hospital death rates associated with cardiogenic shock in patients with acute myocardial infarction: a population-based perspective. Circulation 2009;119(9):1211–9.
4. Gheorghiade M, Pang PS. Acute heart failure syndromes. J Am Coll Cardiol 2009;53(7):557–73.
5. Sochowski RA, Dubbin JD, Naqvi SZ. Clinical and hemodynamic assessment of the hepatojugular reflux. Am J Cardiol 1990;66(12):1002–6.
6. Burch GE, Ray CT. Mechanism of the hepatojugular reflux test in congestive heart failure. Am Heart J 1954;48(3):373–82.
7. Folland ED, Kriegel BJ, Henderson WG, et al. Implications of third heart sounds in patients with valvular heart disease. The veterans affairs cooperative study on valvular heart disease. N Engl J Med 1992;327(7):458–62.

8. Effect of enalapril on survival in patients with reduced left ventricular ejection fractions and congestive heart failure. The SOLVD Investigators. N Engl J Med 1991;325(5):293–302.

9. Drazner MH, Rame JE, Stevenson LW, et al. Prognostic importance of elevated jugular venous pressure and a third heart sound in patients with heart failure. N Engl J Med 2001;345(8):574–81.

10. Nohria A, Tsang SW, Fang JC, et al. Clinical assessment identifies hemodynamic profiles that predict outcomes in patients admitted with heart failure. J Am Coll Cardiol 2003;41(10):1797–804.

11. Stevenson LW. Tailored therapy to hemodynamic goals for advanced heart failure. Eur J Heart Fail 1999;1(3):251–7.

12. Forrester JS, Diamond G, Chatterjee K, et al. Medical therapy of acute myocardial infarction by application of hemodynamic subsets (second of two parts). N Engl J Med 1976;295(25):1404–13.

13. Forrester JS, Diamond G, Chatterjee K, et al. Medical therapy of acute myocardial infarction by application of hemodynamic subsets (first of two parts). N Engl J Med 1976;295(24):1356–62.

14. Stevenson LW, Perloff JK. The limited reliability of physical signs for estimating hemodynamics in chronic heart failure. JAMA 1989;261(6):884–8.

15. Dexter L, Haynes FW, Burwell CS, et al. Studies of congenital heart disease: technique of venous catheterization as a diagnostic procedure. J Clin Invest 1947;26(3):547–53.

16. Swan HJ, Ganz W, Forrester J, et al. Catheterization of the heart in man with use of a flow-directed balloon-tipped catheter. N Engl J Med 1970;283(9):447–51.

17. Connors AF Jr, Speroff T, Dawson NV, et al. The effectiveness of right heart catheterization in the initial care of critically ill patients. SUPPORT Investigators. JAMA 1996;276(11):889–97.

18. Guyatt G. A randomized control trial of right-heart catheterization in critically ill patients. Ontario Intensive Care Study Group. J Intensive Care Med 1991;6(2):91–5.

19. Richard C, Warszawski J, Anguel N, et al. Early use of the pulmonary artery catheter and outcomes in patients with shock and acute respiratory distress syndrome: a randomized controlled trial. JAMA 2003;290(20):2713–20.

20. Dalen JE, Bone RC. Is it time to pull the pulmonary artery catheter? JAMA 1996;276(11):916–8.

21. Koo KK, Sun JC, Zhou Q, et al. Pulmonary artery catheters: evolving rates and reasons for use. Crit Care Med 2011;39(7):1613–8.

22. Tukey MH, Wiener RS. The current state of fellowship training in pulmonary artery catheter placement and data interpretation: a national survey of pulmonary and critical care fellowship program directors. J Crit Care 2013;28(5):857–61.

23. Binanay C, Califf RM, Hasselblad V, et al. Evaluation study of congestive heart failure and pulmonary artery catheterization effectiveness: the ESCAPE trial. JAMA 2005;294(13):1625–33.

24. Cohen MG, Kelly RV, Kong DF, et al. Pulmonary artery catheterization in acute coronary syndromes: insights from the GUSTO IIb and GUSTO III trials. Am J Med 2005;118(5):482–8.

25. Forrester JS, Diamond GA, Swan HJ. Correlative classification of clinical and hemodynamic function after acute myocardial infarction. Am J Cardiol 1977;39(2):137–45.

26. Yancy CW, Jessup M, Bozkurt B, et al. 2013 ACCF/AHA guideline for the management of heart failure: a report of the American College of Cardiology

Foundation/American Heart Association task force on practice guidelines. J Am Coll Cardiol 2013;62:e147–239.

27. Lindenfeld J, Albert NM, Boehmer JP, et al. HFSA 2010 comprehensive heart failure practice guideline. J Card Fail 2010;16(6):e1–194.

28. Killip T 3rd, Kimball JT. Treatment of myocardial infarction in a coronary care unit. A two year experience with 250 patients. Am J Cardiol 1967;20(4):457–64.

29. Granger CB, Goldberg RJ, Dabbous O, et al. Predictors of hospital mortality in the global registry of acute coronary events. Arch Intern Med 2003;163(19):2345–53.

30. Fox KA, Dabbous OH, Goldberg RJ, et al. Prediction of risk of death and myocardial infarction in the six months after presentation with acute coronary syndrome: prospective multinational observational study (GRACE). BMJ 2006; 333(7578):1091.

31. Khot UN, Jia G, Moliterno DJ, et al. Prognostic importance of physical examination for heart failure in non-ST-elevation acute coronary syndromes: the enduring value of Killip classification. JAMA 2003;290(16):2174–81.

32. Knaus WA, Draper EA, Wagner DP, et al. APACHE II: a severity of disease classification system. Crit Care Med 1985;13(10):818–29.

33. Ribeiro M, Carvalho R, Bastos J, et al. Value of APACHE II score to predict mortality in cardiogenic shock patients of a cardiologic ICU. Crit Care 2006; 10(Suppl 1):P402.

34. Mercado-Martinez J, Rivera-Fernandez R, Aguilar-Alonso E, et al. APACHE-II score and Killip class for patients with acute myocardial infarction. Intensive Care Med 2010;36(9):1579–86.

35. Markgraf R, Deutschinoff G, Pientka L, et al. Comparison of acute physiology and chronic health evaluations II and III and simplified acute physiology score II: a prospective cohort study evaluating these methods to predict outcome in a German interdisciplinary intensive care unit. Crit Care Med 2000;28(1):26–33.

36. Vincent JL, Moreno R, Takala J, et al. The SOFA (sepsis-related organ failure assessment) score to describe organ dysfunction/failure. On behalf of the working group on sepsis-related problems of the European Society of Intensive Care Medicine. Intensive Care Med 1996;22(7):707–10.

37. Huang SS, Chen YH, Lu TM, et al. Application of the sequential organ failure assessment score for predicting mortality in patients with acute myocardial infarction. Resuscitation 2012;83(5):591–5.

38. Kirklin JK, Naftel DC, Stevenson LW, et al. INTERMACS database for durable devices for circulatory support: first annual report. J Heart Lung Transplant 2008;27(10):1065–72.

39. The Criteria Committee of the New York Heart Association. Nomenclature and criteria for diagnosis of diseases of the heart and blood vessels. Boston: Little Brown; 1964.

40. Stevenson LW, Pagani FD, Young JB, et al. INTERMACS profiles of advanced heart failure: the current picture. J Heart Lung Transplant 2009;28(6):535–41.

41. Kirklin JK, Naftel DC, Kormos RL, et al. Fifth INTERMACS annual report: risk factor analysis from more than 6,000 mechanical circulatory support patients. J Heart Lung Transplant 2013;32(2):141–56.

42. Stevenson LW. Clinical use of inotropic therapy for heart failure: looking backward or forward? Part I: inotropic infusions during hospitalization. Circulation 2003;108(3):367–72.

43. Cuffe MS, Califf RM, Adams KF Jr, et al. Short-term intravenous milrinone for acute exacerbation of chronic heart failure: a randomized controlled trial. JAMA 2002;287(12):1541–7.

44. Menon V, Webb JG, Hillis LD, et al. Outcome and profile of ventricular septal rupture with cardiogenic shock after myocardial infarction: a report from the SHOCK trial registry. Should we emergently revascularize occluded coronaries in cardiogenic shock? J Am Coll Cardiol 2000;36(3 Suppl A):1110–6.
45. Edwards BS, Edwards WD, Edwards JE. Ventricular septal rupture complicating acute myocardial infarction: identification of simple and complex types in 53 autopsied hearts. Am J Cardiol 1984;54(10):1201–5.
46. French JK, Hellkamp AS, Armstrong PW, et al. Mechanical complications after percutaneous coronary intervention in ST-elevation myocardial infarction (from APEX-AMI). Am J Cardiol 2010;105(1):59–63.
47. Zehender M, Kasper W, Kauder E, et al. Right ventricular infarction as an independent predictor of prognosis after acute inferior myocardial infarction. N Engl J Med 1993;328(14):981–8.
48. Jacobs AK, Leopold JA, Bates E, et al. Cardiogenic shock caused by right ventricular infarction: a report from the shock registry. J Am Coll Cardiol 2003;41(8):1273–9.
49. Mehta SR, Eikelboom JW, Natarajan MK, et al. Impact of right ventricular involvement on mortality and morbidity in patients with inferior myocardial infarction. J Am Coll Cardiol 2001;37(1):37–43.
50. Ketikoglou DG, Karvounis HI, Papadopoulos CE, et al. Echocardiographic evaluation of spontaneous recovery of right ventricular systolic and diastolic function in patients with acute right ventricular infarction associated with posterior wall left ventricular infarction. Am J Cardiol 2004;93(7):911–3.
51. Bursi F, Enriquez-Sarano M, Nkomo VT, et al. Heart failure and death after myocardial infarction in the community: the emerging role of mitral regurgitation. Circulation 2005;111(3):295–301.
52. Thompson CR, Buller CE, Sleeper LA, et al. Cardiogenic shock due to acute severe mitral regurgitation complicating acute myocardial infarction: a report from the SHOCK trial registry. Should we use emergently revascularize occluded coronaries in cardiogenic shock? J Am Coll Cardiol 2000;36(3 Suppl A):1104–9.
53. Davis N, Sistino JJ. Review of ventricular rupture: key concepts and diagnostic tools for success. Perfusion 2002;17(1):63–7.
54. Barbour DJ, Roberts WC. Rupture of a left ventricular papillary muscle during acute myocardial infarction: analysis of 22 necropsy patients. J Am Coll Cardiol 1986;8(3):558–65.
55. Nishimura RA, Schaff HV, Shub C, et al. Papillary muscle rupture complicating acute myocardial infarction: analysis of 17 patients. Am J Cardiol 1983;51(3):373–7.
56. Vlodaver Z, Edwards JE. Rupture of ventricular septum or papillary muscle complicating myocardial infarction. Circulation 1977;55(5):815–22.
57. Wei JY, Hutchins GM, Bulkley BH. Papillary muscle rupture in fatal acute myocardial infarction: a potentially treatable form of cardiogenic shock. Ann Intern Med 1979;90(2):149–52.
58. Nishimura RA, Gersh BJ, Schaff HV. The case for an aggressive surgical approach to papillary muscle rupture following myocardial infarction: "from paradise lost to paradise regained". Heart 2000;83(6):611–3.
59. Russo A, Suri RM, Grigioni F, et al. Clinical outcome after surgical correction of mitral regurgitation due to papillary muscle rupture. Circulation 2008;118(15):1528–34.
60. Vargas-Barron J, Molina-Carrion M, Romero-Cardenas A, et al. Risk factors, echocardiographic patterns, and outcomes in patients with acute ventricular septal rupture during myocardial infarction. Am J Cardiol 2005;95(10):1153–8.

61. Crenshaw BS, Granger CB, Birnbaum Y, et al. Risk factors, angiographic patterns, and outcomes in patients with ventricular septal defect complicating acute myocardial infarction. GUSTO-I (Global Utilization of Streptokinase and TPA for Occluded Coronary Arteries) Trial Investigators. Circulation 2000; 101(1):27–32.

62. Poulsen SH, Praestholm M, Munk K, et al. Ventricular septal rupture complicating acute myocardial infarction: clinical characteristics and contemporary outcome. Ann Thorac Surg 2008;85(5):1591–6.

63. Thiele H, Kaulfersch C, Daehnert I, et al. Immediate primary transcatheter closure of postinfarction ventricular septal defects. Eur Heart J 2009;30(1):81–8.

64. Michel-Behnke I, Ewert P, Koch A, et al. Device closure of ventricular septal defects by hybrid procedures: a multicenter retrospective study. Catheter Cardiovasc Interv 2011;77(2):242–51.

65. Batts KP, Ackermann DM, Edwards WD. Postinfarction rupture of the left ventricular free wall: clinicopathologic correlates in 100 consecutive autopsy cases. Hum Pathol 1990;21(5):530–5.

66. Lopez-Sendon J, Gurfinkel EP, Lopez de Sa E, et al. Factors related to heart rupture in acute coronary syndromes in the global registry of acute coronary events. Eur Heart J 2010;31(12):1449–56.

67. Hochman JS, Sleeper LA, Webb JG, et al. Early revascularization in acute myocardial infarction complicated by cardiogenic shock. SHOCK Investigators. Should we emergently revascularize occluded coronaries for cardiogenic shock. N Engl J Med 1999;341(9):625–34.

68. Hochman JS, Sleeper LA, White HD, et al. One-year survival following early revascularization for cardiogenic shock. JAMA 2001;285(2):190–2.

69. Fox KA, Steg PG, Eagle KA, et al. Decline in rates of death and heart failure in acute coronary syndromes, 1999-2006. JAMA 2007;297(17):1892–900.

70. Yeh RW, Sidney S, Chandra M, et al. Population trends in the incidence and outcomes of acute myocardial infarction. N Engl J Med 2010;362(23):2155–65.

71. Babaev A, Frederick PD, Pasta DJ, et al. Trends in management and outcomes of patients with acute myocardial infarction complicated by cardiogenic shock. JAMA 2005;294(4):448–54.

72. Shah P, Najafi AH, Panza JA, et al. Outcomes and quality of life in patients>or=85 years of age with ST-elevation myocardial infarction. Am J Cardiol 2009;103(2):170–4.

73. O'Gara PT, Kushner FG, Ascheim DD, et al. 2013 ACCF/AHA guideline for the management of ST-elevation myocardial infarction: executive summary: a report of the American College of Cardiology Foundation/American Heart Association task force on practice guidelines. Circulation 2013;127(4):529–55.

74. Berger PB, Holmes DR Jr, Stebbins AL, et al. Impact of an aggressive invasive catheterization and revascularization strategy on mortality in patients with cardiogenic shock in the Global Utilization of Streptokinase and Tissue Plasminogen Activator for Occluded Coronary Arteries (GUSTO-I) trial. An observational study. Circulation 1997;96(1):122–7.

75. Elkayam U, Tasissa G, Binanay C, et al. Use and impact of inotropes and vasodilator therapy in hospitalized patients with severe heart failure. Am Heart J 2007;153(1):98–104.

76. Alousi AA, Johnson DC. Pharmacology of the bipyridines: amrinone and milrinone. Circulation 1986;73(3 Pt 2):III10–24.

77. Givertz MM, Hare JM, Loh E, et al. Effect of bolus milrinone on hemodynamic variables and pulmonary vascular resistance in patients with severe left

ventricular dysfunction: a rapid test for reversibility of pulmonary hypertension. J Am Coll Cardiol 1996;28(7):1775–80.

78. Aranda JM Jr, Schofield RS, Pauly DF, et al. Comparison of dobutamine versus milrinone therapy in hospitalized patients awaiting cardiac transplantation: a prospective, randomized trial. Am Heart J 2003;145(2):324–9.

79. Haikala H, Kaivola J, Nissinen E, et al. Cardiac troponin C as a target protein for a novel calcium sensitizing drug, levosimendan. J Mol Cell Cardiol 1995;27(9): 1859–66.

80. Mebazaa A, Nieminen MS, Packer M, et al. Levosimendan vs dobutamine for patients with acute decompensated heart failure: the survive randomized trial. JAMA 2007;297(17):1883–91.

81. Cohn PF, Gorlin R. Physiologic and clinical actions of nitroglycerin. Med Clin North Am 1974;58(2):407–15.

82. Monrad ES, Baim DS, Smith HS, et al. Milrinone, dobutamine, and nitroprusside: comparative effects on hemodynamics and myocardial energetics in patients with severe congestive heart failure. Circulation 1986;73(3 Pt 2):III168–74.

83. Silver MA, Horton DP, Ghali JK, et al. Effect of nesiritide versus dobutamine on short-term outcomes in the treatment of patients with acutely decompensated heart failure. J Am Coll Cardiol 2002;39(5):798–803.

84. Sackner-Bernstein JD, Kowalski M, Fox M, et al. Short-term risk of death after treatment with nesiritide for decompensated heart failure: a pooled analysis of randomized controlled trials. JAMA 2005;293(15):1900–5.

85. Sackner-Bernstein JD, Skopicki HA, Aaronson KD. Risk of worsening renal function with nesiritide in patients with acutely decompensated heart failure. Circulation 2005;111(12):1487–91.

86. Elkayam U, Ng TM, Hatamizadeh P, et al. Renal vasodilatory action of dopamine in patients with heart failure: magnitude of effect and site of action. Circulation 2008;117(2):200–5.

87. De Backer D, Biston P, Devriendt J, et al. Comparison of dopamine and norepinephrine in the treatment of shock. N Engl J Med 2010;362(9):779–89.

88. Sanborn TA, Sleeper LA, Bates ER, et al. Impact of thrombolysis, intra-aortic balloon pump counterpulsation, and their combination in cardiogenic shock complicating acute myocardial infarction: a report from the SHOCK trial registry. Should we emergently revascularize occluded coronaries for cardiogenic shock? J Am Coll Cardiol 2000;36(3 Suppl A):1123–9.

89. Sjauw KD, Engstrom AE, Vis MM, et al. A systematic review and meta-analysis of intra-aortic balloon pump therapy in ST-elevation myocardial infarction: should we change the guidelines? Eur Heart J 2009;30(4):459–68.

90. Prondzinsky R, Lemm H, Swyter M, et al. Intra-aortic balloon counterpulsation in patients with acute myocardial infarction complicated by cardiogenic shock: the prospective, randomized IABP SHOCK trial for attenuation of multiorgan dysfunction syndrome. Crit Care Med 2010;38(1):152–60.

91. Thiele H, Zeymer U, Neumann FJ, et al. Intraaortic balloon support for myocardial infarction with cardiogenic shock. N Engl J Med 2012;367(14):1287–96.

92. Antman EM, Anbe DT, Armstrong PW, et al. ACC/AHA guidelines for the management of patients with ST-elevation myocardial infarction; a report of the American College of Cardiology/American Heart Association task force on practice guidelines (committee to revise the 1999 guidelines for the management of patients with acute myocardial infarction). J Am Coll Cardiol 2004;44(3):E1–211.

93. Burkhoff D, Cohen H, Brunckhorst C, et al, TandemHeart Investigators Group. A randomized multicenter clinical study to evaluate the safety and efficacy of

the TandemHeart percutaneous ventricular assist device versus conventional therapy with intraaortic balloon pumping for treatment of cardiogenic shock. Am Heart J 2006;152(3):469.e1–8.

94. Thiele H, Sick P, Boudriot E, et al. Randomized comparison of intra-aortic balloon support with a percutaneous left ventricular assist device in patients with revascularized acute myocardial infarction complicated by cardiogenic shock. Eur Heart J 2005;26(13):1276–83.

95. Seyfarth M, Sibbing D, Bauer I, et al. A randomized clinical trial to evaluate the safety and efficacy of a percutaneous left ventricular assist device versus intra-aortic balloon pumping for treatment of cardiogenic shock caused by myocardial infarction. J Am Coll Cardiol 2008;52(19):1584–8.

96. Cheng JM, den Uil CA, Hoeks SE, et al. Percutaneous left ventricular assist devices vs. intra-aortic balloon pump counterpulsation for treatment of cardiogenic shock: a meta-analysis of controlled trials. Eur Heart J 2009; 30(17):2102–8.

97. Shah P, Cowger JA, Haft JW, et al. Percutaneous hemodynamic support for cardiogenic shock prior to left ventricular assist device placement. J Heart Lung Transplant 2013;32(4):S141.

98. Gibbon JH Jr. Artificial maintenance of circulation during experimental occlusion of pulmonary artery. Arch Surg 1937;34:1105–31.

99. Gibbon JH Jr. The development of the heart-lung apparatus. Rev Surg 1970; 27(4):231–44.

100. Clowes GH Jr, Hopkins AL, Neville WE. An artificial lung dependent upon diffusion of oxygen and carbon dioxide through plastic membranes. J Thorac Surg 1956;32(5):630–7.

101. Hill JD, O'Brien TG, Murray JJ, et al. Prolonged extracorporeal oxygenation for acute post-traumatic respiratory failure (shock-lung syndrome). Use of the Bramson membrane lung. N Engl J Med 1972;286(12):629–34.

102. Bartlett RH, Gazzaniga AB, Jefferies MR, et al. Extracorporeal membrane oxygenation (ECMO) cardiopulmonary support in infancy. Trans Am Soc Artif Intern Organs 1976;22:80–93.

103. Pagani FD, Aaronson KD, Swaniker F, et al. The use of extracorporeal life support in adult patients with primary cardiac failure as a bridge to implantable left ventricular assist device. Ann Thorac Surg 2001;71(3 Suppl):S77–81 [discussion: S82–5].

104. Hoefer D, Ruttmann E, Poelzl G, et al. Outcome evaluation of the bridge-to-bridge concept in patients with cardiogenic shock. Ann Thorac Surg 2006; 82(1):28–33.

105. Cheng A, Swartz MF, Massey HT. Impella to unload the left ventricle during peripheral extracorporeal membrane oxygenation. ASAIO J 2013;59(5):533–6.

Hemodynamic Assessment in the Contemporary Intensive Care Unit

A Review of Circulatory Monitoring Devices

Mohamad Kenaan, MD[a],*, Mithil Gajera, MD[b],
Sascha N. Goonewardena, MD[a]

KEYWORDS

- Hemodynamic • Circulatory • Monitoring • Critically ill • Intensive care unit

KEY POINTS

- The ideal circulatory monitoring system would be noninvasive, cost-effective and easy to use.
- As understanding of hemodynamics and critical illness has evolved, more sophisticated circulatory monitoring technologies have been developed.
- The primary hemodynamic goal in the management of critically ill patients includes the assessment and manipulation of the circulatory system to ensure adequate tissue delivery of oxygen and essential metabolic substrates.
- Current monitoring devices should continue to be selected on a patient-specific basis, either alone or in combination with other hemodynamic monitors, until the gold standard hemodynamic monitoring tool is developed.

INTRODUCTION

The primary hemodynamic goal in the management of critically ill patients includes the assessment and manipulation of the circulatory system to ensure adequate tissue delivery of oxygen and essential metabolic substrates. Goals of optimization of the circulatory system in the ICU have met with mixed results. Traditional methods to assess the circulatory system can sometimes be inadequate, particularly in the early stages of shock when compensatory mechanisms may cloud the presentation.[1,2]

[a] Division of Cardiovascular Medicine, Department of Internal Medicine, University of Michigan Medical Center, 1500 East Medical Center Drive, Ann Arbor, MI 48109, USA; [b] Department of Internal Medicine, Christiana Care Health System, 4755 Ogletown-Stanton Road, Newark, DE 19718, USA
* Corresponding author. Division of Cardiovascular Medicine, University of Michigan Cardiovascular Center, 2381 Cardiovascular Center Spc 5853, 1500 East Medical Center Drive, Ann Arbor, MI 48109.
E-mail address: mkenaan@med.umich.edu

Crit Care Clin 30 (2014) 413–445
http://dx.doi.org/10.1016/j.ccc.2014.03.007
0749-0704/14/$ – see front matter © 2014 Elsevier Inc. All rights reserved.

As the understanding of hemodynamics and critical illness has evolved, more sophisticated circulatory monitoring technologies have been developed, including pulmonary artery catheterization (PAC). The introduction of PAC was accompanied with great optimism; unfortunately, clinical studies have failed to show a consistent benefit with routine use of PAC in the ICU. Because of the belief that PAC was inadequate because of technical problems in interpretation and complications associated with its use, a new wave of noninvasive modalities were developed. Traditional methods continue to have a role in assessing critically ill patients but newer technologies have greatly expanded circulatory monitoring systems.

The ideal circulatory monitoring system would be noninvasive, cost-effective, and easy to use. Although such a system remains elusive, several circulatory monitors possess a combination of these characteristics. This article reviews the most commonly available technologies and their underlying physiologic principles as well as their strengths and limitations in the assessment of critically ill patients.

CLINICAL METHODS FOR HEMODYNAMIC ASSESSMENT

Detailed physical examination along with other clinical data provide a framework for assessment of the underlying pathophysiology of the patient against which all information obtained from hemodynamic monitors can be interpreted. These methods are used to infer data about the two major parameters of the circulatory system: intravascular volume and tissue perfusion.

Invasive Blood Pressure Monitoring

Given the unreliability of sphygmomanometers at blood pressure extremes, invasive arterial blood pressure monitoring is often needed in hemodynamically unstable patients. Literature is starting to emerge questioning the use of arterial catheters in critically ill patients. Lakhal and colleagues[3] demonstrated that noninvasive blood pressure monitoring is accurate and reliable compared with invasive monitors. This is particularly when assessing mean arterial blood pressure at the arm level, although limitations at extremes of blood pressure or body mass index were still noted.

Regardless of the method, a mean arterial pressure (MAP) of 60 to 65 mm Hg is the normally accepted target for resuscitative efforts. It is necessary to understand that normalization of blood pressure does not always indicate microcirculatory sufficiency and adequate tissue perfusion. This goal should also be adjusted according to the clinical scenario. For example, a higher MAP may be necessary with untreated critical coronary artery stenosis or elevated intracranial pressure, whereas a lower MAP in the absence of significant tissue hypoperfusion may be tolerated in conditions such as severe aortic insufficiency.

Assessment of filling pressures and left ventricular function using arterial pressure variation

Physiologic variation of arterial blood pressure during the respiratory cycle is driven by the effect of lung inflation and changes in thoracic or abdominal pressure on ventricular loading conditions in the setting of ventricular interdependence. During spontaneous inspiration, the reduction in left ventricular (LV) stroke volume (SV) causes a decrease in systemic blood pressure and pulse pressure (PP) at end-inspiration (**Fig. 1**). During positive pressure ventilation, the right ventricular (RV) preload usually decreases at end-inspiration, shifting the ventricular septum to the right and improving LV compliance. LV preload also increases as the alveolar inflation enhances venous return to the left atrium (LA). This, coupled with the decrease in LV afterload, produces an increase in systemic blood pressure at end-inspiration. A few heart beats later and

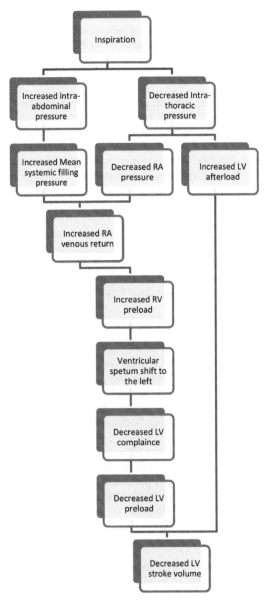

Fig. 1. Physiologic cardiorespiratory interactions in a spontaneously breathing patient.

during expiration, the propagation of the decreased RV SV reaches the LV output and leads to a decrease in systolic blood pressure and PP.[4,5] Appreciating how the venous return changes with the various pathologic states, in addition to its alterations in the setting of positive pressure ventilation, helps in the diagnosis and management of the common hemodynamic profiles encountered in shock.[6]

These variations have been used to predict fluid responsiveness. Michard and colleagues[7] showed that PP variation (PPV) in mechanically ventilated patients was the best predictor of fluid responsiveness. In this study, the optimal cutoff to discriminate fluid responders was a change of 13% in the PP during the respiratory cycle. The respirophasic PPV had a sensitivity of 94%, specificity of 96%, and demonstrated a good correlation with an increase in cardiac index in response to fluid administration.[8] Unfortunately, the usefulness of PPV in spontaneously breathing patients remains unknown.

Central Venous Pressure

Central venous pressure (CVP), a measure of right atrium pressure (RAP), can be estimated noninvasively by measuring the jugular venous pressure or invasively by transducing a central venous catheter with its tip placed in the superior vena cava or right atrium (RA).[9] Normal CVP in a spontaneously breathing patient is 0 to 5 mm Hg, whereas the generally accepted normal upper limit in mechanically ventilated patients is 10 mm Hg. CVP has been suggested as a measure for preload; however, its validity in predicting fluid responsiveness is nonexistent across numerous studies. Except for extremely low values, static levels of CVP are often unreliable in predicting volume expansion responders.[10,11]

Dynamic changes of CVP in response to fluids or in relation to the respiratory cycle have been investigated in evaluating preload responsiveness with some conflicting evidence.[12,13] Caution should be used when using CVP variation because it can be altered by a host of factors independent of volume status, including changes in tidal volumes, abdominal pressure, and vascular tone.[14,15]

Passive Leg Raising Test

The passive leg raising (PLR) maneuver (**Figs. 2** and **3**) returns approximately 200 mL of blood from the lower extremities toward the central circulatory compartment, resulting in an instantaneous increase in right-sided preload.[16] In the setting of fluid responsiveness, this trial would result in an increased pulmonary capillary wedge pressure (PCWP), early mitral inflow, and a resultant augmentation of LV SV. Given the transient nature of improvement in SV, a PLR test should be coupled with real-time monitoring of the aortic blood flow, frequently using Doppler parameters obtained by echocardiography or esophageal Doppler monitor (EDM). A positive PLR test is defined as an increase in aortic blood flow greater than 10% for at least 30 seconds. It predicts preload responsiveness with a sensitivity of 97% and specificity of 94%. Notably, this increase in PCWP is immediate and fully reversible when the legs are laid back down. These studies suggest that the PLR test can help predict fluid responsiveness while avoiding the potentially hazardous effects of unnecessary volume expansion.[12,17]

Laboratory Studies

B-type natriuretic peptide

B-type natriuretic peptide (BNP) is a peptide released by the ventricles when the myocytes are stretched in the setting of increased preload. The role of BNP in assessing intravascular volume has been best studied in stable cardiac and heart failure subjects. In critically ill subjects, many noncardiac conditions are known to increase BNP release,

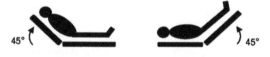

Semirecumbent position   Passive leg raising

Fig. 2. The PLR maneuver. (*From* Teboul JL, Monnet X. Prediction of volume responsiveness in critically ill patients with spontaneous breathing activity. Curr Opin Crit Care 2008;14:334–9; with permission.)

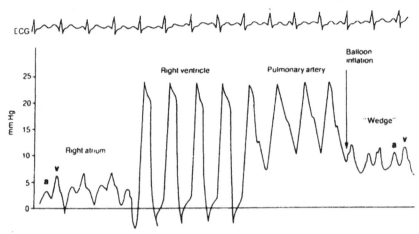

Fig. 3. Normal pulmonary artery catheter tracings in various catheter positions. (*Courtesy of* University of Michigan Health System. Available at: http://www.pathology.med.umich.edu/gynonc/bluebook/treatment/peri/peri2.htm. Accessed August 28, 2013.)

including sepsis, acute lung injury, pulmonary embolism, and intracranial hemorrhage. This makes the interpretation of BNP levels highly unreliable in the ICU.[18–20]

Lactate

Elevated lactate can be caused by a wide range of conditions and medications. Lactate is best used in the ICU as a surrogate of cellular hypoperfusion and is useful for risk stratification in critically ill patients, including cardiac patients. There are also recent data about using lactate as a target endpoint of resuscitation. In septic shock subjects, Jones and colleagues[21] compared resuscitation protocols guided by lactate clearance to goal-central venous oxygen saturation (ScvO2), as suggested by early goal-directed therapy, and found no significant difference in mortality.[22,23] Attana and colleagues[24] also examined the prognostic implications of lactate clearance in subjects developing cardiogenic shock after ST-elevation myocardial infarction. Subjects with 12-hour lactate clearance of less than 10% had lower survival rates.[24] However, clinicians need to be aware of the limitations of monitoring lactate. Not only can lactate be a slowly changing metabolic marker that could lag behind clinical changes, Marik and colleagues[25] also argue that high lactate levels in septic subjects is not always an indication of anaerobic metabolism and, therefore, therapies targeted to treat a nonexistent oxygen debt may be harmful. Rather than targeting therapy to lactate clearance only, understanding and addressing the hemodynamic derangements responsible for elevated lactate levels should be the composite end-point of treatment. In the absence of arterial access, the concentration of central venous lactate can be a reliable substitute for arterial lactate concentration with a good correlation (area under the curve [AUC] 0.98) when lactate concentration is more than 2 mmol/L.[26]

Mixed venous oximetry

Mixed venous oxygen saturation (SvO2) refers to the oxygen saturation of hemoglobin in the proximal pulmonary artery. It is influenced by the balance between oxygen supply and demand, and acts as an indirect measure of oxygen delivery and tissue oxygenation. More specifically, rearrangement of the Fick equation illustrates that venous oxygen content is determined by the arterial oxygen content, oxygen consumption, and cardiac output (CO).

A change in SvO_2 should alert the clinician to a possible alteration in the oxygen supply-demand balance (**Table 1**). SvO_2 values are initially maintained in the normal range by many compensatory mechanisms aimed at increasing oxygen delivery, including an increase in CO. As these mechanisms are exhausted, the venous oxygen reserve is used by increasing oxygen extraction, resulting in a decrease in SvO_2. Beyond this point, when oxygen demand can no longer be met, anaerobic metabolism and lactic acidosis ensues. This point is called critical extraction ratio for oxygen (ERO_2). The critical ERO_2 decreases in several critical illnesses, including sepsis.

Several observational and prospective clinical studies have addressed the diagnostic and prognostic significance of SvO_2 in a variety of critically ill cohorts.[27,28] Despite an extensive amount of research into the clinical usefulness of monitoring SvO_2, its use in guiding therapy remains controversial, especially given its level of invasiveness.

ScvO₂ and its relationship to SvO₂

$ScvO_2$ was introduced as a surrogate for mixed venous oximetry with SvO_2. $ScvO_2$ is a measurement of oxygen saturation in the superior vena cava close to or at the RA junction, whereas SvO_2 is determined in the pulmonary artery. Normally, $ScvO_2$ is lower than SvO_2 but this relationship can be reversed in critically ill patients due to redistribution of the CO and regional variation in oxygen consumption. Data about the correlation between mixed and $ScvO_2$ seem to be highly variable with the greatest discordance in patients with low cardiac index.[29,30] No conclusive evidence exists to support routine use of ScvO2 as a replacement to SvO_2 monitoring and should be used with caution. However, it is clear that, for both markers, recognizing the patient-specific trend is more important than the absolute value.[30,31]

INVASIVE HEMODYNAMIC MONITORING
PAC

Following its introduction into clinical practice in the 1970s, bedside PAC using flow-directed balloon-tipped catheters gradually became a standard of care for critically ill patients. During the PAC era, its widespread use significantly improved the understanding of the physiologic responses and pathophysiologic changes in various conditions. Despite the criticism for the use of PAC generated by the lack of evidence supporting an outcome benefit,[32–36] particularly after the PAC-Man (Assessment of the Clinical Effectiveness of Pulmonary Artery Catheters in Management of Patients in Intensive Care)[37] and ESCAPE (Evaluation Study of Congestive Heart Failure and Pulmonary Artery Catheterization Effectiveness)[38] trials, this invasive hemodynamic tool continues to find a role in the management of a subset of critically ill patients.[39–41] It remains very useful when used for the appropriate indication and interpreted by clinicians with adequate expertise in the analysis and application of data obtained from

Table 1 Interpreting mixed SvO₂	
Decreased SvO₂	**Increased SvO₂**
• Decreased CO	• High CO states (sepsis, cirrhosis, hyperthyroidism)
• Hypoxemia	• Decreased tissue extraction (sepsis)
• Increased metabolic rate (eg, fever)	• Left to right intracardiac shunt
• Anemia	• Severe mitral regurgitation
	• Hypothermia
	• Nitroprusside toxicity or cyanide poisoning
	• Wedged pulmonary artery catheter

PAC. It also is the benchmark against which all new hemodynamic monitors are tested.

Indications and Contraindications

The indications for PAC in critically ill patients include

- Acute myocardial infarction complicated by shock, severe heart failure, or mechanical complications (acute mitral regurgitation, ventricular septal defect)
- Differentiation between various causes of shock
- Severe LV failure to guide therapy, including inotropes, vasodilators, and diuretics
- Cardiac tamponade when clinical and echocardiographic findings are inconclusive
- Assessment of level and magnitude of intracardiac shunt
- Severe acute respiratory distress: to guide the application of positive end-expiratory pressure and use of intravenous fluids
- Severe pulmonary hypertension to guide therapy.

CO Measurements

The PAC provides two methods for the assessment of CO. Thermodilution and Fick principle–derived equations are reliable but are not without limitations.

Thermodilution method

Thermodilution is based on the indicator dilution principle. It is considered the gold standard of CO measurement. It involves the injection of a bolus of cold normal saline through the most proximal port of the PAC followed by measuring the temperature changes by a distal thermistor just proximal to the balloon, allowing the generation of a plot of temperature change against time. CO can then be determined by the modification of the Stewart-Hamilton equation. Measurements obtained by this method average the CO over several cardiac cycles.

The thermodilution method assumes three major conditions: complete mixing of the indicator and blood, constant blood flow, and lack of loss of indicator between the site of injection and place of detection. These assumptions introduce the possibility for inaccurate CO assessment via thermodilution methods with some causes listed in **Table 2**.

Fick principle

CO calculation using the Fick principle is based on the conservation of mass so that the total uptake or release of a substance by an organ is the product of blood flow to that organ multiplied by the arteriovenous concentration difference. Solving for the CO, the equation can be reduced to: $CO = Vo_2/[(SpO_2-SvO_2) \times 1.36 \times 10 \times Hb]$ in which

Table 2 Causes of inaccurate estimation of CO by bolus thermodilution	
Related to patient	• Tricuspid regurgitation • Arrhythmias • Intracardiac shunts • Extremes of CO (very low CO)
Related to injection	• Slow injection (>4 s) • Incorrect volume of injectate • Incorrect temperature of injectate
Related to catheter	• Pulmonary artery catheter is in wedge position • Thermistor impinging on vessel wall • Proximal port within venous sheath

CO is the CO in liters per minute, Vo_2 is the oxygen consumption, SpO_2 is the arterial oxygen saturation, SvO_2 is the oxygen saturation of a mixed venous sample obtained from the distal PAC port, and Hb is hemoglobin in grams per deciliter.

The inaccuracy of the Fick method is mostly related to the oxygen consumption parameter that is often estimated using several formulas ($125 \times$ body surface area [BSA] for men and $110 \times$ BSA for women, or 3 mL O_2/kg $\times$ weight). Even when the Vo_2 is actually measured, subsequent calculations using the same previously measured Vo_2 do not take into account the considerable change in oxygen consumption accompanying the change in clinical status, including fevers, catabolic states, or cooling during induced hypothermia.

Derived Parameters

Once the measured variables are obtained, PAC can be useful in calculating several other hemodynamic parameters that are shown in **Table 3**. It should, however, be noted that the accuracy of these calculated indices is usually affected by the inaccuracies of the multiple measured parameters. Moreover, when an intracardiac shunt is suspected, a saturation run can be performed during the insertion of the PAC. Left to right shunt is suggested by saturation step-up of 7% from an atrial shunt and 5% from a ventricular shunt.

Clinical Scenarios

Using the pressures and CO values obtained from PAC, the data can be integrated into the overall clinical presentation to help establish the diagnosis in several clinical scenarios. A summary of the changes in the filling pressures and CO occurring in the setting of many of various conditions encountered in the critically ill patients is shown in **Table 4**.

Table 3
Measured and derived hemodynamic parameters from pulmonary artery catheter

Measured Hemodynamic Variable		Normal Value
RAP		0–7 mm Hg
RV	Systolic pressure	15–30 mm Hg
	Diastolic pressure	0–8 mm Hg
Pulmonary artery	Systolic pressure	15–30 mm Hg
	Diastolic pressure	4–12 mm Hg
	Mean pressure (MPAP)	10–20 mm Hg
PCWP		8–15 mmHg
CO		5.0–8.0 $L.min^{-1}$

Derived Hemodynamic Variable	Normal Value
Cardiac index = CO/BSA	2.8–4.2 $L.min^{-1}.m^{-2}$
SVR SVR = [(MAP−RAP) × 80]/CO	700–1600 $dyne.s.cm^{-5}$ 9–20 Wood units
Pulmonary vascular resistance (PVR) PVR = [(MPAP−PCWP) × 80]/CO	20–130 $dyne.s.cm^{-5}$ 0.25–1.6 Wood units
Stroke volume index (SVI) = cardiac index/heart rate	35–70 $mL.m^{-2}$ per beat
Left ventricular stroke work index (LVSWI) LVSWI = (MAP−PCWP) × SVI × 0.0136	44–68 $g-m/m^2$
RV stroke work index (RVSWI) RVSWI = (MPAP−RAP) × SVI × 0.0136	4–8 $g-m/m^2$

Abbreviations: MPAP, mean pulmonary artery pressure; SVR, systemic vascular resistance.

Table 4
Changes of pulmonary artery catheter parameters in various clinical scenarios

Condition		RA	RV	PA	PCWP	CO	SVR	Comments
Shock	Hypovolemic	↓	↓	↓	↓	↓	↑	—
	Cardiogenic	-/↑	-/↑	-/↑	↑	↓	↑	
	Distributive	↓	↓	↓	↓	↑/↓	↓	
RV infarct		↑	↓ RVSP ↑ RVDP	—	-/↓	↓	↑	• RA >PCWP • Steep Y-descent • Square root sign in RV tracing
Acute mitral regurgitation		—	—	—	↑	↓	↑	• Prominent v-wave in PCWP tracing (v-wave >2 PCWP)
Tamponade		↑	↑	↑	↑	↓	↑	• Diastolic equalization of pressure • RA has steep X-descent and absent Y-descent
Massive pulmonary embolism		↑	↑ RVSP ↑ RVDP	↑	↓	↓	↑	• Ventricularization of PA waveform with rapid diastolic descent • Absent dicrotic notch
Acute VSD		↑	↑	↑	↑	↓	↑	• O$_2$ saturation step-up • Prominent v-wave
Constriction		↑	↑	↑	↑	↓	↑	• Dip and plateau in RV • M- or W-shaped RA tracing

Abbreviations: PA, pulmonary artery; RVDP, RV diastolic pressure; RVSP, RV systolic pressure; SVR, systemic vascular resistance; VSD, ventricular septal defect.

MINIMALLY INVASIVE HEMODYNAMIC MONITORING AND IMAGING

The major reservations and concerns about the use of PAC given its level of invasiveness and the lack of evidence supporting improved outcomes, as well as the decreased familiarity and training in PAC, have triggered the search for less invasive hemodynamic monitoring methods. As a result, many imaging modalities and minimally invasive monitors have surfaced as potential alternatives to invasive catheterization.

Echocardiography

Echocardiography has been established as an essential tool in the evaluation of critically ill patients. It can assist in the rapid, accurate, and noninvasive diagnosis of a broad range of acute cardiovascular diseases. The availability of echocardiography has appropriately decreased the need for invasive procedures needed to diagnosis life-threatening conditions such as acute mitral regurgitation and tamponade. A comprehensive echocardiographic evaluation has a high sensitivity and specificity for defining cardiac causes of shock when performed by a trained sonographer and interpreted by an experienced cardiologist.[42]

General indications in the ICU
The general indications for an echocardiogram in the ICU can be fairly extensive (**Table 5**). Some of these indications and limitations of transthoracic echocardiography (TTE) necessitate the performance of transesophageal echocardiography (TEE).

| Table 5 |
| ICU indications for echocardiographic examination |

Indication	Assessment
Hemodynamic compromise	• Ventricular function • Valvular function • Hemodynamically significant pericardial effusion • Volume status • Findings suggestive of pulmonary embolism • Cardiothoracic surgical complications
Unexplained hypoxemia	• Shunt • Ventricular function • Findings suggestive of pulmonary embolism
Infective endocarditis	• Valves • Hardware
Source of emboli	• LV function • LV apical thrombi • Atrial appendage and atrial body thrombi • Shunt
Aortic dissection	• Diagnosis of dissection flap and aortic enlargement • Complications of dissection including pericardial effusion and aortic regurgitation

Echocardiographic assessment of hemodynamic parameters

Several hemodynamic parameters can be evaluated using the different modalities of echocardiography, including two-dimensional (2D)-echo, color, and spectral Doppler interrogation.

Assessment of preload and volume responsiveness Accurate estimation of preload, volume status, and fluid responsiveness is essential for the proper management of patients with circulatory insufficiency. Using filling pressures to infer LV preload can be inaccurate in conditions that affect LV compliance or in the presence of dynamic LV outflow obstruction. Defining preload as LV end-diastolic volume (EDV) establishes echocardiography as a potentially useful tool in assessing preload.

Subjective assessment of LV volume by visual inspection may be helpful at extremes of cardiac filling. Systolic obliteration of a small LV cavity is often suggestive of hypovolemia. More quantitative measures are usually available by using endocardial border tracing. LV end-diastolic area (EDA) and EDV are commonly used to estimate LV preload.[43,44] Such findings should be interpreted within the clinical context because a large EDA or EDV would not necessarily equate to adequate preload in patients with chronic severe LV dysfunction and dilation. As a result, single-point estimations of LV dimensions have, at best, a modest correlation to fluid responsiveness.[45–47] Alternatively, changes in EDA can be better at predicting changes in CO in response to fluid challenges. This parameter should be used judiciously because it has been validated in small studies and can be affected by multiple factors that can render it less useful.[48]

Echocardiograms also provide estimates of right-sided and left-sided filling pressures. Several echocardiogram-derived parameters have also been assessed in predicting volume responsiveness.

RAP

- Measuring inferior vena cava (IVC) diameter and its respirophasic response can be used to estimate RA pressure as shown in **Table 6**.[49,50]

Table 6 **Echocardiographic estimation of RA pressure**		
IVC Size (cm)	**Respiratory Collapsibility of IVC[a]**	**Estimated RA Pressure (mm Hg)**
<2.1	>50% collapse	0–5
	<50% collapse	5–10
>2.1	>50% collapse	
	<50% collapse	>15

[a] (maximum expiratory diameter−minimum inspiratory diameter)/maximum diameter × 100%.

- IVC is best viewed in the subcostal or subxiphoid window and is usually measured at 2 cm from its junction with the RA, usually at the level of the hepatic vein.
- This technique faces many limitations, including unpredictable variation with positive pressure ventilation and questionable reliability in patients with elevated right heart pressures, intra-abdominal pressures, or pulmonary hypertension.

LA pressure
- Spectral Doppler used to determine mitral valve inflow variables and pulmonary vein flow patterns in addition to tissue Doppler imaging (TDI) and LA volume can be used to help estimate LA pressure (LAP) (**Fig. 4**).

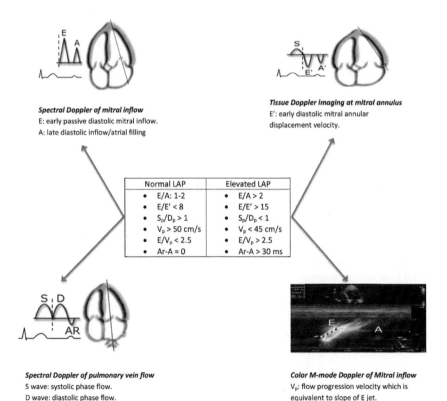

Spectral Doppler of mitral inflow
E: early passive diastolic mitral inflow.
A: late diastolic inflow/atrial filling

Tissue Doppler imaging at mitral annulus
E′: early diastolic mitral annular displacement velocity.

Normal LAP	Elevated LAP
• E/A: 1-2	• E/A > 2
• E/E′ < 8	• E/E′ > 15
• $S_p/D_p > 1$	• $S_p/D_p < 1$
• $V_p > 50$ cm/s	• $V_p < 45$ cm/s
• $E/V_p < 2.5$	• $E/V_p > 2.5$
• Ar-A = 0	• Ar-A > 30 ms

Spectral Doppler of pulmonary vein flow
S wave: systolic phase flow.
D wave: diastolic phase flow.
Ar: atrial reversal wave

Color M-mode Doppler of Mitral inflow
V_p: flow progression velocity which is equivalent to slope of E jet.

Fig. 4. Echocardiographic assessment of left atrial pressure (LAP).

- In hypovolemia, the LV early diastolic filling (mitral inflow E wave) decreases in comparison to the late LV filling during atrial contraction (mitral inflow A wave) leading to a lower E to A ratio, as does the systolic phase of pulmonary vein flow.
- As LAP becomes significantly elevated, the E wave increases out of proportion to the A wave leading to an increased E/A ratio together with elevated E/E' (E' being the early diastolic mitral annular displacement velocity obtained using TDI) and predominance of diastolic pulmonary vein blood flow (in the absence of mitral regurgitation). Specific thresholds that have been found to be supportive of elevated LAP include E/E' greater than 15, E/A greater than 2, and pulmonary vein systolic to diastolic wave ratio of less than 1, especially if they occur in the setting of LA dilation. Other supportive but more technically difficult and, therefore, less commonly preformed measures include (1) a color M-mode Doppler flow propagation velocity through the mitral valve (Vp) less than 45 cm per second, (2) E/Vp greater than 2.5 (in patients with depressed LV ejection fraction), and (3) the time difference between the duration of the atrial reversal wave of pulmonary vein flow and the mitral inflow A-wave duration (Ar-A) greater than 30 milliseconds. These variables are illustrated in **Fig. 4**.
- The reliability of these measures decrease in the setting of positive pressure ventilation by altering venous pulmonary return to the LA and affecting early passive filling. They can also be difficult to assess in the setting of tachyarrhythmia, along with other limiting factors.

Volume responsiveness
- IVC dispensability index defined as (IVC maximum diameter−IVC minimum diameter) per IVC minimum diameter has been evaluated in small studies. In mechanically ventilated patients, an IVC dispensability index in excess of 12% to 18% has been suggested to predict volume responsiveness, as would a value exceeding 40% in spontaneously breathing patients.[51–53] This parameter should be used cautiously in the appropriate clinical setting because it remains subject to many of the limitations encountered with CVP measurements and has not been validated in large trials.
- A more promising dynamic measure for assessing fluid responsiveness is the respiratory variation of peak aortic velocity by more than 12% indicating preload responsiveness. This measure is most reliable in mechanically ventilated patients without asynchrony or arrhythmias.[54,55]

Cardiac output
Several methods to measure the CO using 2D and Doppler echocardiography have been described. These techniques focus on combining Doppler-derived instantaneous blood flow velocity through a conduit with a cross-sectional area (CSA) of the conduit to obtain an estimate of the SV from which CO can be deduced. Of these structures, the LV-outflow tract (LVOT) conduit and aortic valve measurements are the most commonly used. The LVOT CSA is calculated from the LVOT diameter assuming a circular shape of the LVOT. Multiplying this CSA with the LVOT flow velocity time integral from spectral Doppler tracings will yield SV (**Fig. 5**), which is then multiplied by heart rate to obtain CO with good correlation with thermodilution-obtained CO.[56–58]

Ventricular function
Clinical examination is often insufficient to provide adequate assessment of biventricular function in the ICU where timely and accurate estimation of systolic function is an integral part of the management of most patients:

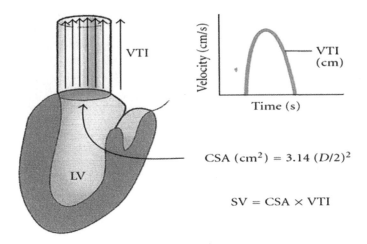

$$CSA\ (cm^2) = 3.14\ (D/2)^2$$

$$SV = CSA \times VTI$$

CSA represents the cross sectional area of the left ventricular outflow tract (LVOT) obtained by measuring the LVOT radius usually on the long axis views. LVOT velocity time integral (VTI) is then obtained using pulsed wave spectral Doppler imaging.

Fig. 5. Echocardiographic estimation of SV using LVOT flow. (*From* Otto CM. Textbook of clinical echocardiography. 3rd edition. Philadelphia: Elsevier Saunders, 2004; with permission.)

- LV function: Echocardiography can provide adequate information of LV function in most ICU patients. Global ventricular function can be reliably qualitatively assessed by visual inspection. Several quantitative measures could be used to estimate LV systolic function, including fractional shortening percentage and Teichholz equation (only reliable in the absence of focal wall motion abnormalities), the modified Simpson method, and wall motion score.[43,44,59,60]
- RV function: Another essential part of ventricular assessment is the RV function, which can be compromised in a variety of conditions. Echocardiographic evaluation of the RV requires an assessment of size, kinetics of the cavity, septal interaction, and other sequelae of RV disease.[61,62]
  - Assessment of RV function is primarily subjective by visual inspection. Measures of tricuspid annular plane systolic excursion less than 1.6 cm and use of TDI can be helpful in quantitative measures of RV function.
  - RV size is often evaluated by visual comparison to LV. Quantitatively, the ratio of diastolic RV area to that of the LV can be used to assess RV dilation with moderate enlargement suggested by a ratio greater than 0.6 and severe RV dilation when the ratio is greater than 1.
  - Septal motion: Systolic septal flattening (D-sign) is consistent with RV pressure overload and diastolic septal bowing into the LV implies RV volume overload (**Fig. 6**).
  - RA-IVC dilation, opening of the foramen ovale as the RA pressure exceeds that of the LA, and presence of TR are all useful in the assessment of the RV.

Assessment of pulmonary artery pressure

Pulmonary hypertension is common in critically ill patients and is defined as resting pulmonary systolic pressure of greater than 30 mm Hg, diastolic pressure of 15 mm Hg, or a mean of 25 mm Hg. Using continuous wave spectral Doppler, an

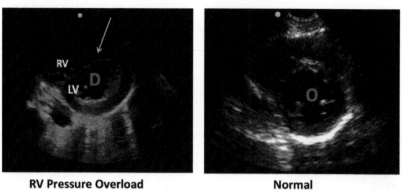

RV Pressure Overload   **Normal**

Fig. 6. Echocardiographic D-sign consistent with RV pressure overload. Ventricular short axis view. Right panel shows a normal circular left ventricle with crescenteric right ventricular shape during ventricular systole. Left panel shows a D-shaped left ventricle due to septal flattening and shift (*blue arrow*) to the left caused by right ventricular pressure overload during ventricular systole. (*Data from* Goldhaber Z. Echocardiography in the management of pulmonary embolism. Ann Intern Med 2002;136:691–700.)

echocardiogram can estimate pressures using the modified Bernoulli equation, which is simplified to[63]

- Systolic pressure = $4(V_{TR\ max})^2$ + RAP, where $V_{TR\ max}$ is the maximum tricuspid regurgitant velocity
- Diastolic pressure = $4(V_{PI\ end\text{-}diastolic})^2$ + RAP, where $V_{PI\ end\text{-}diastolic}$ is the end-diastolic pulmonary regurgitant velocity.

To calculate the systolic and diastolic pulmonary artery pressures, tricuspid and pulmonary regurgitation, respectively, must be present. Some investigators have questioned the accuracy of pulmonary artery pressure estimation by echocardiography in patients with underlying WHO Group III pulmonary hypertension.[64,65] This can partially be attributed to the difficulty in obtaining an accurate Doppler signal in the setting of pulmonary abnormalities.

Evaluation of cardiac tamponade

Recognizing cardiac tamponade in the critically ill patients is necessary. Most intensivists rely on echocardiography as the primary diagnostic tool. The parasternal and apical windows will usually show the effusion but it is not uncommon for critically ill patients to have suboptimal image quality with the only adequate images through the subcostal windows. The subcostal window is also useful in assessing the feasibility of pericardiocentesis because the needle will follow a similar tract.

Several parameters are used to assess for echocardiographic evidence of tamponade[59]:

- RV diastolic collapse is highly specific for cardiac tamponade. M-mode in the parasternal windows can make it easier to detect diastolic collapse of the RV.
- RA collapse is less specific and should not be confused with RA systolic contraction. The specificity of RA collapse improves if it last for more than one-third the PR interval.
- It is important to recognize that these findings can be absent in the setting of compartmentalized effusions or hematomas, particularly in poststernotomy patients with localized chamber compression.

- Doppler evaluation of atrioventricular valve inflow respiratory variation is the echocardiographic equivalent of pulsus paradoxus. It is based on the exaggerated interventricular dependence and can be helpful in confirming the hemodynamic significance of an effusion (**Fig. 7**). Mitral valve E wave respiratory variation by more than 25% and, to a lesser extent, tricuspid valve variation of 40% can be suggestive of hemodynamic compromise. These parameters should be used more cautiously in patients on positive pressure mechanical ventilators and in patients with arrhythmias or significant bronchospasm.
- Evidence of filling pressure elevation suggested by a distended IVC with minimal respirophasic collapse is a prerequisite for tamponade. Conditions causing significantly decreased right-sided filling pressures can be associated with right atrial collapse in the absence of actual tamponade. In these circumstances, a fluid challenge followed by repeating the echocardiogram would be helpful.

Other applications of echocardiography in the hemodynamically unstable patient
In addition to the usefulness of echocardiography in providing discrete hemodynamic measures related to filling pressure and perfusion, it is also useful in establishing the cause of circulatory insufficiency in some patients. Echocardiography can provide information about valvular dysfunction. It is also useful in assessing for postmyocardial infarction or cardiac surgery mechanical complications as causes of shock or intracardiac shunts as causes of refractory hypoxemia.

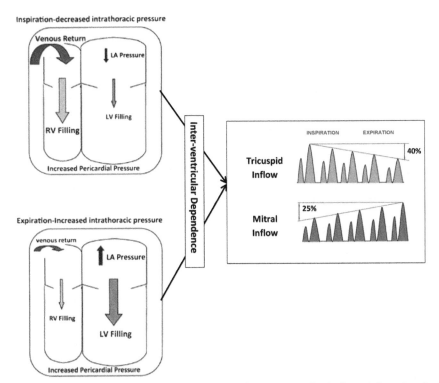

Fig. 7. Echocardiographic pulsus paradoxus in cardiac tamponade. (*Adapted from* Stanford University. Echocardiography in the ICU. Available at: http://www.stanford.edu/group/ccm_echocardio/cgi-bin/mediawiki/index.php/Tamponade. Accessed September 15, 2013.)

Comparison to PAC and Effects of Echocardiography on Management

In critically ill patients, echocardiography is useful in clarifying the diagnosis and defining the underlying pathophysiologic process in a different and complementary way to other circulatory monitoring modalities. The correlation between hemodynamic parameters assessed by PAC and echocardiography can be variable.[54–57,63] Available evidence suggests that bedside echo is of considerable benefit in management of patients with unexplained hemodynamic instability. Several studies have shown that either formal TTE or TEE can result in a change in the management of up to 50% of the study population.[42,66,67] Poelaert and colleagues[68] showed that 44% of subjects with a PAC underwent therapeutic changes after a TEE was performed in both cardiac and septic groups. However, there have been no convincing data to demonstrate that echocardiographic-guided management improves clinical outcomes.

Emerging Trends in ICU Echocardiography

The role of goal-directed echocardiography performed by intensivists who are not trained in cardiology is constantly growing due to its immediate availability and diagnostic value. The literature continues to confirm that brief, goal-directed TTE performed by intensivists are feasible and reliable in assessing some causes of shock.[69–71] Vieillard-Baron and colleagues[72] also demonstrated that qualitative assessment of hemodynamics using TEE can be accurate and useful in managing circulatory failure in septic shock. The development of a new generation of portable, lightweight, battery-powered, hand-carried ultrasound (HCU) has further strengthened this role of echocardiography. The accuracy of images created by these devices has shown good agreement with standard echocardiography when using standard 2D imaging.[71,73–76] Nevertheless, intensivist-performed, brief echocardiographic examinations using HCU should not be used to replace formal echocardiograms but, instead, as an adjunct to physical examination.[77] One of the current limitations of echocardiography compared with the other commonly used circulatory monitoring devices is that it does not provide continuous data. A single-use, miniaturized, indwelling 2D-TEE has been developed to allow continuous hemodynamic assessment with good promise in improving the usefulness of echocardiography in monitoring the response to therapy in the ICU.[78] With the decreased use of PAC and the obvious value of echocardiography in critically-ill patients, many training programs have already started shifting some attention to provide trainees sufficient education and experience with using this modality.

ESOPHAGEAL DOPPLER MONITOR

EDM was initially introduced in 1971 by Side and Gosling and subsequently modified by Singer in 1998. An esophageal Doppler monitor is a minimally invasive hemodynamic device that evaluates the CO and fluid status based on the assessment of descending aortic blood flow.[79–81] Using a Doppler probe inserted into the esophagus, the velocity of the descending aortic blood flow can be determined by the frequency shift as the waves get reflected of the moving red blood cells. The spectral analysis of the Doppler shift provides the velocity waveforms. This waveform is used to estimate SV and CO.

Insertion and Placement

The EDM probe is about 6 to 7 mm in diameter. Two types of probes are available: CardioQ (Deltex Medical, Chichester, UK) probe and HemoSonic (Arrown

International, USA) probe, the latter of which has M-mode capabilities. The probe is inserted orally or nasally in intubated patients. The probe is usually inserted to the distal esophagus where it is closest and most parallel to the aorta. Contraindications to EDM placement include pharyngeal and esophageal disease (pharyngeal pouch, esophageal stent, cancer, stricture, surgery) or significant systemic coagulopathy.

Safety and advantages
- Ease of use
- Speed: it requires about 5 minutes to place and obtain a clear signal[82,83]
- Absence of major complications associated with other invasive techniques
- Provides continuous monitoring
- Short period of training for the operator to develop efficiency and accuracy.[84]

Measured Parameters and Waveform Analysis

The pulsatile blood flow in the aorta translates to a change in velocity over time, allowing the calculation of a stroke distance in the descending aorta (SDa). SDa is the distance a column of blood travels along the aorta with each ventricular systole. The SDa is estimated by integrating the derivative of the velocity over time from the start of ejection to the end of flow that equates to the AUC of the velocity-time curve. The shape of the waveform and several other parameters obtained from the velocity-time curve allow the assessment of preload, afterload, and contractility (**Fig. 8**).

Corrected flow time
Flow time (FT) in milliseconds, equivalent to LV-ejection time, is measured from the base of the waveform starting from the beginning of the aortic pulse upstroke to its return to baseline. Corrected FT (FTc) is calculated by correcting for a heart rate of 60 beats per minute using the Bazzett correction formula. The normal range of FTc is generally 330 to 360 ms.[82] EDM uses FTc as a measure of LV preload. Some data suggest using SV, as opposed to FTc, as a more reliable indicator for preload because FTc can be directly affected by changes in afterload and contractility. Other factors, such as left bundle branch block, can affect LV-ejection time independent of hemodynamics. It is important to recognize conditions when the patient may be volume overloaded and yet have a low FTc due to pathologic limitation to LV preload (pulmonary embolism, mitral stenosis, tamponade).

Mean acceleration and peak velocity
Mean acceleration (MA) is the slope of the upstroke of the aortic pulse velocity waveform. MA, often used as a surrogate for peak acceleration which in turn, is a good measure of LV contractility independent of afterload. The height of the velocity curve is the peak velocity (PV), calculated as centimeters per second that, together with MA, can be used to infer information about LV contractility and afterload. The normal PV normally declines with age and a good estimate of the lower end of normal PV in adults is 120 minus age.

CO
The SDa is estimated by the area under the velocity-time curve. Using a built-in nomogram for age, height, and weight or using the M-mode capabilities of the HemoSonic probe, the distal aortic CSA (A) is obtained. The product of these two parameters provides the aortic SV ($SVa = SDa \times A$), which is multiplied by a correction factor, to account for the cephalic circulation, to estimate the SV (SV). The CO is calculated as CO equals SV multiplied by heart rate.

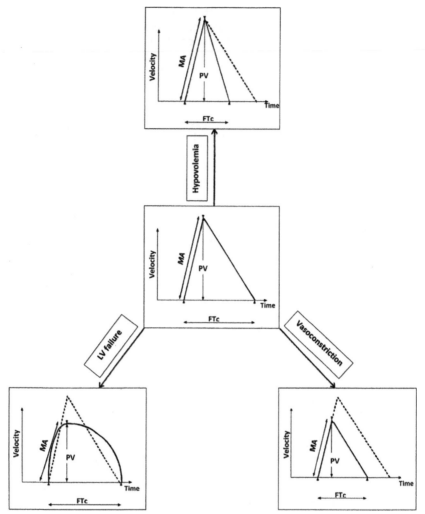

Fig. 8. EDM-measured parameters and their change in various clinical scenarios. (*Modified from* King SL, Lim MS. The use of the esophageal Doppler monitor in the intensive care unit. Crit Care Resusc 2004;6:113–22.)

Additional hemodynamic measures

The force and kinetic energy associated with each cardiac cycle have been assessed as potential contractility indices and seem to have a more discriminative power compared with MA and PV.[85] Similarly, the total systemic vascular resistance index and compliance can also be calculated and could be useful in patients being treated with vasoactive agents.

Clinical Scenarios

The EDM waveform shape and the measured or derived parameters are often helpful in identifying the various hemodynamic profiles encountered in the ICU, particularly in the setting of intravascular hypovolemia. These various profiles are summarized in **Table 7** and **Fig. 8.**

Table 7
EDM profiles in various hemodynamic states

Clinical Scenario	FTc	PV	MA	Comments
Hypovolemia	↓	Normal	Normal	• Narrower waveform
LV failure	-/↑	↓	↓	• Dome-shaped as opposed to triangular waveform • FTc >360 ms
Vasoconstriction	↓	↓	-/↑	• Shorter and narrower waveform

Assumptions and Limitations of EDM

Two major assumptions are the basis of CO measurements using EDM. Because the probe measures blood flow in the descending aorta, it presumes a fixed percentage of CO to supply the coronary, cerebral, and brachiocephalic circulation, and adjusts for it with a correction factor. This percentage is reliable in young healthy patients but can be highly variable depending on the metabolic activity of different organs or the pathologic state. The second assumption is the cross-sectional area of the descending aorta because using the nomogram might not be applicable to all patients. The M-mode option does not completely resolve this problem because the diameter of the aorta is dynamic and changes with alterations in vascular tone, volume status, and PP.[86,87]

Other limitations in the use of EDM include

- Operator dependence, accurate probe position, and issues with dislodgement
- Inaccurate in aortic regurgitation, aneurysm, or coarctation, and in patients with IABP
- Cannot provide SvO_2
- Most studies were done in subjects with hypovolemic shock (it is less extensively studied in cardiogenic and distributive shocks).

Validity and Clinical Evidence

There has been a sizable body of evidence to evaluate the validity of EDM-derived measures and to support their clinical value in critically ill patients. Most of the studies were performed in hemodynamically stable patients. More recent data have provided evidence for its use in hemodynamically unstable cohorts.[80,88–90]

Several studies have compared FTc to other measures of preload, including PCWP and LV EDA index, with good agreement.[91–94] One study followed FTc and PCWP in subjects whose ventricular preload was being manipulated.[95] The results showed matched changes in FTc and PCWP in hypovolemic and normovolemic subjects. In hypervolemic subjects receiving nitrates PCWP decreased, whereas FTc initially increased, reflecting optimal CO before decreasing. This showed that FTc is a useful measure to direct optimal ventricular loading.[91,92] Ventilator-induced variations in PV and SV accurately correlate with fluid responsiveness.[96,97]

In contrast, reviews on the ability of EDM to accurately assess CO and contractility have been variable in hemodynamically unstable subjects. Some studies have shown a good correlation between the CO derived from EDM compared with thermodilution (r as high as 0.89), whereas other trials have demonstrated EDM can underestimate CO by as much as 40%.[83,89,98–100] Most of these studies found a good agreement between changes in CO noticed on EDM and thermodilution with correlation coefficients of 0.90 to 0.94, with significantly lower interobserver variability in EDM CO compared with thermodilution.[80,84,98] This suggests that EDM is highly useful in accurately reflecting the direction and magnitude of change in CO over time but less useful in measuring absolute CO. The data on the use of EDM-derived measures to guide the administration and titration of inotropes remain limited.[101]

Effect on Outcomes

Numerous studies have appraised the effect of EDM-guided fluid management on outcomes. Those trials have primarily included surgical subjects with fluid replenishment using EDM, resulting in improved outcomes varying from shorter ICU stay, ability to tolerate diet earlier, and shorter hospital stays.[102–104] On closer examination of the data, it seems that EDM subjects received more fluids, which might explain the effect on outcome. These studies were not completely blinded and were restricted to the surgical cohort. Further studies to determine the effect on other outcomes, including mortality, that examine medical and cardiac ICU subjects with vasoactive medications are necessary.

Clinical Value

Compared with PAC, EDM is a minimally invasive, safe, and easy means to continuous, real-time circulatory monitoring that requires minimal training and can safely be used for a prolonged period of time without significant complications. In clinical practice, EDM has been best studied and shown to be most useful in goal-directed optimization of preload[84,91,95] in intravascularly volume-depleted patients. This is especially true when emphasis is placed on the trend of change in SV and CO as opposed to absolute values. Further studies are needed to confirm the same level of reliability in cardiac patients and its usefulness in guiding vasoactive and inotropic agents use.

PULSE CONTOUR ANALYSIS OR PULSE WAVE ANALYSIS

Newly emerging technologies based on pulse wave analysis (PWA) can be helpful in the measurement and optimization of flow. These devices have gained attention because they are relatively less invasive. They are all based on a similar basic principle of continuously estimating SV by analyzing arterial pressure waveforms but they use different techniques with varying proprietary algorithms. Understanding the physiology and technology used in PWA is important for the correct measurement and interpretation of the hemodynamic variables obtained.

Principles

The Windkessel effect describes the interaction between SV and the compliance of the arterial tree and can be evaluated using the shape of the arterial pressure waveform. In 1974, Wesseling and colleagues[105,106] developed a basic algorithm for monitoring SV by measuring the area under the systolic portion of the arterial pressure waveform and then dividing the area by aortic impedance. CO is calculated by multiplying the derived SV by the heart rate (**Fig. 9**). A modification to the formula, adding a correction factor for individual aortic impedance that was lacking in the earlier formula, remains in use today.

Devices

Several devices, available commercially, use the PWA for continuous CO measurement. Three are most commonly used and are the focus of this review. These systems can be broadly divided into two groups, those requiring calibration (PiCCO and lithium dilution CO [LiDCO]) and the uncalibrated systems (Flo-Trac).

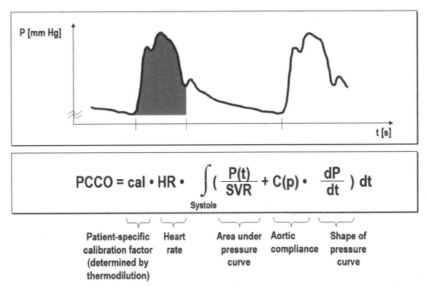

Fig. 9. Principle of PW analysis using the PiCCO system.

PiCCO system (Pulsion Medical Systems, Germany)
- PiCCO requires a thermistor-tipped arterial line to measure downstream temperature changes after the injection of a cold indicator via a central venous catheter.
- It uses PWA according to a modified Wesseling algorithm with periodic thermodilution calibration to continuously measure SV and calculate the CO, SV variation (SVV), PPV, and systemic vascular resistance.
- It is useful in periodically measuring several other parameters, including intrathoracic blood volume (ITBV), global EDV (GEDV), and extravascular lung water (EVLW), all of which are measures of cardiac preload, pulmonary edema, and contractility that together provide a global indication of cardiac performance.

LiDCO system (LiDCO Ltd, UK)
- LiDCO uses PWA along with dye dilution (lithium) calibration to measure CO.
- For calibration, a small dose of lithium is injected into a vein, where an ion selective electrode sensor mounted on a peripheral arterial line plots the concentration of lithium over time to calculate the CO.
- For PWA, this system uses an algorithm based on the law of conservation of power for continuous CO calculations. It assumes that the net power change in the arterial tree is equal to the amount of blood entering (SV) minus that of blood leaving. Once calibrated for compliance, the linear relationship between power and flow can be obtained and converted to nominal SV that is then converted to an actual SV.

Flo-Trac or Vigileo system (Edwards Lifesciences, California, USA)
- Flo-Trac is designed around the application of advanced statistical principles to the arterial pressure tracing, resulting in the creation of a proprietary algorithm that recalibrates itself constantly, rending external calibration unnecessary.

- It is based on a principle of the linear relation between PP and SV. The arterial pressure waveform is sampled every 20 seconds at 100 Hz, allowing the arterial pulsatility to be derived from the standard deviation of the pressure wave over 20 seconds, which is then multiplied by the patient-specific aortic compliance to obtain SV.
- It can be unreliable with arterial waveform artifact, aortic regurgitation, intense peripheral vasoconstriction, severe cardiac dysfunction, and irregular pulse or tachycardia.

Clinical Value and Reliability

Literature about the reliability and clinical value of PWA monitors has been variable. A high degree of correlation between CO obtained by the PWA method and PAC has been demonstrated in different clinical settings, including cardiac surgery, burn surgery, neurosurgery, and septic patients.[107–112] In a study by Hamzaoui and colleagues,[113] the reliability of PiCCO in subjects with rapidly changing vascular tone was found to be good with frequent calibrations. Similar results have been demonstrated for the LiDCO system.[111,114,115] In contrast, the earlier generation of Flo-Trac was associated with significant bias with a percentage error of greater than 30% compared with PAC. The third generation of Flo-Trac claims to have overcome these problems but the literature supporting this claim is conflicting.[116–119] There is a sizable body of evidence suggesting that, although PAC, Flo-Trac, LiDCO, and PiCCO display similar mean CO values, they often trend differently in response to therapy and show different interdevice agreement.[120]

Besides CO monitoring, PWA methods can be used for evaluating volume status and fluid responsiveness. Although GEDV and ITBV have some value,[121–123] SVV and PPV during the inspiratory and expiratory phases of mechanical ventilation are the most promising dynamic variables to optimize fluid therapy. Applicable thresholds of this parameter differ depending on the device used. The PiCCO technical specifications list SVV and PPV of less than 10% as being normal, with an optimal threshold values greater than 12% for SVV and greater than 13.5% for PPV for predicting a 25% increase in SV when assessing fluid responsiveness. The LiDCO product information states that an SVV or PPV less than 10% is normal, whereas values greater than 13% to 15% predict fluid responsiveness. The major limitation with these dynamic variables is the limited trials regarding their usefulness in spontaneously breathing patients. To reliably use these parameters in clinical practice, patients need to be synchronous on mechanical ventilation with tidal volume greater than 8 mL/kg.[124–126]

Effect on Outcomes

Regarding its effect on clinical outcomes, trials supporting PWA methods to guide goal-directed therapy are limited and variable. A prospective study comparing PiCCO with PAC showed no effect on mortality but an association with greater positive fluid balance and fewer ventilator-free days. After the correction for confounders, the choice of the monitoring system had no influence on the major outcomes, whereas a positive fluid balance was a significant independent predictor of examined outcomes.[127,128] On the other hand, the use of PiCCO-based hemodynamic optimization was found to be associated with improved outcomes in decompensated liver cirrhosis and subjects with subarachnoid hemorrhage.[128,129] Hemodynamic optimization with LiDCO was also associated with improved outcomes in high-risk surgical and critically ill patients. Nevertheless, these systems should be used cautiously in hemodynamically unstable patients.

THORACIC ELECTRICAL BIOIMPEDANCE OR IMPEDANCE CARDIOGRAPHY

Impedance cardiography (thoracic electrical bioimpedance [TEB]) in the measurement of cardiovascular performance was introduced in the late 1960s.[90] Its appeal was that is was the least invasive method to continuously monitor SV and CO. It is based on the measurement of changes in the thoracic impedance to an electrical current that is produced by the fluctuations in thoracic blood volume with each cardiac cycle.

Depending on the equation used, the theory behind impedance cardiography models the thorax as a cylinder[130] or a truncated cone[131] that is homogenously perfused with blood of a specific resistivity based on the hematocrit. The thorax has a steady state mean base impedance. Spot or band electrodes placed on the patient's thorax are used to emit and sense a low-voltage (2.5–4.0 mA), high-frequency (70–100 kHz), alternating electrical current through the thorax.[90] The electrical impedance is inversely proportional to the volume of thoracic fluids, implying that the pulsatile decrease in total thoracic impedance can be used in several mathematical models to estimate the beat-to-beat SV as well as CO.

Limitations and Pitfalls

The models used for estimating hemodynamic parameters from impedance cardiography are based on multiple assumptions that introduce a margin of inaccuracy. These limitations, and other pitfalls of impedance cardiography, are summarized in **Table 8**. Newer generation TEB methods have overcome some of these limitations by having faster signal processing,[132] better signal filters, improved EKG triggering, and respiratory filtering.

Clinical Value

The apparent advantages offered by TEB when it comes to noninvasiveness and ease of use have resulted in extensive testing to establish its effectiveness and applicability. Trials using TEB, in comparison with thermodilution[133–136] and direct and indirect Fick methods,[137–139] have shown TEB to be reliable in young healthy volunteers. Results have been highly inconsistent in the critically ill population with problems including

Table 8
Limitation and pitfalls of impedance cardiography

Limitations and Pitfalls	Examples
Ignores the effects of other factors beside aortic blood flow on thoracic bioimpedance	• Changes in tissue fluid volume • Respiratory-induced changes in pulmonary and venous blood flow • Pulmonary edema • Pleural effusion • Chest wall edema
Alteration in electrode position can drastically change CO measurements	—
Bases the measurement of ventricular ejection time on distance between QRS on EKG	• Precludes use in patients with arrhythmias.
Subject to interference from mechanical ventilation	—
Uses nomograms based on age, height, weight, and gender to estimate the volume of electrically participating tissue	• Inaccurate in patients who do not fit nomogram criteria • Inaccurate with sternal wire or other cases of presence of metal in the chest

underestimation of high CO and overestimation of low CO, particularly in the setting of positive pressure ventilation, arrhythmias, and pulmonary disorders (due to changes in thoracic cavity configuration and surface area). It is also highly unreliable in the presence of valvular disease and intracardiac shunts.

As a result, ICG remains controversial with regard to its accuracy and use in clinical practice. However, many investigators who question its ability to estimate absolute CO values, suggest usefulness in following hemodynamic trends within individuals.[140–143] Without further improvements in signal processing and accuracy in hemodynamically unstable patients, it is unlikely that TEB will become a standard monitor in the critical care setting. New advancements have produced three new monitors that show some promise in the unstable patients (**Table 9**).

Indirect Fick Method

A new noninvasive monitor called the NICO system (Novametrix Medical Systems, Wallingford, CT) can be used in mechanically ventilated patients to estimate pulmonary artery blood flow that, in the absence of a significant shunt, should be equal to the CO. The NICO system is based on carbon dioxide (CO_2) elimination by the lungs using a technique called the differential CO_2 Fick partial rebreathing method. It involves adding 150 mL of dead space to the ventilator circuit by opening a rebreathing valve and then measuring the change in CO_2 elimination and end-tidal CO_2 made during a period of no rebreathing and a subsequent rebreathing period. This allows the calculation of CO.

Promising advantages of the NICO systems include its noninvasiveness, ease of use, and the ability to provide capillary blood flow and several other ventilation parameters. It is constructed on several assumptions that can affect its accuracy in CO measurement. This system is less reliable in patients with diffusion abnormalities or in the setting of pulmonary shunting[144] and heterogeneous ventilation encountered in acute lung injury.[145,146] Changes in ventilation affecting dead space can have significant artificial effects on CO estimations. Another important limitation of the NICO system is the inability to assess volume status and fluid responsiveness. It can only be used in mechanically ventilated patients.

FUTURE DIRECTIONS FOR HEMODYNAMIC MONITORING IN THE ICU

Despite all the controversy regarding the use of PAC, there has been no argument against the limitations of physical examination in critically ill patients and the need

Table 9 Thoracic electrical bioimpedance monitors	
Aesculon (Osypka Medical, LA Jolla, CA, USA)	• Uses electrical velocimetry • Interprets maximum rate of change in TEB to calculate CO
ECOM (CONMED, Utica, NY, USA)	• Places electrode on endotracheal tube cuff due to proximity to aorta eliminating many assumptions • Preliminary data suggest adequate reliability
Bioreactance (NICOM, Cheetah TEB, Vancouver, WA, USA)	• Analyzes frequency variations of the delivered oscillating current • Higher signal-to-noise ratio resulting in improved performance • High agreement with other monitors (PAC, PiCCO, Flo-Trac)

for better hemodynamic assessment to provide a better understanding of the underlying pathophysiologic state and, as important, help in the development of goal-directed management strategies. To achieve these goals and to overcome the perceived limitations of PAC, alternative hemodynamic assessments have evolved. These new technologies have their own strengths and limitations and patient-specific variables cannot be ignored with the use of these technologies.

The noninvasive, easy-to-use, cost-effective, and reliable hemodynamic monitor remains elusive. Perhaps, just as important, there is paucity of large, clinical studies comparing these newer modalities with each other and traditional hemodynamic assessments, making it difficult to define the patient populations that clearly would benefit from these technologies. Correspondingly, more trials are constantly being performed to validate promising parameters such as ITBV, GEDV, and EVLW in clinical use. Further studies to assess the effect of current and developing devices on clinical outcomes remain in progress. Likewise, data on the efficacy and outcome improvement using a combination of two modalities seem to be lacking and need further investigation, which could be the focus of future studies. In the meantime, current monitoring devices should continue to be selected on a patient-specific basis, either alone or in combination with other hemodynamic monitors, until the gold standard hemodynamic monitoring tool is developed.

REFERENCES

1. Rodriguez RM, Berumen KA. Cardiac output measurement with an esophageal Doppler in critically ill Emergency Department patients. J Emerg Med 2000; 18(2):159–64.
2. Saugel B, Ringmaier S, Holzapfel K, et al. Physical examination, central venous pressure and chest radiography for the prediction of transpulmonary thermodilution-derived hemodynamic parameters in critically ill patients: a prospective trial. J Crit Care 2011;26(4):402–10.
3. Lakhal K, Macq C, Ehrmann S, et al. Noninvasive monitoring of blood pressure in the critically ill: reliability according to the cuff site (arm, thigh or ankle). Crit Care Med 2012;40:1207–13.
4. Feihl F, Broccard A. Interaction between respiration and systemic hemodynamics. Part I: basic concepts. Intensive Care Med 2009;35:45–54.
5. Broccard A. Cardiopulmonary interactions and volume status assessment. J Clin Monit Comput 2012;26:383–91.
6. Funk DJ, Jacobsohn E, Kumar A. The role of venous return in critical illness and shock: part II-shock and mechanical ventilation. Crit Care Med 2013;41: 573–9.
7. Michard F, Boussard S, Chemla D, et al. Relation between respiratory changes in arterial pulse pressure and fluid responsiveness in septic patients with acute circulatory failure. Am J Respir Crit Care Med 2000; 162(1):134–8.
8. Marik P, Cavallazzi R, Vasu T, et al. Dynamic changes in arterial waveform derived variables and fluid responsiveness in mechanically ventilated patients: a systematic review of the literature. Crit Care Med 2009;37:2642–7.
9. Cook DJ, Simel DL. Does this patient have abnormal central venous pressure? JAMA 1996;275(8):630–4.
10. Marik PE, Baram M, Vahid B. Does central venous pressure predict fluid responsiveness? A systematic review of the literature and the tale of seven mares. Chest 2008;134:172–8.

11. Marik PE, Cavallazzi R. Does the central venous pressure predict fluid responsiveness. An updated meta-analysis and a plea for some common sense. Crit Care Med 2013;41:1774–81.
12. Teboul JL, Monnet X. Prediction of volume responsiveness in critically ill patients with spontaneous breathing activity. Curr Opin Crit Care 2008;14:334–9.
13. Magder S, Lagonidis D, Erice F. The use of respiratory variations in right atrial pressure to predict the cardiac output response to PEEP. J Crit Care 2001;16:108–14.
14. Magder S. How to use central venous pressure measurements. Curr Opin Crit Care 2005;11:264–70.
15. Barnes GE, Laine GA, Giam PY, et al. Cardiovascular response to elevation of intra-abdominal hydrostatic pressure. Am J Physiol 1985;248:R208–13.
16. Rutlen DL, Wackers FJ, Zaret BL. Radionuclide assessment of peripheral intravascular capacity: a technique to measure intravascular volume changes in the capacitance circulation in man. Circulation 1981;64:146–52.
17. Monnett X, Reinzo M, Osman D, et al. Passive leg raising predicts fluid responsiveness in the critically ill. Crit Care Med 2006;34:1402–7.
18. Rudiger A, Gasser S, Fischler M, et al. Comparable increase of B-type natriuretic peptide and amino-terminal pro-B-type natriuretic peptide levels in patients with severe sepsis, septic shock and acute heart failure. Crit Care Med 2006;34:2140–4.
19. Forfia PR, Watkins SP, Rame JE, et al. Relationship between B-type natriuretic peptides and pulmonary wedge pressure in the intensive care unit. J Am Coll Cardiol 2005;45:1667–71.
20. Dixon J, Philips B. The interpretation of brain natriuretic peptide in critical care patients; will it ever be useful? Crit Care 2010;14:184–5.
21. Jones AE, Shapiro NI, Trzeciak S, et al. Lactate clearance vs. central venous oxygen saturation as goals of early sepsis therapy: a randomized clinical trial. JAMA 2010;303:739–46.
22. Fuller B, Dellinger RP. Lactate as a hemodynamic marker in the critically ill. Curr Opin Crit Care 2012;18(3):267–72.
23. Nguyen HB, Rivers EP, Knoblich EP, et al. Early lactate clearance is associated with improved outcome in severe sepsis and septic shock. Crit Care Med 2004;32:1637–42.
24. Attana P, Lazzeri C, Chiostri M, et al. Lactate clearance in cardiogenic shock following ST elevation myocardial infarction: a pilot study. Acute Card Care 2012;14:20–6.
25. Marik PE, Bellomo R, Delma V. Lactate clearance as a target of therapy in sepsis: a flawed paradigm. OA Crit Care 2013;1(1):3–8.
26. Reminiac F, Saint-Etienne C, Runge I, et al. Are central venous lactate and arterial lactate interchangeable? A human retrospective study. Anesth Analg 2012;115(3):605–10.
27. Van B, Wietasch G, Scheeren T, et al. Clinical review: use of venous oxygen saturations as a goal - a yet unfinished puzzle. Crit Care 2011;15:232.
28. Walley KR. Use of central venous oxygen saturation to guide therapy. Am J Respir Crit Care Med 2001;184:514–20.
29. Chawla L, Zia H, Gutierrez G, et al. Lack of equivalence between central and mixed venous oxygen saturation. Chest 2004;126:1891–6.
30. Yazigi A, El Khoury C, Jebara S, et al. Comparison of central venous to mixed venous oxygen saturation in patients with low cardiac index and filling pressures after coronary artery surgery. J Cardiothorac Vasc Anesth 2008;22:77–83.

31. Dueck MH, Klimek M, Appenrodt S, et al. Trends but not individual values of central venous oxygen saturation agree with mixed venous oxygen saturation during varying hemodynamic conditions. Anesthesiology 2005;103: 249–57.
32. Bender JS, Smith-Meek MA, Jones CE. Routine pulmonary artery catheterization does not reduce morbidity and mortality of elective vascular surgery: results of a prospective randomized trial. Ann Surg 1997;226(3):229–37.
33. Connors AF, Speroff T, Dawson NV, et al. The effectiveness of right heart catheterization in the initial care of critically ill patients. JAMA 1996;276:889–97.
34. Rhodes A, Cusack RJ, Newman PJ, et al. A randomized controlled trial of the pulmonary artery catheter in critically ill patients. Intensive Care Med 2002;28: 256–64.
35. Isaacson IJ, Lowdon JD, Berry AJ, et al. The value of pulmonary artery catheter and central venous monitoring in patients undergoing abdominal aortic reconstruction surgery: a comparative study of two selected, randomized, groups. J Vasc Surg 1990;12:754–60.
36. Soni N. Swan song for the Swan-Ganz catheter? the use of pulmonary artery catheters probably needs re-evaluation-but they should not be banned. BMJ 1996;3313:763–4.
37. Harvey S, Harrison D, Singer M, et al. Assessment of the clinical effectiveness of pulmonary artery catheters in management of patients in intensive care (PAC-Man): a randomized controlled trial. Lancet 2005;366:472–7.
38. Binanay C, Califf RM, Hasselblad V, et al. Evaluation study of congestive heart failure and pulmonary artery catheterization effectiveness. JAMA 2005;294(13): 1625–33.
39. Morris AM, Chapman RH, Gardner RM. Frequency of wedge pressure errors in the ICU. Crit Care Med 1985;13:705–8.
40. Iberti TJ, Fischer EP, Leibowitz AB, et al. A multicenter study of physicians' knowledge of the pulmonary artery catheter. JAMA 1990;264:2928–32.
41. Gnaegi A, Feihl F, Perret C. Intensive care physicians' insufficient knowledge of right heart catheterization at the bedside: time to act? Crit Care Med 1997;25: 213–20.
42. Joseph MX, Disney PJ, Da Costa R, et al. Transthoracic echocardiography to identify or exclude cardiac cause of shock. Chest 2004;126:1592–7.
43. Schiller NB, Shah PM, Crawford M, et al. Recommendations for quantitation of the left ventricle by two-dimensional echocardiography. American Society of Echocardiography Committee on Standards, Subcommittee on Quantitation of Two-Dimensional Echocardiograms. J Am Soc Echocardiogr 1989;2:358–67.
44. Lang RM, Bierig M, Devereux RB. Recommendations for chamber quantification: a report from the American society of echocardiography's guidelines and standards committee and the chamber quantification writing group. J Am Soc Echocardiogr 2005;18:1440–63.
45. Tousignant CP, Walsh F, Mazer CD. The use of transesophageal echocardiography for preload assessment in critically ill patients. Anesth Analg 2000;90: 351–5.
46. Thys DM, Hillel Z, Goldman ME, et al. A comparison of hemodynamic indices derived by invasive monitoring and two dimensional echocardiography. Anesthesiology 1987;67:630–4.
47. Douglas PS, Edmonds HL, Sutton MS, et al. Unreliability of hemodynamic indexes of left ventricular size during cardiac surgery. Ann Thorac Surg 1987; 44:31–4.

48. Swenson JD, Harkin C, Pace NL, et al. Transesophageal echocardiography: an objective tool in defining maximum ventricular response to intravenous fluid therapy. Anesth Analg 1996;83:1149–53.

49. Jue J, Chung W, Schiller NB. Does inferior vena cava size predict right atrial pressures in patients receiving mechanical ventilation? J Am Soc Echocardiogr 1992;5:613–9.

50. Nagueh SF, Kopelen HA, Zoghbi WA. Relation of mean right atrial pressure to echocardiographic and Doppler parameters of right atrial and right ventricular function. Circulation 1996;93:1160–9.

51. Feissel M, Michard F, Faller JP, et al. The respiratory variation in inferior vena cava diameter as a guide to fluid therapy. Intensive Care Med 2004;30:1834–7.

52. Barbier C, Loubieres Y, Schmidt C, et al. Respiratory changes in inferior vena cava diameter are helpful in predicting fluid responsiveness in ventilated septic patients. Intensive Care Med 2004;30:1740–6.

53. Muller L, Bobbia X, Toumi M, et al. Respiratory variations of inferior vena cava diameter predict fluid responsiveness in spontaneously breathing patients with acute circulatory failure: need for a cautious use. Crit Care 2012;16:R188.

54. Benjamin E, Griffin K, Leibowitz AB, et al. Goal-directed transesophageal echocardiography performed by intensivist to assess left ventricular function: comparison with pulmonary artery catheterization. J Cardiothorac Vasc Anesth 1998;12:10–5.

55. Costachescu T, Denault A, Guimond JG, et al. The hemodynamically unstable patient in the intensive care unit: hemodynamic vs. transesophageal echocardiographic monitoring. Crit Care Med 2002;30:1214–23.

56. Feinberg MS, Hopkins WE, Davila-Roman VG, et al. Multiplane transesophageal echocardiographic Doppler imaging accurately determines cardiac output measurements in critically ill patients. Chest 1995;107:769–73.

57. Mclean AS, Needham A, Stewart D, et al. Estimation of cardiac output by noninvasive echocardiographic techniques in the critically ill subject. Anaesth Intensive Care 1997;25:250–4.

58. Ihlen H, Amlie JP, Dale J, et al. Determination of cardiac output by Doppler echocardiography. Br Heart J 1984;51:54–60.

59. Stamos TD, Soble JS. The use of echocardiography in the critical care setting. Crit Care Clin 2001;17:253–70.

60. Troianos CA, Porembka DT. Assessment of left ventricular function and hemodynamics with transesophageal echocardiography. Crit Care Clin 1996;12:253–72.

61. Jardin F, Dubourg O, Bourdarias JP. Echocardiographic pattern of acute cor pulmonale. Chest 1997;111:209–17.

62. Vieillard-Baron A, Prin S, Chergui K, et al. Echo-Doppler demonstration of acute cor pulmonale at the bedside in the medical intensive care unit. Am J Respir Crit Care Med 2002;166:1310–9.

63. Stevenson JG. Comparison of several noninvasive methods for estimation of pulmonary artery pressure. J Am Soc Echocardiogr 1989;2:157–71.

64. Taleb M, Khuder S, Tinkel J, et al. The diagnostic accuracy of Doppler echocardiography in assessment of pulmonary artery systolic pressure: a meta-analysis. Echocardiography 2013;30:258–65.

65. Fisher MR, Criner GJ, Fishman AP, et al. Estimating pulmonary artery pressures by echocardiography in patients with emphysema. Eur Respir J 2007;30:914–21.

66. Bruch C, Comber M, Schmermund A, et al. Diagnostic usefulness and impact on management of transesophageal echocardiography in surgical intensive care units. Am J Cardiol 2003;91:510–3.

67. Hwang JJ, Shyu KG, Chen JJ, et al. Usefulness of transesophageal echocardiography in the treatment of critically ill patients. Chest 1993;104:861–6.
68. Poelaert JI, Trouerbach J, De Buyzere M, et al. Evaluation of transesophageal echocardiography as a diagnostic and therapeutic aid in a critical care setting. Chest 1995;107:774–9.
69. Counselman FL, Sanders A, Slovis CM, et al. The status of bedside ultrasonography training in emergency medicine residency programs. Acad Emerg Med 2003;10:37–42.
70. Mandavia DP, Aragona J, Chan L, et al. Ultrasound training for emergency physicians: a prospective study. Acad Emerg Med 2000;7:1008–14.
71. Manasia AR, Nagaraj HM, Kodali RB, et al. Feasibility and potential clinical utility of goal directed transthoracic echocardiography performed by noncardiologist intensivists using a small hand-carried device (SonoHeart) in critically ill patients. J Cardiothorac Vasc Anesth 2005;19:155–9.
72. Vieillard-Baron A, Charron C, Chergui K, et al. Bedside echocardiographic evaluation of hemodynamics in sepsis: is a qualitative evaluation sufficient? Intensive Care Med 2006;32:1547–52.
73. Spevack DM, Tunick PA, Kronzon I. Hand carried echocardiography in the critical care setting. Echocardiography 2003;20:455–61.
74. Vignon P, Chastanger C, Francois B, et al. Diagnostic ability of hand-held echocardiography in ventilated critically ill patients. Crit Care 2003;7:R84–91.
75. Goodkin GM, Spevack DM, Tunick PA, et al. How useful is hand-carried bedside echocardiography in critically ill patients? J Am Coll Cardiol 2001;37:2019–22.
76. Beaulieu Y, Marik P. Bedside ultrasonography in the ICU: Part 1. Chest 2005;128:881–95.
77. DeCara JM, Lang RM, Spencer KT. The hand-carried ultrasound device as an aid to the physical examination. Echocardiography 2003;20:477–85.
78. Vieillard-Baron A, Slama M, Charron C, et al. A pilot study on safety and clinical utility of a single-use 72-hour indwelling transesophageal echocardiography probe. Intensive Care Med 2013;39:629–35.
79. Singer M. Oesophageal doppler. Curr Opin Crit Care 2009;15(3):244–8.
80. Dark PM, Singer M. The validity of trans-esophageal Doppler ultrasonography as a measure of cardiac output in critically ill adults. Intensive Care Med 2004;30:2060–6.
81. Schober P, Loer SA, Schwarte LA. Perioperative hemodynamic monitoring with trans-esophageal Doppler technology. Anesth Analg 2009;109(2):340–53.
82. Singer M. Esophageal Doppler monitoring of aortic blood flow: beat-by-beat cardiac output monitoring. Int Anesthesiol Clin 1993;31:99–125.
83. Klein G, Emmerich M, Maisch O, et al. Clinical evaluation of non-invasive monitoring aortic blood flow by a transesophageal echo-Doppler Device. Anesthesiology 1998;89:A446.
84. Lefrant J, Bruelle P, Aya A, et al. Training is required to improve the reliability of esophageal Doppler to measure cardiac output in critically ill patients. Intensive Care Med 1998;24:347–52.
85. Atlas G, Brealey D, Dhar S, et al. Additional hemodynamic measurements with an esophageal Doppler monitor: a preliminary report of compliance, force, kinetic energy and afterload in the clinical setting. J Clin Monit Comput 2012;26:473–82.
86. Kamal GD, Symreng T, Starr J. Inconsistent esophageal Doppler cardiac output during acute blood loss. Anesthesiology 1990;72:95–9.

87. List W, Gravenstein N, Banner T, et al. Interaction in sheep between mean arterial pressure and cross sectional area of the descending aorta: implications for esophageal Doppler monitoring. Anesthesiology 1987;67:178A.
88. Seoudi HM, Perkal MF, Hanrahan A, et al. The esophageal Doppler monitor in mechanically ventilated surgical patients: does it work? J Trauma 2003;55(4):720–5.
89. Valtier B, Cholley BP, Belot JP, et al. Noninvasive monitoring of cardiac output in critically ill patients using transesophageal Doppler. Am J Respir Crit Care Med 1998;158:77–83.
90. Jensen L, Yakimets J, Teo K. A review of impedance cardiography. Heart Lung 1995;24:183–93.
91. Madan AK, UyBarreta VV, Aliabadi-Wahle S, et al. Esophageal Doppler ultrasound monitor versus pulmonary artery catheter in the hemodynamic management of critically ill surgical patients. J Trauma 1999;46(4):607–11.
92. Kincaid EH, Fly MG, Chang MC. Noninvasive measurements of preload using esophageal Doppler are superior to pressure-based estimates in critically injured patients. Crit Care Med 1999;27(Suppl):A111.
93. Singer M, Clarke J, Bennett ED. Continuous hemodynamic monitoring by esophageal Doppler. Crit Care Med 1989;17:447–52.
94. King SL, Lim MS. The use of the oesophageal Doppler Monitor in the intensive care unit. Crit Care Resusc 2004;6:113–22.
95. Singer M, Bennett ED. Noninvasive optimization of left ventricular filling using esophageal Doppler. Crit Care Med 1991;19(9):1132–7.
96. Vallee F, Fourcade O, De Soyres O, et al. Stroke output variations calculated by esophageal Doppler is a reliable predictor or fluid response. Intensive Care Med 2005;31:1388–93.
97. Slama M, Masson H, Teboul JL, et al. Monitoring of respiratory variations of aortic blood flow velocity using esophageal Doppler. Intensive Care Med 2004;30(6):1182–7.
98. Laupland KB, Brands CJ. Utility of esophageal Doppler as a minimally invasive hemodynamic monitor: a review. Can J Anaesth 2002;49(4):393–401.
99. Spahn DR, Schmid ER, Tornic M, et al. Noninvasive versus invasive assessment of cardiac output after cardiac surgery: clinical validation. J Cardiothorac Vasc Anesth 1990;4:46–59.
100. Penny JA, Anthony J, Shennan AH, et al. A comparison of hemodynamic data derived by pulmonary artery flotation catheter and the esophageal Doppler monitor in preeclampsia. Am J Obstet Gynecol 2000;183:658–61.
101. Singer M, Allen MJ, Webb AR, et al. Effects of alterations in left ventricular filling, contractility, and systemic vascular resistance on the ascending aortic blood velocity waveform of normal subjects. Crit Care Med 1991;19:1138–45.
102. Mythen MG, Webb AR. Perioperative plasma volume expansion reduces the indices of gut musical hypoperfusion during cardiac surgery. Arch Surg 1995; 130:423–9.
103. Sinclair S, James S, Singer M. Intraoperative intravascular volume optimization and length of hospital stay after repair of proximal femoral fracture: randomised controlled trial. BMJ 1997;315:909–12.
104. Conway DH, Mayall R, Abdul-Latif MS, et al. Randomised controlled trial investigating the influence of intravenous fluid titration using esophageal Doppler monitoring during bowel surgery. Anaesthesia 2002;57:845–9.
105. Wesseling KH, Jansen JR, Settels JJ, et al. Computation of aortic flow from pressure in humans using a nonlinear, three element model. J Appl Physiol (1985) 1993;74:2566–73.

106. Wesseling KH, De Wit B, Weber JA, et al. A simple device for continuous measurement of cardiac output. Adv Cardiovasc Physiol 1983;5:16–52.
107. Della Rocca GC, Coccia C. Cardiac output monitoring: aortic transpulmonary thermodilution and pulse contour analysis agree with standard thermodilution methods in patients undergoing lung transplantation. Can J Anaesth 2003;50: 707–11.
108. Bendjelid K, Marx G, Kiefer N, et al. Performance of a new pulse contour method for continuous cardiac output monitoring: validation in critically ill patients. Br J Anaesth 2013;111(4):573–9.
109. McCoy JV, Hollenberg SM, Dellinger RP, et al. Continuous cardiac index monitoring: a prospective observational study of agreement between a pulmonary artery catheter and a calibrated minimally invasive technique. Resuscitation 2009; 80(8):893–7.
110. Chakravarthy M, Patil TA, Jayaprakash K, et al. Comparison of simultaneous estimation of cardiac output by four techniques in patients undergoing off-pump coronary artery bypass surgery-a prospective observational study. Ann Card Anaesth 2007;10(2):121–6.
111. Costa MG, Della Rocca G, Chiarandini P, et al. Continuous and intermittent cardiac output measurement in hyperdynamic conditions: pulmonary artery catheter vs. lithium dilution technique. Intensive Care Med 2008;34:257–63.
112. Hofer CK, Button D, Weibel L, et al. Uncalibrated radial and femoral arterial pressure waveform analysis for continuous cardiac output measurement: an evaluation in cardiac surgery patients. J Cardiothorac Vasc Anesth 2010; 24(2):257–64.
113. Hamzaoui O, Monnet X, Richard C, et al. Effects of changes in vascular tone on the agreement between pulse contour and transpulmonary thermodilution cardiac output measurements within an up to 6-hour calibration-free period. Crit Care Med 2008;36(2):434–40.
114. Cecconi M, Dawson D, Grounds RM, et al. Lithium dilution cardiac output measurement in the critically ill patient: determination of precision of the technique. Intensive Care Med 2009;35(3):498–504.
115. Cecconi M, Fawcett J, Grounds RM. A prospective study to evaluate the accuracy of pulse power analysis to monitor cardiac output in critically ill patients. BMC Anesthesiol 2008;8:3–12.
116. Button D, Weibel L, Reuthebuch O, et al. Clinical evaluation of the FloTrac/Vigileo system and two established continuous cardiac output monitoring devices in patients undergoing cardiac surgery. Br J Anaesth 2007;99(3): 329–36.
117. McGee WT, Horswell JL, Calderon J, et al. Validation of a continuous, arterial pressure-based cardiac output measurement: a multicenter, prospective clinical trial. Crit Care 2007;11(5):R105.
118. Breukers RM, Sepehrkhouy S, Spiegelenberg SR, et al. Cardiac output measured by a new arterial pressure waveform analysis method without calibration compared with thermodilution after cardiac surgery. J Cardiothorac Vasc Anesth 2007;21(5):632–5.
119. Compton FD, Zukunft B, Hoffmann C, et al. Performance of a minimally invasive uncalibrated cardiac output monitoring system (Flotrac/Vigileo) in haemodynamically unstable patients. Br J Anaesth 2008;100:451–6.
120. Haidan M, Kim HK, Severyn DA, et al. Cross-comparison of cardiac output trending accuracy of LiDCO, PiCCO, FloTrac and pulmonary artery catheters. Crit Care 2010;14(6):R212.

121. Hofer CK, Furrer L, Matter-Ensner S, et al. Volumetric preload measurement by thermodilution: a comparison with transoesophageal echocardiography. Br J Anaesth 2005;94(6):748–55.
122. Tomicic V, Graf J, Echevarría G, et al. Intrathoracic blood volume versus pulmonary artery occlusion pressure as estimators of cardiac preload in critically ill patients. Rev Med Chil 2005;133(6):625–31.
123. Sakka SG, Bredle DL, Reinhart K, et al. Comparison between intrathoracic blood volume and cardiac filling pressures in the early phase of hemodynamic instability of patients with sepsis or septic shock. J Crit Care 1999;14(2): 78–83.
124. Zhang Z, Lu B, Sheng X, et al. Accuracy of stroke volume variation in predicting fluid responsiveness: a systematic review and meta-analysis. J Anesth 2011; 25(6):904–16.
125. Reuter DA, Felbinger TW, Schmidt C, et al. Stroke volume variations for assessment of cardiac responsiveness to volume loading in mechanically ventilated patients after cardiac surgery. Intensive Care Med 2002;28(4):392–8.
126. Belloni L, Pisano A, Natale A, et al. Assessment of fluid-responsiveness parameters for off-pump coronary artery bypass surgery: a comparison among LiDCO, transesophageal echocardiography, and pulmonary artery catheter. J Cardiothorac Vasc Anesth 2008;22(2):243–8.
127. Uchini S, Bellomo R, Morimatsu H, et al. Pulmonary artery catheter versus pulse contour analysis: a prospective epidemiological study. Crit Care 2006;10(6): R174.
128. Mutoh T, Kazumata K, Ishikawa T, et al. Performance of bedside transpulmonary thermodilution monitoring for goal-directed hemodynamic management after subarachnoid hemorrhage. Stroke 2009;40(7):2368–74.
129. Manglitz C, Encke J, Stremmel W, et al. Hemodynamic monitoring-guided therapy using the PiCCO-technology in decompensated liver cirrhosis. Z Gastroenterol 2009;47:5–18.
130. Kubicek WG, Karnegis JN, Patterson RP, et al. Development and evaluation of an impedance cardiac output system. Aerosp Med 1966;37:1208–12.
131. Sramek BB, Rose DM, Miyamoto A. Stroke volume equation with a linear base impedance model and its accuracy, as compared to thermodilution and magnetic flow meter techniques in humans and animals. Proceedings of Sixth International Conference on electrical Bioimpedance. Zadar (Yugoslavia), 1983. p. 38–41.
132. Nagel JG, Shyu LY, Reddy SP, et al. New signal processing techniques for improved precision of noninvasive impedance cardiography. Ann Biomed Eng 1989;17:517–34.
133. Donovan KD, Dobb GJ, Woods PD, et al. Comparison of thoracic electrical impedance and thermodilution methods for measuring cardiac output. Crit Care Med 1986;14:1038–44.
134. Costello GT, Edwards WL, Bumb KL. Impedance cardiography in open thorax patients. Crit Care Med 1987;15:363.
135. Fuller HD. The validity of cardiac output measurement by thoracic impedance: a meta-analysis. Clin Invest Med 1992;15:103–12.
136. Mehlsen J, Bonde J, Stadeager C, et al. Reliability of impedance cardiography in measuring central hemodynamics. Clin Physiol 1991;11:579–88.
137. Du Quesnay MC, Stoute GJ, Hughson RL. Cardiac output in exercise by impedance cardiography during breathing holding and normal breathing. J Appl Physiol (1985) 1987;62:101–7.

138. Niizeki K, Miyamoto Y, Doi K. A comparison between cardiac output determined by impedance cardiography and the rebreathing method during exercise in man. Jpn J Physiol 1989;39:441–6.

139. Salandin V, Zussa C, Risica G, et al. Comparison of cardiac output estimation by thoracic electrical bioimpedance, thermodilution and Fick methods. Crit Care Med 1988;16:1157–8.

140. Lopez-Saucedo A, Hirt M, Appel PL, et al. Feasibility of noninvasive physiologic monitoring in resuscitation of trauma patients in the emergency department. Crit Care Med 1988;16:482–90.

141. Gastfriend RG, Van De Water JM, Leonard ML, et al. Impedance cardiography: current status and clinical application. Am Surg 1986;52:636–40.

142. Meguid MM, Lukaski HC, Tripp MD, et al. Rapid bedside method to assess changes in post-operative fluid status with bioelectrical impedance analysis. Surgery 1992;112:502–8.

143. Spinale FG, Reines HD, Cook MC, et al. Noninvasive estimation of extravascular lung water using bioimpedance. J Surg Res 1989;47:535–40.

144. Rocco M, Spadetta G, Morelli A, et al. A comparative evaluation of thermodilution and partial CO2 rebreathing techniques for cardiac output assessment in critically ill patients during assisted ventilation. Intensive Care Med 2004;30: 82–7.

145. de Abreu MG, Quintel M, Ragaller M, et al. Partial carbon dioxide rebreathing: a reliable technique for noninvasive measurement of non-shunted pulmonary capillary blood flow. Crit Care Med 1997;25(4):675–83.

146. Green DW. Comparison of cardiac outputs during major surgery using the Deltex CardioQ oesophageal Doppler monitor and the Novametrix-Respironics NICO: a prospective observational study. Int J Surg 2007;5(3):176–82.

Submassive Pulmonary Embolism

Laurence W. Busse, MD*, Jason S. Vourlekis, MD

KEYWORDS

- Pulmonary embolism • Submassive • Risk stratification • Thrombolysis
- Intermediate-risk pulmonary embolism • Right ventricular dysfunction

KEY POINTS

- Acute pulmonary embolism (PE) is common and associated with a high degree of morbidity and mortality.
- PE can present silently or with hemodynamic collapse and cardiac arrest, is difficult to diagnose, and treatment options depend on accurate and timely risk stratification.
- Severity in PE depends on the amount of clot burden as well as physiologic response to the clot, and is stratified into low risk, submassive, and massive, with increasing levels of mortality.

INTRODUCTION

Acute pulmonary embolism (PE) is part of the spectrum comprising venous thromboembolic disease. In the United States alone there are estimated to be 350,000 to 600,000 cases of venous thromboembolism (VTE) annually with 100,000 to 200,000 related deaths.[1,2] PE is associated with a high rate of morbidity and mortality, depending on the clinical presentation and underlying cardiopulmonary status. Mortality ranges from low in the hemodynamically stable patient to being almost a certainty in severe cases. In all risk groups, combined in-hospital mortality is estimated at 15%.[3] Arguably the single biggest contributor to mortality in PE is failure of diagnosis.[4] Long-term morbidity including recurrence, chronic venous insufficiency, and chronic thromboembolic pulmonary hypertension can occur in up to 12.9%, 7.3%, and 35% of patients, respectively, at 1 year.[5–7]

VTE is common in the critical care setting. The frequency depends on the method of surveillance. Systematic screening for deep vein thrombosis (DVT) by ultrasonography identifies thrombus in as many as 40% of patients.[8–10] Patel and colleagues[11]

Disclosures: The authors have no disclosures to report.
Section of Critical Care Medicine, Department of Medicine, Inova Fairfax Medical Center, 3300 Gallows Road, Falls Church, VA 22042, USA
* Corresponding author.
E-mail address: laurence.busse@inova.org

Crit Care Clin 30 (2014) 447–473
http://dx.doi.org/10.1016/j.ccc.2014.03.006
0749-0704/14/$ – see front matter © 2014 Elsevier Inc. All rights reserved.

conducted a multicenter, retrospective study of VTE incidence in patients in established intensive care units (ICUs) based on clinical diagnosis. The incidence of DVT was 1.0% and the incidence of PE was 0.5%, despite most patients having received pharmacologic prophylaxis. ICU admission is an independent risk factor for the presence of VTE.[12] The economic burden of VTE is considerable, contributing an average additional hospital cost of $8763 per patient (not accounting for severity of PE) and an attributable length of stay increase of 3 to 4 days.[13] PE is considered preventable and in 2008 the Centers for Medicare and Medicaid Services (CMS) stopped reimbursing hospitals for nosocomial VTE following certain orthopedic procedures. The Federal Agency for Healthcare Quality and Research adopted postoperative VTE as patient safety indicator, which requires mandatory reporting of all such events. Given such scrutiny and emphasis, much effort has been spent on identifying risk factors, educating patients and health care providers, and putting into place procedures and protocols designed to minimize the occurrence of VTE.

The presentation of PE is complex and variable, and can range from asymptomatic to fatal. Therefore, much research has gone into the development of clinical decision tools to aid in the diagnosis of PE. Given the heterogeneity of outcomes, similar attention has been given to the development of risk stratification tools and treatment algorithms that take into account the estimated morbidity and mortality.

DEFINITIONS

PE can be categorized into low-risk, submassive, and massive PE, which correlate well with increasing levels of mortality and are readily identified with available technology. Massive PE, which accounts for 5% of all PE-related admissions, is characterized by shock, typically defined as systolic blood pressure less than 90 mm Hg or a reduction of 40 mm Hg in systolic blood pressure from baseline for at least 15 minutes.[14] Patients manifest typical signs of organ hypoperfusion including encephalopathy, oliguria, cold and clammy extremities, or frank cardiac arrest.[15,16]

Submassive PE denotes the important subset of patients who seem hemodynamically stable, but have evidence of right ventricular strain or dysfunction. Right ventricular dysfunction results from right ventricular pressure overload, and findings include hypokinesis and dilatation of the right ventricle, flattening and paradoxical motion of the interventricular septum toward the left ventricle, tricuspid regurgitation, severe right ventricular free wall hypokinesis and apical sparing (McConnell sign), loss of respiratory variation in the diameter of the inferior vena cava, and pulmonary hypertension as identified by a peak tricuspid valve pressure gradient greater than 30 mm Hg or tricuspid regurgitant peak flow velocity greater than 2.5 m/s.[17-19] These findings are supported by varying levels of evidence, and no single finding can predict death. Hence, a combination of findings is routinely used to diagnose right ventricular dysfunction.[20,21] Transthoracic echocardiography has long been established as a valid tool in determining evidence of right ventricular dysfunction, as has computed tomography (CT) angiography (CTA).[19,22] Right ventricular strain is a function of increased wall tension, which results in myocardial cell damage and necrosis. Myocardial damage can be elucidated by several different criteria, with varying levels of supporting evidence. Electrocardiographic findings (including complete and incomplete right bundle branch block and $S_1Q_3T_3$ pattern) as well as several biomarkers (troponin, brain natriuretic peptide [BNP] and N-terminal proBNP [NT-proBNP], heart-type fatty acid binding protein [H-FABP]) have been studied. Although right ventricular dysfunction and strain can be identified easily with the aforementioned tests, there is no gold standard in the diagnosis of submassive PE, and the clinician is often left to decide which test or combination of tests is most meaningful. **Table 1** shows the various tests that can be used to identify the presence of right ventricular dysfunction or strain, and hence submassive PE. These data show that no single test clearly outperforms any other, which is why no dominant approach to diagnosis and risk stratification exists.

Patients with submassive PE have an in-hospital mortality of up to 30% compared with low-risk patients with PE who have an estimated in-hospital mortality of only

Table 1
Sensitivity, specificity, predictive values, and areas under the curve for the various risk stratification modalities

Modality	Outcomes	Sensitivity	Specificity	PPV	NPV	AUC
TTE	Mortality[75,76,79]	0.52–0.70	0.44–0.58	0.05–0.58	0.60–0.91	—
Troponin	Mortality, major complication, detection of RVD from PE[51,56,57,76,82,84,129]	0.22–0.81	0.11–0.90	0.12–0.75	0.65–1.0	0.58–0.94
BNP	Mortality, major complication, detection of RVD from PE[54,56,57,76,77,82,129]	0.75–0.93	0.25–0.70	0.23–0.67	0.76–1.0	0.67–0.81
H-FABP	Mortality, major complication[56,57]	0.89–1.0	0.82	0.28–0.41	0.99–1.0	0.89–0.99
CTA	Mortality, complicated course, severe PE requiring lysis or embolectomy, detection of RVD from PE[60–64,67,76,82–84]	0.38–0.92	0.30–0.98	0.10–0.90	0.58–0.1	0.51–0.87
ECG	Severe PH from PE, identification of massive PE by Miller index or PH, detection of RVD, pulmonary perfusion defect ≥50[42,45,68,72,73]	0.07–0.85	0.61–1.0	0.70–1.0	0.26–0.73	0.62
SS	Mortality dichotomized between low-risk and high-risk classes, pulmonary perfusion defect ≥50%[42–44]	0.33–0.96	0.44–0.55	0.11–0.14	0.98–0.99	0.42–0.87
BM + CTA	Mortality, complicated course, detection of RVD from PE[82–84]	0.47–0.94	0.74–0.95	0.64–0.90	0.72–0.97	0.64–0.96
ECG + SS	Pulmonary perfusion defect ≥50%[42]	0.41	0.73	—	—	0.582
TTE + BM	Mortality, major in-hospital complication[77,80]	0.61–0.61	0.75–0.80	0.37–0.38	0.86–0.91	—

Abbreviations: BM, biomarkers (troponin and/or BNP); BNP and its analogues; CTA, computed tomography angiography; ECG, electrocardiography; PH, pulmonary hypertension; RVD, right ventricular dysfunction; SS, scoring systems; TTE, transthoracic echocardiography.

0.4% to 0.9% (**Fig. 1**).[14,23,24] Submassive PE may require more aggressive forms of treatment, such as thrombolysis or catheter-directed therapy (CDT), so prompt recognition of the patients with submassive PE can facilitate appropriate treatment and transfer (ie, the ICU) for monitoring. Moreover, the intensivist may need to design and implement proper protocols for the timely and appropriate management of submassive PE, because the complex landscape can be difficult to navigate if a patient decompensates and is on the verge of cardiovascular collapse.

PATHOGENESIS AND PATHOPHYSIOLOGY

Most pulmonary emboli start out as lower extremity or pelvic DVTs.[25] In a large autopsy series of patients with known PE, 83% had clots in the lower extremity venous circulation, whether clinically suspected or not.[26] A combination of intrinsic and external factors contributes to the initiation and propagation of clot, which is highlighted by the classic Virchow triad of circulatory stasis, hypercoagulability, and endothelial injury. Not all DVTs embolize to the pulmonary circulation. Approximately 20% of calf DVTs migrate to the thighs, and only 50% of these embolize to the lungs.[27] Once in the lungs, the degree of clot burden and circulatory occlusion determines the physiologic consequences of a PE. Approximately 25% occlusion of the pulmonary vasculature is enough to cause an increase in pulmonary arterial pressure and a decrease in arterial oxygen tension, and a 35% to 40% occlusion is associated with increased right atrial pressure.[28]

PE initiates a cascade of increasing hypoxemia, pulmonary vasoconstriction, and obstruction, all of which increase pulmonary vascular resistance (PVR). The increase in PVR and ensuing increase in pulmonary artery pressures cause a decrease in right ventricular stroke volume, which is initially compensated by a catecholamine-induced tachycardia.[24] Continued increase of right ventricular afterload leads to increased wall stress and oxygen demand on the ventricular tissue and can ultimately lead to ischemia, infarction, and right ventricular dilatation. The circulatory failure seen in PE is mediated through a decrease in left ventricular preload, which is the direct result

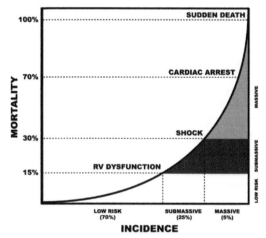

Fig. 1. Estimated mortality for PE, indexed by severity. The presence of shock indicates massive PE. A subgroup of patients with right ventricle (RV) dysfunction are deemed submassive, and can have mortality in excess of 30%. Thus, accurate and timely risk stratification and treatment are important.

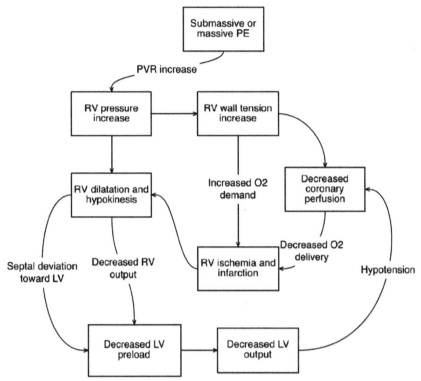

Fig. 2. The pathophysiology of massive and submassive PE. LV, left ventricle; PE, acute pulmonary embolism; PVR, pulmonary vascular resistance; RV, right ventricle.

of pulmonary outflow obstruction from clot burden and a reduced left ventricular compliance from shifting of the interventricular septum into the left ventricular cavity (**Fig. 2**).[29]

Concomitant systemic hypoxemia and hypocapnia exist as a result of the ventilation-perfusion mismatch, right-to-left shunt, reduced venous oxygen content, and increased physiologic dead space.[24] Most patients present with clinical evidence of alveolar hyperventilation manifested by tachypnea and a low arterial carbon dioxide tension. The presence of hypercapnia may signify a particularly large PE or limited ventilatory reserve, and is a poor prognostic sign.[20] In submassive PE, tachycardia may be the only sign of right ventricular strain.

RISK STRATIFICATION

The diagnosis of PE can be complex and challenging and the reader is referred to several excellent resources in the literature.[3,30–34] Once the diagnosis is made, efforts should be undertaken to risk stratify PE into low-risk, submassive, or massive categories. Signs and symptoms of PE, such as dyspnea, pleurisy, hypoxia, tachycardia, encephalopathy, and seizure, are nonspecific and of little assistance in risk stratification.[34,35] There are several tools available to assist in quantifying the amount of clot burden and corresponding risk of mortality and morbidity, including clinical decision tools, biomarkers, CTA, electrocardiography (ECG), echocardiography, and ventilation-perfusion scintigraphy, and these are discussed later.

CLINICAL DECISION TOOLS

The Geneva score, as originally described in 2001 and simplified in 2008, is used to calculate the probability of PE as low, intermediate, or high based on several risk factors combined with clinical signs and symptoms.[31,36,37] The Wells score likewise evaluates the presence of PE based on pretest probability and a combination of objective (physical examination) and subjective criteria.[38,39] These scoring systems have been evaluated against each other, other scoring systems, and clinical gestalt in several studies, and perform equally well.[40] However, these clinical decision rules were developed and validated in the assessment of the probability of PE, not the severity of PE. Nonetheless, some efforts have been made to evaluate these clinical decision rules in risk stratification of PE. Bova and colleagues[41] evaluated several prognostic markers in 201 normotensive patients with known PE, including echocardiography, biomarker analysis, blood gas, and the Geneva score. Hypoxemia, troponin, and the Geneva score predicted in-hospital mortality, and the Geneva score was an independent predictor of mortality in multivariate analysis. In contrast, the Wells score was evaluated in conjunction with ECG and was nonpredictive of anatomic severity of PE in a retrospective evaluation of patients.[42]

One objective index that may be used in risk stratification is the Pulmonary Embolism Severity Index (PESI). The PESI was derived via regression analysis of 11 known patient characteristics that were independently associated with adverse outcome or death. Patients are stratified into a risk category based on the PESI score, with mortality ranging from 0% to 1.6% in class I to between 10.0% and 24.5% in class V.[43] **Table 2** shows the originally derived independent risk factors for mortality in the PESI score. PESI has been evaluated in risk stratification.[44] Jimenez and colleagues[45] examined the PESI score along with troponin in 318 hemodynamically stable patients with PE, and the PESI score was associated with death. However, this analysis included both the submassive and low-risk group, and the study was not designed to test the PESI score a priori as an identifier of submassive PE. The PESI score was further examined in a series of 89 patients with nonmassive PE and it predicted mortality when patients were classified according to PESI classification. A higher PESI score correlated with the presence of right ventricular dysfunction. In fatal events, a higher PESI score correlated with the presence of increased troponin. These results suggest that the PESI score has value in identifying the submassive group.[46]

BIOMARKERS
Troponin

Troponin is a sensitive and specific marker for myocardial injury, and has been shown to be increased in patients with submassive or massive PE. Both troponin I and troponin T have been studied in this population and perform similarly. However, many other disease processes can present with increased troponins (such as myocardial infarction, myocarditis, sepsis, and brain injury), so increased troponin must be interpreted with caution. Several studies have found that, in patients with PE, both troponin I and troponin T levels correlate well with right ventricular overload and dilatation.[47–49] In addition, increased troponin in the setting of PE is associated with prolonged hypotension; cardiogenic shock; and the need for resuscitation, mechanical ventilation, and inotropic support.[50] Most importantly, troponin has been shown to be an independent predictor of mortality. The 2002 MAPPET 2 (Management Strategy and Prognosis of Pulmonary Embolism Trial) study showed that high troponin levels correlated with increased in-hospital mortality, PE-related complications, and the incidence of recurrence.[51] A more recent 2007 meta-analysis of 1985 patients from 20 studies concluded

Table 2
The PESI score, which stratifies patients into increasing levels of mortality. The PESI may aid the clinician in risk stratifying in submassive PE

Prognostic Variables	Points Assigned
Demographics	
Age (y)	Age
Male sex	+10
Comorbid Conditions	
Cancer	+30
Heart failure	+10
Chronic lung disease	+10
Critical Findings	
Pulse ≥110 beats per min	+20
Systolic blood pressure <100 mm Hg	+30
Respiratory rate ≥30 breaths per min	+20
Temperature <36°C	+20
Altered mental status[a]	+60
Arterial oxygen saturation <90%[b]	+20

Total point score obtained by summing the patient's age with the points given for each applicable prognostic variable.

Risk based on total point score and predicted mortality: class I (very low risk), fewer than 65 points, mortality 0% to 1.6%; class II (low risk), 66 to 85 points, mortality 1.7% to 3.5%; class III (intermediate risk), 86 to 105 points, mortality 3.2% to 7.1%; class IV (high risk), 106 to 125 points, mortality 4.0% to 11.4%; class V (very high risk), more than 125 points, mortality 10.0% to 24.5%.

[a] Disorientation, lethargy, stupor, or coma.

[b] With or without supplemental oxygen.

Adapted from Aujesky D, Obrosky DS, Stone RA, et al. Derivation and validation of a prognostic model for pulmonary embolism. Am J Respir Crit Care Med 2005;172(8):1041–6.

than increased troponin was associated with a higher risk of short-term mortality, with an odds ratio of 5.24.[52] Increased troponin was also able to identify normotensive patients with VTE who were at higher risk of dying, with an odds ratio for mortality of 5.90.[52] Troponin can be normal in patients with low-risk pulmonary emboli, and has been studied as a predictor of survival with a negative predictive value of 92%.[51]

BNP and NT-proBNP

BNP (and the analogue NT-proBNP, hereafter referred to as BNP) is a neuroprotein that is synthesized and secreted by the myocardium in response to ventricular strain. BNP acts to regulate blood pressure by manipulation of systemic vascular resistance, urine output, and blood plasma volume.[53] Like troponin, BNP is a nonspecific marker of cardiac injury and its specificity in the diagnosis of PE is limited. BNP has greater use in risk stratification in established PE. BNP is associated with a higher risk of all-cause mortality, death, or serious complication attributed to PE. In their comprehensive review, Coutance and colleagues[54] found that increased BNP was associated with a higher short-term risk of death (odds ratio, 6.57), with a sensitivity and specificity to predict death of 93% and 48%, respectively. Moreover, low BNP had a negative predictive value of 99% in excluding adverse outcome. A separate systematic review analyzed BNP in a subgroup of patients with acute submassive PE based on echocardiographic assessment and also found an increased odds ratio of 7.63 for in-hospital mortality.[55]

H-FABP

H-FABP is a novel biomarker that has recently been evaluated as an early prognosticator of poor outcomes in acute PE. It is a small cytoplasmic protein that is present in tissues with active fatty acid metabolism, such as myocardium, and is released into the circulation (within 90 minutes) during myocardial injury. Much like troponin and BNP, abnormal H-FABP has been associated with a complicated hospital course. H-FABP was able to outperform troponin and BNP in prognosticating outcome in acute PE.[56] In submassive PE, H-FABP also has been shown to be a valuable prognosticator of adverse outcome.[57] Despite these data, H-FABP is not routinely used in most institutions as a diagnostic tool or for risk stratification.

CTA

CTA has emerged in the last decade as the gold standard in the diagnosis of PE, essentially replacing pulmonary angiography. Its low cost and 24-hour availability make it an ideal screening and diagnostic test. Increasing sensitivity, specificity, and prognostic value have paralleled technological advances in radiographic methods. In a 2005 systematic review of 15 studies, a negative CTA was able to predict the absence of acute PE, with a negative predictive value of 99.1%.[58] In the more recent PIOPED II (Prospective Investigation of Pulmonary Embolism Diagnosis II) study, CTA showed a sensitivity and specificity of 83% and 96%, respectively, with a positive predictive value of 92% to 96%, depending on pretest probability.[59] CTA may also elucidate alternative diagnoses. With regard to risk stratification, CTA can show right ventricular overload in submassive and massive PE via the measurement of the size of the right ventricle in a cross-sectional picture. CTA has been found to have a sensitivity, specificity, negative predictive value, and positive predictive value for diagnosing right ventricular overload of 92%, 44%, 80%, and 67%, respectively.[4] A ratio of right ventricle/left ventricle (RV/LV) size ratio of more than 1.0 was representative of right ventricular dilatation, but there is no standardized value, and ratios of 0.9 to as high as 1.6 have also been proposed (**Fig. 3**).[60–63]

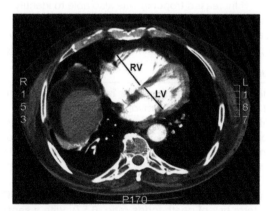

Fig. 3. Measurement of right ventricular dilatation via CTA. Ventricular diameters are measured as the maximal distance between the ventricular endocardium and the intraventricular septum, perpendicular to the long axis of the heart. (*From* Becattini C, Agnelli G, Vedovati MC, et al. Multidetector computed tomography for acute pulmonary embolism: diagnosis and risk stratification in a single test. Eur Heart J 2011;32(13):1658; with permission.)

CTA in risk stratification has been validated in several studies, and right ventricular enlargement and increased RV/LV ratio on CTA correlate with increased mortality and clinical deterioration.[61,64] In a recent analysis of 457 patients with acute PE, the absence of right ventricular dysfunction on CTA had a negative predictive value for death of 100%.[64] CTA-elucidated clot burden was also studied in 516 patients with submassive PE. Central (as opposed to lobar or distal) embolization was associated with death or clinical deterioration (hazard ratio, 8.3), whereas distal embolization was associated with benign outcome (hazard ratio, 0.12).[65] Okada and colleagues[66] used three-dimensionally reconstructed images of 64-section dual-energy CT to compare volumetric assessment of clot burden with pulmonary artery pressure, pulmonary artery diameter, and D-dimer and found them to be highly correlated. The prognostic value of CTA-calculated volumetric assessment of clot burden was examined by Apfaltrer and colleagues,[67] who compared perfusion defect volume (PDvol) with CTA-obstruction scores, CTA-elucidated right ventricular dilatation, and adverse events (ICU admission or death). Patients with adverse events were more likely to have higher PDvol, evidence of right ventricular dilatation, and higher CTA-obstruction scores.

ECG

Electrocardiographic abnormalities during PE arise from changes in the impedance of the myocardium and vector of electrical currents through the heart caused by anatomic and functional changes. The most common ECG pattern in PE is sinus tachycardia, which is neither sensitive nor specific. Other findings on ECG, such as an S1Q3T3 pattern (an S wave in lead I, a Q wave in lead III, and an inverted T wave in lead III), right precordial T-wave inversions, and right bundle branch block are less common, but equally insensitive and nonspecific.[68] ECG has been extensively analyzed in risk stratification of PE, with variable results. Some analyses of ECG tracings in cases of non–risk-stratified pulmonary emboli showed virtually no correlation with hemodynamic compromise.[69,70] However, in patients with known massive PE, T-wave inversions in the precordial leads have been shown to be predictive of the severity of PE.[68] In a review of 90 patients with submassive or massive PE, ECG patterns were abnormal in 78% and 94% respectively and neither atrial flutter nor fibrillation was detected in any patient.[71] More recently, ECG was compared with biomarkers in the detection of right ventricular dysfunction in a retrospective study of 48 patients with acute PE, and was highly sensitive and specific (75% and 95%). ECG also outperformed the biomarkers in diagnostic accuracy.[72] ECG scoring systems have been shown to be predictors of right ventricular overload or death.[73,74] However, these scoring systems are usually complicated and difficult to recall, limiting their use. At present, ECG is used adjunctively in risk stratification as supporting evidence of right ventricular dysfunction in submassive PE and to evaluate for alternative diagnoses.

ECHOCARDIOGRAPHY

Transthoracic echocardiography (TTE) has a dual role in PE both as a diagnostic study and as a risk stratification tool. TTE is primarily used in the evaluation of right and left ventricular function, valvular disease, possible right-to-left shunt via patent foramen ovale, and measurement of pulmonary artery systolic pressure via regurgitant flow across the tricuspid valve. In PE, direct visualization of clot is rare and is only seen with very large main pulmonary arteries or intracardiac thrombus.[20] Most evidence for diagnosis is indirect (right ventricular dilatation or hypokinesis, tricuspid regurgitation, or paradoxic septal movement) and is largely caused by the presence of right ventricular strain seen in submassive or massive PE. Hence TTE is most valuable as a tool for risk stratification, and can be performed either by a trained echocardiographer or the clinician (using a point-of-care ultrasound device). The role of TTE in risk stratification has been extensively studied in the subset of patients in whom submassive PE is suspected. An analysis of more than 1000 normotensive patients from the International Cooperative Pulmonary Embolism Registry (ICOPER) registry with TTE found that right ventricular hypokinesis was an independent predictor of 30-day mortality.[75] A 2008 meta-analysis of hemodynamically stable patients examined the prognostic value of TTE-identified right ventricular dysfunction in predicting death, compared with CTA-identified right ventricular dysfunction or biomarker-identified right ventricular strain. In the 5 studies evaluating TTE, the unadjusted mortality risk ratio of right ventricular dysfunction was 2.5. TTE was moderately accurate in predicting mortality in the setting of right ventricular dysfunction, with a sensitivity and specificity of 70% and 57%, respectively. The prognostic value of TTE exceeded that of CTA (with sensitivity and specificity of 65% and 56%, respectively), but was inferior to the biomarkers BNP, NT-proBNP, and troponin (with sensitivity and specificity of 81%–93% and 58%–84%, respectively).[76] In contrast, Binder and colleagues[77] compared TTE with cardiac biomarkers as a means for predicting death from PE, and right ventricular dysfunction on echocardiogram was associated with a 12-fold increased risk of adverse outcome from PE compared with increased BNP, which did not predict adverse outcome. Furthermore, no appreciable benefit was gained when TTE and biomarkers were combined. Other studies have evaluated TTE as a predictor of death from PE with similarly equivocal results.[78–80]

RISK STRATIFICATION STRATEGIES AND GUIDELINES

Because of the mortality implications associated with submassive PE, risk stratification (ie, identifying and differentiating the hemodynamically stable patient with subclinical evidence of right ventricular overload from the hemodynamically stable patient without right ventricular overload) remains an important aspect of management. Numerous efforts have been undertaken to improve the yield on risk stratification by combining biomarkers and radiology. Tulevski and colleagues[81] were able to show that the combination of increased troponin and BNP in normotensive patients predicted death, and that discordant biomarkers (increased BNP and normal troponin) correlated poorly with mortality. In a population of non–risk-stratified patients with PE, an algorithm combining the presence of increased troponin ($\geq$0.04 ng/mL) or BNP ($\geq$1000 pg/mL) with TTE evidence of right ventricular dysfunction was able to identify those with a higher risk of death or major adverse event.[77] CTA in combination with either increased troponin or BNP has been shown to predict right ventricular dilatation better than either CTA or biomarker tests alone and, more importantly, can predict death and adverse outcome.[82–84]

Current guidelines recommend that efforts be made to identify patients with submassive PE, in whom more aggressive treatment (ie, thrombolysis) may be beneficial. However, there is no single recommended strategy for this, and clinicians are left to decide which test or combination of tests is best.[85,86] According to current American College of Chest Physicians (ACCP) guidelines, in the presence of clinical evidence of instability and failure to improve on anticoagulant therapy, right ventricular dysfunction as seen on biomarker, ECG, echocardiography, or CT should inform the overall clinical assessment, but the decision of thrombolytic therapy should not be made on this determination alone. The ACCP recommends that tests of right ventricular overload not be routinely measured.[85] The American College of Emergency Physicians (ACEP) endorses the use of the PESI as a way to risk stratify patients in the submassive group, but stops short of committing to treatment decisions based on this analysis.[40] According to American Heart Association (AHA) guidelines, clinical scores, echocardiography, CTA, ECG, biomarkers, and hybrid studies (combined tools) may all be used in identifying right ventricular dysfunction, but clinical judgment is required to determine which method is appropriate for the individual patient.[87] The European Society of Cardiology (ESC) recommends risk stratification of non–high-risk (submassive or low-risk) patents via the use of clinical decision rules, ECG, imaging, or biochemical markers, but stops short of endorsing one method rather than another (class IIa, level B).[86] Some risk stratification algorithms that have been proposed and can be found in the literature.[15,20,88]

The evidence and guidelines show that no gold standard has emerged for risk stratification in PE. Although right ventricular dysfunction can easily be identified using TTE, CTA, or ECG, this finding does not always correlate with outcome (see **Table 1**). The same argument can be made for biomarkers and right ventricular strain. However, the authors propose an algorithm for risk stratification in **Fig. 4**. When PE is diagnosed and shock is absent (indicating low-risk or submassive PE), the clinician should seek to identify high-risk features, including right ventricular enlargement on CTA, increased biomarkers, or an increased PESI score. Because CTA is typically completed as part of the initial diagnostic work-up, this study is usually readily available. Moreover, troponin, BNP, and ECG are also usually part of the initial diagnostic evaluation of PE, which typically presents with chest pain and shortness of breath. In the authors' opinion, PESI calculation is an easy noninvasive test and should be completed for all confirmed cases of PE. If any of the aforementioned tests indicate right ventricular dysfunction or strain, the authors recommend TTE as a confirmatory test. Confirmation of right ventricular dysfunction on TTE indicates submassive PE and the corresponding treatment algorithm (**Fig. 5**).

TREATMENT

Treatment of PE focuses on 3 major efforts: supportive care, prevention of subsequent clot formation, and the reversal of obstructive shock. Treatment pathways of low-risk PE and massive PE are well defined, and are discussed elsewhere. However, treatment of submassive PE is not as clear-cut, and is discussed later.

Anticoagulation

The mainstay of treatment of PE is anticoagulation. In the acute setting, this is typically accomplished with intravenous heparin administered continuously, low-molecular-weight heparin (LMWH), or fondaparinux. Initiation with an oral anticoagulant, such as warfarin or rivaroxaban, is begun soon thereafter. The duration of therapy depends on clinical factors, such as underlying comorbidities and propensity of recurrence. Only 1 randomized trial comparing unfractionated heparin with placebo was performed in 1960, and was stopped early when a dramatic reduction in adverse outcome was seen in the heparin group.[89] LMWH is an alternative to heparin and has the added benefit of being dosed by weight once or twice per day, with no required coagulation profile monitoring. LMWH has been compared with unfractionated heparin in 2 studies of more than 1600 patients with VTE as well as a meta-analysis and it showed no differences in major thromboembolic events or major bleeding.[90–92] Fondaparinux, a newer parenteral synthetic antithrombotic agent with specific anti–factor Xa activity, performed similarly to unfractionated heparin with respect to mortality, recurrent

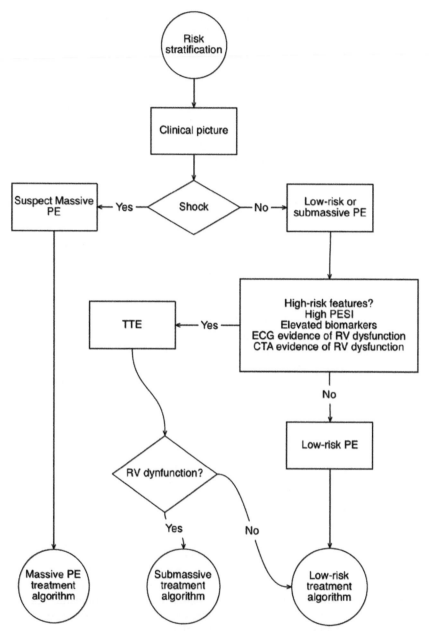

Fig. 4. Proposed algorithm for risk stratification of PE. PE, acute pulmonary embolism; PESI, pulmonary embolism severity index; TTE, transthoracic echocardiography.

thrombotic events, and bleeding complications in a large, open-label randomized trial of hemodynamically stable patients.[93] The newer oral anticoagulants (dabigatran, rivaroxaban, and apixaban) are appealing compared with unfractionated heparin and LMWH in their route of administration and lack of monitoring. Dabigatran, which recently received a US Food and Drug Administration (FDA) indication for DVT and PE,

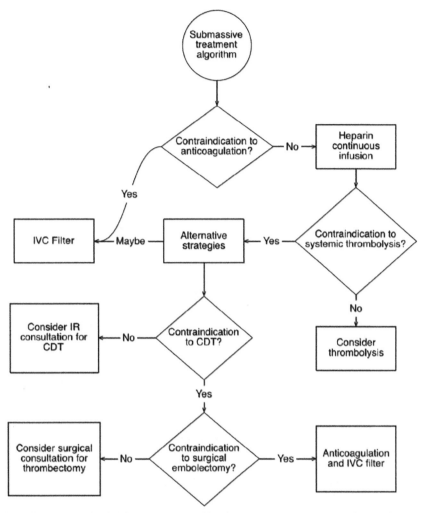

Fig. 5. Proposed algorithm for treatment of submassive PE. CDT, catheter-directed therapy; IR, interventional radiology; IVC, inferior vena cava.

has been compared with warfarin in a noninferiority trial of more than 2500 patients with acute PE, and it was equally effective in preventing recurrence with a similar bleeding risk.[94] Rivaroxaban versus enoxaparin and warfarin was studied in a noninferiority trial of more than 4800 patients and was as efficacious as the standard therapy in preventing symptomatic recurrence with a similar bleeding risk.[95] In the recently published AMPLIFY (Apixaban for the Initial Management of Pulmonary Embolism and Deep-Vein Thrombosis as First-Line Therapy) study, apixaban, which is also under review by the FDA for a venous thromboembolism indication, was noninferior to the conventional therapy (LMWH and warfarin) for recurrence of thromboembolic disease or death and was superior in bleeding risk.[96] The use of LMWH and fondaparinux and the novel oral anticoagulant rivaroxaban in submassive PE is controversial.[87] To date, no studies have compared the various anticoagulants specifically in the setting of submassive PE, and most clinicians agree that, if there is a possibility of thrombolysis, it may be prudent to use short-acting unfractionated heparin. Unfractionated heparin is the only anticoagulant that has been studied in conjunction with thrombolytic therapy.[85] The AHA recommends the use of heparin for submassive PE.[87] The British Thoracic Society (BTS) and the ACCP both recommend that unfractionated heparin be used preferentially rather than LMWH when rapid reversal of effect may be needed (grade C and not rated, respectively).[97,98] The ESC recommends unfractionated heparin for patients with massive PE in whom thrombolysis may be used (class I, level A), but takes no stance on this in patients with submassive PE, because it does not recommend thrombolysis in this group.[86]

Thrombolysis

Thrombolysis of PE is accomplished via intravenous administration of the thrombolytic agent alteplase (recombinant tissue plasminogen activator [tPA]). Alternatives to tPA include streptokinase, urokinase, reteplase, and tenecteplase, and the choice of thrombolytic agent is usually institution specific and beyond the scope of this article. In the United States, only alteplase has an FDA indication for use in submassive and massive PE. Thrombolytics activate plasminogen to plasmin, resulting in the accelerated lysis of thrombi. They have been shown in several trials to reduce clot burden and improve hemodynamics.[99–101] However, after 1 week the reduction in vascular obstruction and ventricular dilatation achieved with tPA is no different from that achieved with heparin alone.[99,102] Clinical outcomes after thrombolysis have also been extensively studied in numerous randomized trials. A 2004 meta-analysis compared mortality and bleeding in 748 non–risk-stratified patients with PE who received thrombolysis versus anticoagulation. In this study, patients with massive PE experienced a dramatic reduction in recurrent PE and mortality (9.4% vs 19%) but also a 2-fold greater risk of major bleeding (odds ratio, 1.98). However, when all patients (massive and nonmassive) were included, mortality and major bleeding differences were eliminated, but there was a significant increase in nonmajor bleeding.[103] Given the high morbidity and mortality of hemodynamically unstable patients with PE, most authorities recommend the use of thrombolytics.[40,85–87,97]

Subclinical right ventricular dysfunction in a normotensive patient (submassive PE) is associated with higher mortality, which may be mitigated with a more aggressive treatment approach, such as thrombolysis. Because of the risk of major adverse events, use of thrombolysis in submassive PE is controversial. Early studies showed increased mortality in a group of patients with submassive PE treated with thrombolytics.[104] In contrast, Konstantinides and colleagues[105] randomized patients with submassive PE to either heparin alone or alteplase plus heparin, and the combined end point of death or clinical deterioration was significantly higher in the heparin alone group, and no fatal or cerebral bleeding occurred in the thrombolytic group. Becattini and colleagues[106] randomized 58 hemodynamically stable patients with PE and right ventricular dysfunction to single-dose bolus tenecteplase versus placebo and noted a higher rate of resolution of right ventricular dilatation in the thrombolytic group (30% vs 10%). Another study randomized 72 hemodynamically stable patients with PE with TTE-proven right ventricular dysfunction to tenecteplase plus heparin versus heparin alone, and found significantly improved right ventricular size and function, as well as reduced clinical end points at a 6-month interval.[107] Based on these and prior results, current ACCP, AHA, and ESC guidelines indicate that thrombolysis may be used in hemodynamically stable patients in certain situations when the risk of bleeding is low and the potential for decompensation is high (ACCP grade 2C, AHA class IIb level C, ESC class IIb level B).[85–87] The BTS and ACEP recommend against thrombolysis in nonmassive PE situations (grade B and level B, respectively).[40,97]

The large prospective, multicenter, randomized, placebo-controlled Pulmonary Embolism Thrombolysis (PEITHO) trial evaluating the use of thrombolytics in submassive PE was recently published. One thousand and five normotensive patients with intermediate-risk PE (characterized by the presence of right ventricular dysfunction and myocardial injury) were randomized to thrombolysis or placebo with end points of death, hemodynamic decompensation (or collapse), bleeding, stroke, recurrent pulmonary embolism, and serious adverse events, with the primary endpoint being a composite of death from any cause or hemodynamic decompensation within 7 days of randomization.[108] The primary endpoint occurred in 13 patients (2.6%) in the thrombolytic arm compared with 28 patients (5.6%) in the placebo arm ($P = .02$). There was no difference in all-cause mortality at 7 days ($P = .42$ or at 30 days ($P = .42$). However, patients in the thrombolysis arm experienced less hypotension and need for catecholamine vasopressors ($P = .002$). Nonintracranial major bleeding ($P < .001$) and hemorrhagic strokes ($P = .003$) were more common in the thrombolysis arm. In addition, when stratified by age older than 75 years versus 75 years or younger, mortality and morbidity benefits were only seen in the younger group.

Other trials of thrombolysis have reported intracranial hemorrhage in up to 3% of patients and major bleeding in up to 20%.[88] ICU monitoring is important and clinicians must be vigilant in surveying for complications that warrant prompt reversal of coagulopathy or emergent consultation (eg, neurosurgery). Thrombolysis must be given with caution, and informed consent is required in many settings. Absolute and relative contraindications are mainly related to bleeding risk, and are listed in **Table 3**. Because of the high risks associated with thrombolysis, alternatives to this therapy exist, and are discussed later.

Surgical Embolectomy

Surgical embolectomy is usually reserved for patients with massive PE who have contraindications to thrombolytics, failed thrombolytic therapy, paradoxic embolism, right heart thrombus, or a clot in transit. Patients are placed on cardiopulmonary bypass and a median sternotomy is required for access to the heart and central vessels, with clot removed mechanically under direct visualization. Embolectomy has never

Table 3	
Absolute and relative contraindications to thrombolytic therapy	
Absolute Contraindications	**Relative Contraindications**
Major trauma within 3 wk	Cancer at more than the age of 75 y
Major surgery within 3 wk	TIA within 6 mo
Major head trauma within 3 wk	Oral anticoagulation therapy
Prior hemorrhagic CVA	Noncompressible punctures
Ischemic CVA within 6 mo	Traumatic resuscitation
CNS neoplasm	Refractory hypertension
GI bleeding within 1 mo	Advanced liver disease
Active bleeding	Infective endocarditis
	Active peptic ulcer
	Pregnancy
	Postpartum state within 1 wk

Abbreviations: CNS, central nervous system; CVA, cardiovascular accident; GI, gastrointestinal; TIA, transient ischemic attack.

been compared with medical management in a randomized, controlled trial, but was evaluated in a series of patients with massive PE assigned to medical or surgical management. There were significant differences among the groups, but 77% (10 of 13) survived embolectomy, and 67% (16 of 24) survived thrombolysis. Hemorrhage was higher in the medical therapy group and sepsis was higher in the surgical therapy group.[109] Embolectomy compared favorably with repeated thrombolysis with regard to hospital course in a series of 488 patients who failed original thrombolysis (with no statistically significant difference in mortality).[110] In a case series of patients with PE at a single center, Sukhija and colleagues[111] reported a lower mortality in 18 unstable patients (massive PE) who underwent embolectomy (2 of 18, or 11%) compared with 6 hemodynamically stable patients (submassive PE) who underwent thrombolysis (2 of 6, or 33%).

Mortality in pulmonary embolectomy has traditionally been high, but has decreased over the past 5 decades, from more than 50% in the 1960s to 26% in the 1990s to between 10% and 20% currently, primarily as a result of improved surgical technique and a shift toward a healthier patient population.[112] Pulmonary embolectomy is indicated in select patients with massive PE and cardiovascular collapse, but this practice is changing as clinicians gain a better understanding of the mortality implications of subclinical right ventricular failure. A 2005 series of patients with combined massive (N = 28) and submassive (N = 15) PE cited a postprocedure 1-year survival of 86%.[112] Another series of 29 patients with submassive PE calculated an 89% survival rate after pulmonary embolectomy.[113] Based on similar results, Sareyyupoglu and colleagues[114] concluded that embolectomy should be considered earlier in the course of the disease, including during submassive PE.

Current guidelines regarding embolectomy are discordant, but the procedure may regain some of its favor as mortality decreases and patient selection continues to improve. The AHA recommends that surgical embolectomy only be considered in submassive PE if the patient is deemed to have clinical evidence of adverse prognosis (class IIb level C), whereas the ACCP and ESC recommend pulmonary embolectomy only for patients with massive PE who have contraindications to, or have failed, thrombolysis or CDTs (grade 2C and class I level C, respectively).[85–87]

Inferior Vena Cava Filter

Inferior vena cava (IVC) filters disrupt the embolization to the lungs of thrombus originating in the deep veins of the lower extremities and pelvis. The 2 major indications for IVC filter placement are contraindication to anticoagulation and recurrent DVT formation despite anticoagulation.[115] IVC filters also play an important adjunctive role in surgical embolectomy, in which a 5% recurrence rate may be expected.[20] There are currently no data on the role of IVC filters in submassive PE, and placement should be considered on a case-by-case basis, on weighing the associated prothrombotic effects against the possibility of recurrent or fatal PE. Current guidelines call for routine IVC filter use when readily available (BTS grade C), only if there is recurrent PE (AHA class I level C, ESC class IIb level B) or if there is a contraindication to anticoagulation (ACCP grade 1B, AHA class I level B, ESC class IIb level B). In addition, IVC filter may be considered for patients with acute PE and very poor cardiopulmonary reserve (AHA class IIb level C), and should not be used routinely as an adjunct to anticoagulation or fibrinolysis (AHA class III level C).[85–87,97]

Outcomes with IVC filters are equivocal. In conjunction with thrombolysis, IVC filter placement may be associated with a reduction in early PE and death, although this finding was associated with a small (N = 10) subset of patients of the ICOPER trial and may have been confounded by selection bias.[98,116] There was no observed difference in mortality between permanent IVC filters and no filters in an early study by Decousus and colleagues,[117] with the lower incidence of early PE in the IVC filter group contrasted by an increase in late incidence. Retrievable filters, designed to mitigate the prothrombotic characteristics of permanent filters, have been examined in a multitude of case series, registries, and cohort studies, but have never been compared with permanent filters or no filters in a randomized manner. Retrievable filters have been associated with similar complication rates and outcomes as permanent filters.[118,119]

Catheter-Directed Therapy

Catheter-directed therapy (CDT) includes an array of therapies including pharmacologic thrombolysis, clot fragmentation, embolectomy, balloon angioplasty, and percutaneous thrombectomy. CDT typically is performed by specialists in either interventional radiology or cardiology. CDT is thought to mitigate risks associated with systemic thrombolysis or surgical embolectomy. The use of CDT to perform combination procedures (eg, embolectomy and pharmacologic thrombolysis) may potentiate the effectiveness of the thrombolytics alone, because smaller doses of pharmacologic thrombolytics may be exposed to a larger surface area of clot.[120] Moreover, CDT serves as both a diagnostic and therapeutic procedure, and resolution of hemodynamic compromise can often be observed in real time. Historical mortality for CDT ranges from 0% to 25%, and incidence of bleeding ranges from 0% to 17%.[121] However, old techniques (such as the 12-French Greenfield suction catheter embolectomy) have largely been replaced by newer techniques that take advantage of smaller devices and improvements in design, and mortality and the number of complications have improved. At present, the only product indicated for use in PE is the Greenfield system, and the FDA has issued a black-box warning for the new AngioJet device, citing several procedure-related complications or deaths, most commonly hemoptysis.[122] The type of procedure available to a patient is usually institution specific, and can include any or all of the options discussed earlier, alone or in combination (ie, local thrombolysis and thrombectomy in 1 procedure). To date, data on these techniques are sparse, and mainly consist of case series. No controlled trials have ever compared surgical embolectomy with CDT, for example.[121] Systemic thrombolysis was compared with intrapulmonary thrombolysis during pulmonary angiography in an old study (before widespread adoption of CTA for diagnosis), and outcomes were equivocal.[123] A 2009 meta-analysis comparing modern CDT (<10-French catheter size) with systemic thrombolysis in 594 patients with massive PE (retrospectively, and all uncontrolled) found an 86.5% success rate (hemodynamic stabilization, improvement of hypoxia, or survival from PE) and 7.9% complication rate with CDT.[120]

Most data on CDT are in the massive PE population, but there are some studies of the submassive population. The Greenfield system was evaluated in a case series of 46 patients, 4 of whom had submassive PE. All 4 patients were weaned from ventilatory assistance within 6 to 8 hours after the procedure.[124] A 2007 case series evaluated rheolytic thrombectomy (clot dissolution via a high-pressure stream of fluid) with the AngioJet system in addition to local thrombolysis (N = 1) and IVC filter placement (N = 4) in 4 patients with submassive PE. Improved flow, symptoms, hemodynamics, and survival were noted in all 4 patients.[125] Ferrigno and colleagues[126] evaluated AngioJet (plus local thrombolytics and IVC filter placement) in 11 patients with submassive PE, and noted improved hemodynamics (N = 11) but transient hemoptysis (N = 3). Other individual cases and series have been reported with similar findings.[127,128] However, to date, no randomized, controlled trials have evaluated CDT against other therapies in reducing clot burden or improving clinical outcome in submassive PE. As such, guidelines are vague and noncommittal. For massive PE, the ACCP recommends the use of CDT over no such treatment in patients who have contraindications to, or have failed, systemic thrombolysis, provided that expertise and resources are available (grade 2C). There is no mention of this therapy for submassive PE, however.[85] The AHA recommends that catheter embolectomy may be considered for patients with submassive PE who are judged to have clinical evidence of poor prognosis (new hemodynamic instability, worsening respiratory failure, severe right ventricular dysfunction, or major myocardial necrosis) (class IIb level C).[87] The BTS recommends the consideration of invasive approaches (thrombus fragmentation and IVC filter insertion) when facilities and expertise are readily available, but does not clarify a patient population (grade C).[97] In addition, the ESC recommends that CDT may be considered as an alternative to surgical treatment in patients with high-risk (massive) PE when thrombolysis is absolutely contraindicated or has failed, but does not mention the submassive population (class IIb level C).[86]

TREATMENT ALGORITHMS

Algorithm-based management strategies can assist the clinician in navigating the complexity and variability of presentation of PE and the multitude of treatment options available. These algorithms should include a multidisciplinary team approach (including radiology, interventional radiology, cardiothoracic surgery, pulmonary and internal medicine, emergency medicine, nursing, and ancillary services), around-the-clock availability of resources, and referral and transfer contingency plans to appropriate PE centers.[115] Submassive PE in particular has been shown to be associated with increased morbidity and mortality, and thus early and accurate risk stratification must be made based on some or all of the aforementioned tools. Initial diagnostic results can often assist in risk stratification (CTA for initial diagnosis and evaluation of right ventricular dilatation, cardiac enzymes and BNP for initial diagnosis of dyspnea or chest pain and as a marker of myocardial damage), but are not universally obtained. Once diagnosis is made, appropriate additional risk stratification tools, such as echocardiography, should be used. In addition, specific treatment strategies must be implemented based on the diagnosis and risk stratification (ie, systemic thrombolysis for submassive PE with features of decompensation or CDT when systemic thrombolysis is contraindicated). The authors propose the management algorithm presented later (see **Fig. 5**).

The optimal treatment of submassive PE relies on appropriate clinical assessment of risk versus benefit of thrombolytics, including obtaining evidence of (1) pending respiratory or circulatory collapse and (2) right ventricular failure.[87] Clinical evidence of cardiopulmonary collapse may include hypotension, a shock index (heart rate in beats per minute divided by systolic blood pressure in millimeters of mercury) of more than 1, hypoxemia, an increased Borg score, right ventricular hypokinesis or McConnell sign, septal dysfunction, increased right ventricular systolic pressure, or increased biomarkers.[87] If, in the clinician's judgment, the benefits of thrombolysis outweigh the risks, systemic thrombolytics should be administered. CDT or pulmonary embolectomy should be considered if there is a contraindication to systemic thrombolysis or when systemic thrombolysis has failed. Hybrid CDT therapies (thrombectomy or fragmentation with thrombolysis) are the subject of an emerging field of research.

SUMMARY

PE is common and is associated with a high degree of morbidity and mortality. It can present silently or with hemodynamic collapse and cardiac arrest, is difficult to diagnose, and treatment options depend on accurate and timely risk stratification. Diagnosis begins with a high index of suspicion and a physical examination, followed by the possible application of one of many validated clinical decision rules. Ancillary tests, including CTA, laboratory markers, V/Q scan, and lower extremity ultrasonography, can assist in excluding or confirming the diagnosis, as well as playing a role in risk stratification. Severity in PE depends on the amount of clot burden as well as physiologic response to the clot, and is stratified into low risk, submassive, and massive, with increasing levels of mortality. Submassive PE is a diagnostic and management challenge and requires evaluation of subclinical hemodynamic parameters to identify right ventricular strain or impending cardiopulmonary failure. Patients are normotensive, but have radiographic, ECG, or biomarker evidence of ventricular failure. Clinicians are obligated to implement a more aggressive treatment plan, including consideration of thrombolysis or CDT. Guideline recommendations from 4 major subspecialties in Europe and the United States are presented herein and include the current opinions on diagnosis, risk stratification, and management. Algorithmic protocols for the management of PE can assist in complex medical decisions, and should highlight specific institutional capabilities. Forthcoming and future research should be designed to answer the many controversial management questions about submassive PE, including the role of thrombolytics, CDT, and hybrid therapies.

REFERENCES

1. Dalen JE, Alpert JS. Natural history of pulmonary embolism. Prog Cardiovasc Dis 1975;17(4):259–70.
2. Office of the Surgeon General (US). National Heart, Lung, and Blood Institute (US). The Surgeon General's Call to Action to Prevent Deep Vein Thrombosis and Pulmonary Embolism. Rockville (MD): Office of the Surgeon General (US) 2008. Available at: http://www.ncbi.nlm.nih.gov/books/NBK44178/.
3. Konstantinides S. Clinical practice. Acute pulmonary embolism. N Engl J Med 2008;359(26):2804–13. http://dx.doi.org/10.1056/NEJMcp0804570.
4. Shujaat A, Shapiro JM, Eden E. Utilization of CT pulmonary angiography in suspected pulmonary embolism in a major urban emergency department. Pulm Med 2013;2013:915213. http://dx.doi.org/10.1155/2013/915213.
5. Haythe J. Chronic thromboembolic pulmonary hypertension: a review of current practice. Prog Cardiovasc Dis 2012;55(2):134–43. http://dx.doi.org/10.1016/j.pcad.2012.07.005.
6. Heit JA, Mohr DN, Silverstein MD, et al. Predictors of recurrence after deep vein thrombosis and pulmonary embolism: a population-based cohort study. Arch Intern Med 2000;160(6):761–8.
7. Mohr DN, Silverstein MD, Heit JA, et al. The venous stasis syndrome after deep venous thrombosis or pulmonary embolism: a population-based study. Mayo Clin Proc 2000;75(12):1249–56.
8. Hirsch DR, Ingenito EP, Goldhaber SZ. Prevalence of deep venous thrombosis among patients in medical intensive care. JAMA 1995;274(4):335–7.
9. Ibrahim EH, Iregui M, Prentice D, et al. Deep vein thrombosis during prolonged mechanical ventilation despite prophylaxis. Crit Care Med 2002;30(4):771–4.
10. Marik PE, Andrews L, Maini B. The incidence of deep venous thrombosis in ICU patients. Chest 1997;111(3):661–4.
11. Patel R, Cook DJ, Meade MO, et al. Burden of illness in venous thromboembolism in critical care: a multicenter observational study. J Crit Care 2005;20(4):341–7. http://dx.doi.org/10.1016/j.jcrc.2005.09.014.

12. Edelsberg J, Hagiwara M, Taneja C, et al. Risk of venous thromboembolism among hospitalized medically ill patients. Am J Health Syst Pharm 2006;63(20 Suppl 6):S16–22. http://dx.doi.org/10.2146/ajhp060389.
13. Fanikos J, Rao A, Seger AC, et al. Hospital costs of acute pulmonary embolism. Am J Med 2013;126(2):127–32. http://dx.doi.org/10.1016/j.amjmed.2012.07.025.
14. Kucher N, Goldhaber SZ. Management of massive pulmonary embolism. Circulation 2005;112(2):e28–32. http://dx.doi.org/10.1161/CIRCULATIONAHA.105.551374.
15. Lankeit M, Konstantinides S. Thrombolytic therapy for submassive pulmonary embolism. Best Pract Res Clin Haematol 2012;25(3):379–89. http://dx.doi.org/10.1016/j.beha.2012.06.005.
16. Kasper W, Konstantinides S, Geibel A, et al. Management strategies and determinants of outcome in acute major pulmonary embolism: results of a multicenter registry. J Am Coll Cardiol 1997;30(5):1165–71.
17. Goldhaber SZ. Echocardiography in the management of pulmonary embolism. Ann Intern Med 2002;136(9):691–700.
18. Piazza G. Submassive pulmonary embolism. JAMA 2013;309(2):171–80. http://dx.doi.org/10.1001/jama.2012.164493.
19. Nazeyrollas P, Metz D, Jolly D, et al. Use of transthoracic Doppler echocardiography combined with clinical and electrocardiographic data to predict acute pulmonary embolism. Eur Heart J 1996;17(5):779–86.
20. Marshall PS, Matthews KS, Siegel MD. Diagnosis and management of life-threatening pulmonary embolism. J Intensive Care Med 2011. http://dx.doi.org/10.1177/0885066610392658.
21. Vieillard-Baron A, Page B, Augarde R, et al. Acute cor pulmonale in massive pulmonary embolism: incidence, echocardiographic pattern, clinical implications and recovery rate. Intensive Care Med 2001;27(9):1481–6. http://dx.doi.org/10.1007/s001340101032.
22. Kasper W, Meinertz T, Kersting F, et al. Echocardiography in assessing acute pulmonary hypertension due to pulmonary embolism. Am J Cardiol 1980;45(3):567–72.
23. Kreit JW. The impact of right ventricular dysfunction on the prognosis and therapy of normotensive patients with pulmonary embolism. Chest 2004;125(4):1539–45.
24. Wood KE. Major pulmonary embolism: review of a pathophysiologic approach to the golden hour of hemodynamically significant pulmonary embolism. Chest 2002;121(3):877–905.
25. Bell WR, Simon TL. Current status of pulmonary thromboembolic disease: pathophysiology, diagnosis, prevention, and treatment. Am Heart J 1982;103(2):239–62.
26. Sandler DA, Martin JF. Autopsy proven pulmonary embolism in hospital patients: are we detecting enough deep vein thrombosis? J R Soc Med 1989;82(4):203–5.
27. Alpert JS, Dalen JE. Epidemiology and natural history of venous thromboembolism. Prog Cardiovasc Dis 1994;36(6):417–22.
28. McIntyre KM, Sasahara AA. The hemodynamic response to pulmonary embolism in patients without prior cardiopulmonary disease. Am J Cardiol 1971;28(3):288–94.
29. Jardin F, Dubourg O, Gueret P, et al. Quantitative two-dimensional echocardiography in massive pulmonary embolism: emphasis on ventricular interdependence and leftward septal displacement. J Am Coll Cardiol 1987;10(6):1201–6.

30. Fedullo PF, Tapson VF. Clinical practice. The evaluation of suspected pulmonary embolism. N Engl J Med 2003;349(13):1247–56. http://dx.doi.org/10.1056/NEJMcp035442.
31. Le Gal G, Righini M, Roy PM, et al. Prediction of pulmonary embolism in the emergency department: the revised Geneva score. Ann Intern Med 2006; 144(3):165–71.
32. Magana M, Bercovitch R, Fedullo P. Diagnostic approach to deep venous thrombosis and pulmonary embolism in the critical care setting. Crit Care Clin 2011;27(4):841–67. http://dx.doi.org/10.1016/j.ccc.2011.08.003, vi.
33. Wells PS, Anderson DR, Rodger M, et al. Excluding pulmonary embolism at the bedside without diagnostic imaging: management of patients with suspected pulmonary embolism presenting to the emergency department by using a simple clinical model and D-dimer. Ann Intern Med 2001;135(2):98–107.
34. Stein PD, Woodard PK, Weg JG, et al. Diagnostic pathways in acute pulmonary embolism: recommendations of the PIOPED II investigators. Radiology 2007; 242(1):15–21. http://dx.doi.org/10.1148/radiol.2421060971.
35. Stein PD, Henry JW. Clinical characteristics of patients with acute pulmonary embolism stratified according to their presenting syndromes. Chest 1997; 112(4):974–9. http://dx.doi.org/10.1378/chest.112.4.974.
36. Wicki J, Perneger TV, Junod AF, et al. Assessing clinical probability of pulmonary embolism in the emergency ward: a simple score. Arch Intern Med 2001;161(1):92–7.
37. Klok FA, Mos IC, Nijkeuter M, et al. Simplification of the revised Geneva score for assessing clinical probability of pulmonary embolism. Arch Intern Med 2008; 168(19):2131–6. http://dx.doi.org/10.1001/archinte.168.19.2131.
38. Wells PS, Ginsberg JS, Anderson DR, et al. Use of a clinical model for safe management of patients with suspected pulmonary embolism. Ann Intern Med 1998; 129(12):997–1005.
39. Wells PS, Anderson DR, Rodger M, et al. Derivation of a simple clinical model to categorize patients probability of pulmonary embolism: increasing the models utility with the SimpliRED D-dimer. Thromb Haemost 2000;83(3):416–20.
40. Fesmire FM, Brown MD, Espinosa JA, et al. Critical issues in the evaluation and management of adult patients presenting to the emergency department with suspected pulmonary embolism. Ann Emerg Med 2011;57(6):628–52.e75. http://dx.doi.org/10.1016/j.annemergmed.2011.01.020.
41. Bova C, Greco F, Misuraca G, et al. Diagnostic utility of echocardiography in patients with suspected pulmonary embolism. Am J Emerg Med 2003;21(3):180–3.
42. Kanbay A, Kokturk N, Kaya MG, et al. Electrocardiography and Wells scoring in predicting the anatomic severity of pulmonary embolism. Respir Med 2007; 101(6):1171–6. http://dx.doi.org/10.1016/j.rmed.2006.11.009.
43. Aujesky D, Obrosky DS, Stone RA, et al. Derivation and validation of a prognostic model for pulmonary embolism. Am J Respir Crit Care Med 2005; 172(8):1041–6. http://dx.doi.org/10.1164/rccm.200506-862OC.
44. Aujesky D, Roy PM, Le Manach CP, et al. Validation of a model to predict adverse outcomes in patients with pulmonary embolism. Eur Heart J 2006; 27(4):476–81. http://dx.doi.org/10.1093/eurheartj/ehi588.
45. Jimenez D, Diaz G, Molina J, et al. Troponin I and risk stratification of patients with acute nonmassive pulmonary embolism. Eur Respir J 2008;31(4):847–53. http://dx.doi.org/10.1183/09031936.00113307.
46. Palmieri V, Gallotta G, Rendina D, et al. Troponin I and right ventricular dysfunction for risk assessment in patients with nonmassive pulmonary embolism in the

emergency department in combination with clinically based risk score. Intern Emerg Med 2008;3(2):131–8. http://dx.doi.org/10.1007/s11739-008-0134-2.

47. Amorim S, Dias P, Rodrigues RA, et al. Troponin I as a marker of right ventricular dysfunction and severity of pulmonary embolism. Rev Port Cardiol 2006;25(2): 181–6.

48. Mehta NJ, Jani K, Khan IA. Clinical usefulness and prognostic value of elevated cardiac troponin I levels in acute pulmonary embolism. Am Heart J 2003;145(5): 821–5. http://dx.doi.org/10.1016/S0002-8703(02)94704-6.

49. Meyer T, Binder L, Hruska N, et al. Cardiac troponin I elevation in acute pulmonary embolism is associated with right ventricular dysfunction. J Am Coll Cardiol 2000;36(5):1632–6. http://dx.doi.org/10.1016/S0735-1097(00)00905-0.

50. Giannitsis E, Müller-Bardorff M, Kurowski V, et al. Independent prognostic value of cardiac troponin T in patients with confirmed pulmonary embolism. Circulation 2000;102(2):211–7. http://dx.doi.org/10.1161/01.CIR.102.2.211.

51. Konstantinides S, Geibel A, Olschewski M, et al. Importance of cardiac troponins I and T in risk stratification of patients with acute pulmonary embolism. Circulation 2002;106(10):1263–8.

52. Becattini C, Vedovati MC, Agnelli G. Prognostic value of troponins in acute pulmonary embolism: a meta-analysis. Circulation 2007;116(4):427–33. http://dx. doi.org/10.1161/CIRCULATIONAHA.106.680421.

53. Levin ER, Gardner DG, Samson WK. Natriuretic peptides. N Engl J Med 1998; 339(5):321–8. http://dx.doi.org/10.1056/NEJM199807303390507.

54. Coutance G, Le Page O, Lo T, et al. Prognostic value of brain natriuretic peptide in acute pulmonary embolism. Crit Care 2008;12(4):R109. http://dx.doi.org/10. 1186/cc6996.

55. Cavallazzi R, Nair A, Vasu T, et al. Natriuretic peptides in acute pulmonary embolism: a systematic review. Intensive Care Med 2008;34(12):2147–56. http://dx. doi.org/10.1007/s00134-008-1214-5.

56. Puls M, Dellas C, Lankeit M, et al. Heart-type fatty acid-binding protein permits early risk stratification of pulmonary embolism. Eur Heart J 2007;28(2):224–9. http://dx.doi.org/10.1093/eurheartj/ehl405.

57. Dellas C, Puls M, Lankeit M, et al. Elevated heart-type fatty acid-binding protein levels on admission predict an adverse outcome in normotensive patients with acute pulmonary embolism. J Am Coll Cardiol 2010;55(19):2150–7. http://dx. doi.org/10.1016/j.jacc.2009.10.078.

58. Quiroz R, Kucher N, Zou KH, et al. Clinical validity of a negative computed tomography scan in patients with suspected pulmonary embolism: a systematic review. JAMA 2005;293(16):2012–7. http://dx.doi.org/10.1001/jama.293.16.2012.

59. Stein PD, Fowler SE, Goodman LR, et al. Multidetector computed tomography for acute pulmonary embolism. N Engl J Med 2006;354(22):2317–27. http:// dx.doi.org/10.1056/NEJMoa052367.

60. Quiroz R, Kucher N, Schoepf UJ, et al. Right ventricular enlargement on chest computed tomography: prognostic role in acute pulmonary embolism. Circulation 2004;109(20):2401–4. http://dx.doi.org/10.1161/01.CIR.0000129302.90476.BC.

61. Schoepf UJ, Kucher N, Kipfmueller F, et al. Right ventricular enlargement on chest computed tomography: a predictor of early death in acute pulmonary embolism. Circulation 2004;110(20):3276–80. http://dx.doi.org/10.1161/01.CIR. 0000147612.59751.4C.

62. Collomb D, Paramelle PJ, Calaque O, et al. Severity assessment of acute pulmonary embolism: evaluation using helical CT. Eur Radiol 2003;13(7):1508–14. http://dx.doi.org/10.1007/s00330-002-1804-5.

63. van der Meer RW, Pattynama PM, van Strijen MJ, et al. Right ventricular dysfunction and pulmonary obstruction index at helical CT: prediction of clinical outcome during 3-month follow-up in patients with acute pulmonary embolism. Radiology 2005;235(3):798–803. http://dx.doi.org/10.1148/radiol.2353040593.

64. Becattini C, Agnelli G, Vedovati MC, et al. Multidetector computed tomography for acute pulmonary embolism: diagnosis and risk stratification in a single test. Eur Heart J 2011;32(13):1657–63. http://dx.doi.org/10.1093/eurheartj/ehr108.

65. Vedovati MC, Becattini C, Agnelli G, et al. Multidetector CT scan for acute pulmonary embolism: embolic burden and clinical outcome. Chest 2012;142(6): 1417–24. http://dx.doi.org/10.1378/chest.11-2739.

66. Okada M, Nakashima Y, Kunihiro Y, et al. Volumetric evaluation of dual-energy perfusion CT for the assessment of intrapulmonary clot burden. Clin Radiol 2013;68(12):e669–75. http://dx.doi.org/10.1016/j.crad.2013.07.018.

67. Apfaltrer P, Bachmann V, Meyer M, et al. Prognostic value of perfusion defect volume at dual energy CTA in patients with pulmonary embolism: correlation with CTA obstruction scores, CT parameters of right ventricular dysfunction and adverse clinical outcome. Eur J Radiol 2012;81(11):3592–7. http://dx.doi.org/10.1016/j.ejrad.2012.02.008.

68. Ferrari E, Imbert A, Chevalier T, et al. The ECG in pulmonary embolism. Predictive value of negative T waves in precordial leads–80 case reports. Chest 1997; 111(3):537–43.

69. McIntyre KM, Sasahara AA, Littmann D. Relation of the electrocardiogram to hemodynamic alterations in pulmonary embolism. Am J Cardiol 1972;30(3):205–10.

70. Sreeram N, Cheriex EC, Smeets JL, et al. Value of the 12-lead electrocardiogram at hospital admission in the diagnosis of pulmonary embolism. Am J Cardiol 1994;73(4):298–303.

71. Stein PD, Dalen JE, McIntyre KM, et al. The electrocardiogram in acute pulmonary embolism. Prog Cardiovasc Dis 1975;17(4):247–57.

72. Kim SE, Park DG, Choi HH, et al. The best predictor for right ventricular dysfunction in acute pulmonary embolism: comparison between electrocardiography and biomarkers. Korean Circ J 2009;39(9):378–81. http://dx.doi.org/10.4070/kcj.2009.39.9.378.

73. Daniel KR, Courtney DM, Kline JA. Assessment of cardiac stress from massive pulmonary embolism with 12-lead ECG. Chest 2001;120(2):474–81.

74. Kukla P, Dlugopolski R, Krupa E, et al. Electrocardiography and prognosis of patients with acute pulmonary embolism. Cardiol J 2011;18(6):648–53.

75. Kucher N, Rossi E, De Rosa M, et al. Prognostic role of echocardiography among patients with acute pulmonary embolism and a systolic arterial pressure of 90 mm Hg or higher. Arch Intern Med 2005;165(15):1777–81. http://dx.doi.org/10.1001/archinte.165.15.1777.

76. Sanchez O, Trinquart L, Colombet I, et al. Prognostic value of right ventricular dysfunction in patients with haemodynamically stable pulmonary embolism: a systematic review. Eur Heart J 2008;29(12):1569–77. http://dx.doi.org/10.1093/eurheartj/ehn208.

77. Binder L, Pieske B, Olschewski M, et al. N-terminal pro-brain natriuretic peptide or troponin testing followed by echocardiography for risk stratification of acute pulmonary embolism. Circulation 2005;112(11):1573–9. http://dx.doi.org/10.1161/CIRCULATIONAHA.105.552216.

78. Gibson NS, Sohne M, Buller HR. Prognostic value of echocardiography and spiral computed tomography in patients with pulmonary embolism. Curr Opin Pulm Med 2005;11(5):380–4.

Ishmael

79. ten Wolde M, Sohne M, Quak E, et al. Prognostic value of echocardiographically assessed right ventricular dysfunction in patients with pulmonary embolism. Arch Intern Med 2004;164(15):1685–9. http://dx.doi.org/10.1001/archinte.164.15.1685.

80. Scridon T, Scridon C, Skali H, et al. Prognostic significance of troponin elevation and right ventricular enlargement in acute pulmonary embolism. Am J Cardiol 2005;96(2):303–5. http://dx.doi.org/10.1016/j.amjcard.2005.03.062.

81. Tulevski II, ten Wolde M, van Veldhuisen DJ, et al. Combined utility of brain natriuretic peptide and cardiac troponin T may improve rapid triage and risk stratification in normotensive patients with pulmonary embolism. Int J Cardiol 2007; 116(2):161–6. http://dx.doi.org/10.1016/j.ijcard.2006.03.030.

82. Henzler T, Roeger S, Meyer M, et al. Pulmonary embolism: CT signs and cardiac biomarkers for predicting right ventricular dysfunction. Eur Respir J 2012;39(4): 919–26. http://dx.doi.org/10.1183/09031936.00088711.

83. Kang DK, Sun JS, Park KJ, et al. Usefulness of combined assessment with computed tomographic signs of right ventricular dysfunction and cardiac troponin T for risk stratification of acute pulmonary embolism. Am J Cardiol 2011;108(1):133–40. http://dx.doi.org/10.1016/j.amjcard.2011.03.009.

84. Meyer M, Fink C, Roeger S, et al. Benefit of combining quantitative cardiac CT parameters with troponin I for predicting right ventricular dysfunction and adverse clinical events in patients with acute pulmonary embolism. Eur J Radiol 2012;81(11):3294–9. http://dx.doi.org/10.1016/j.ejrad.2012.06.023.

85. Kearon C, Akl EA, Comerota AJ, et al. Antithrombotic therapy for VTE disease: antithrombotic therapy and prevention of thrombosis. 9th edition: American college of chest physicians evidence-based clinical practice guidelines. Chest 2012;141(Suppl 2):e419S–94S. http://dx.doi.org/10.1378/chest.11-2301.

86. Torbicki A, Perrier A, Konstantinides S, et al. Guidelines on the diagnosis and management of acute pulmonary embolism: the Task Force for the Diagnosis and Management of Acute Pulmonary Embolism of the European Society of Cardiology (ESC). Eur Heart J 2008;29(18):2276–315. http://dx.doi.org/10.1093/eurheartj/ehn310.

87. Jaff MR, McMurtry MS, Archer SL, et al. Management of massive and submassive pulmonary embolism, iliofemoral deep vein thrombosis, and chronic thromboembolic pulmonary hypertension: a scientific statement from the American Heart Association. Circulation 2011;123(16):1788–830. http://dx.doi.org/10.1161/CIR.0b013e318214914f.

88. Piazza G, Goldhaber SZ. Fibrinolysis for acute pulmonary embolism. Vasc Med 2010;15(5):419–28. http://dx.doi.org/10.1177/1358863X10380304.

89. Barritt DW, Jordan SC. Anticoagulant drugs in the treatment of pulmonary embolism. A controlled trial. Lancet 1960;1(7138):1309–12.

90. Quinlan DJ, McQuillan A, Eikelboom JW. Low-molecular-weight heparin compared with intravenous unfractionated heparin for treatment of pulmonary embolism: a meta-analysis of randomized, controlled trials. Ann Intern Med 2004;140(3):175–83.

91. The Columbus Investigators. Low-molecular-weight heparin in the treatment of patients with venous thromboembolism. The Columbus Investigators. N Engl J Med 1997;337(10):657–62. http://dx.doi.org/10.1056/NEJM199709043371001.

92. Simonneau G, Sors H, Charbonnier B, et al. A comparison of low-molecular-weight heparin with unfractionated heparin for acute pulmonary embolism. The THESEE study group. Tinzaparine ou heparine standard: evaluations dans l'embolie pulmonaire. N Engl J Med 1997;337(10):663–9. http://dx.doi.org/10.1056/NEJM199709043371002.

93. Buller HR, Davidson BL, Decousus H, et al. Subcutaneous fondaparinux versus intravenous unfractionated heparin in the initial treatment of pulmonary embolism. N Engl J Med 2003;349(18):1695–702. http://dx.doi.org/10.1056/NEJMoa035451.

94. Schulman S, Kearon C, Kakkar AK, et al. Dabigatran versus warfarin in the treatment of acute venous thromboembolism. N Engl J Med 2009;361(24):2342–52. http://dx.doi.org/10.1056/NEJMoa0906598.

95. EINSTEIN-PE Investigators, Buller HR, Prins MH, et al. Oral rivaroxaban for the treatment of symptomatic pulmonary embolism. N Engl J Med 2012;366(14): 1287–97. http://dx.doi.org/10.1056/NEJMoa1113572.

96. Agnelli G, Buller HR, Cohen A, et al. Oral apixaban for the treatment of acute venous thromboembolism. N Engl J Med 2013;369(9):799–808. http://dx.doi.org/10.1056/NEJMoa1302507.

97. British Thoracic Society Standards of Care Committee Pulmonary Embolism Guideline Development Group. British Thoracic Society guidelines for the management of suspected acute pulmonary embolism. Thorax 2003;58(6):470–83.

98. Kearon C, Kahn SR, Agnelli G, et al. Antithrombotic therapy for venous thromboembolic disease: American College of Chest Physicians evidence-based clinical practice guidelines (8th edition). Chest 2008;133(Suppl 6):454S–545S. http://dx.doi.org/10.1378/chest.08-0658.

99. Dalla-Volta S, Palla A, Santolicandro A, et al. PAIMS 2: Alteplase combined with heparin versus heparin in the treatment of acute pulmonary embolism. Plasminogen activator Italian multicenter study 2. J Am Coll Cardiol 1992;20(3):520–6.

100. Goldhaber SZ, Haire WD, Feldstein ML, et al. Alteplase versus heparin in acute pulmonary embolism: randomised trial assessing right-ventricular function and pulmonary perfusion. Lancet 1993;341(8844):507–11.

101. The PIOPED Investigators. Tissue plasminogen activator for the treatment of acute pulmonary embolism. A collaborative study by the PIOPED investigators. Chest 1990;97(3):528–33.

102. Konstantinides S, Tiede N, Geibel A, et al. Comparison of alteplase versus heparin for resolution of major pulmonary embolism. Am J Cardiol 1998;82(8): 966–70.

103. Wan S, Quinlan DJ, Agnelli G, et al. Thrombolysis compared with heparin for the initial treatment of pulmonary embolism: a meta-analysis of the randomized controlled trials. Circulation 2004;110(6):744–9. http://dx.doi.org/10.1161/01.CIR.0000137826.09715.9C.

104. Hamel E, Pacouret G, Vincentelli D, et al. Thrombolysis or heparin therapy in massive pulmonary embolism with right ventricular dilation: results from a 128-patient monocenter registry. Chest 2001;120(1):120–5.

105. Konstantinides S, Geibel A, Heusel G, et al. Management strategies and prognosis of Pulmonary Embolism-3 trial investigators. Heparin plus alteplase compared with heparin alone in patients with submassive pulmonary embolism. N Engl J Med 2002;347(15):1143–50. http://dx.doi.org/10.1056/NEJMoa021274.

106. Becattini C, Agnelli G, Salvi A, et al. Bolus tenecteplase for right ventricle dysfunction in hemodynamically stable patients with pulmonary embolism. Thromb Res 2010;125(3):e82–6. http://dx.doi.org/10.1016/j.thromres.2009.09.017.

107. Fasullo S, Scalzo S, Maringhini G, et al. Six-month echocardiographic study in patients with submassive pulmonary embolism and right ventricle dysfunction: comparison of thrombolysis with heparin. Am J Med Sci 2011;341(1):33–9. http://dx.doi.org/10.1097/MAJ.0b013e3181f1fc3e.

108. Meyer G, Vicaut E, Danays T, et al. Fibrinolysis for patients with intermediate-risk pulmonary embolism. N Engl J Med 2014;370(15):1402–11.
109. Gulba DC, Schmid C, Borst HG, et al. Medical compared with surgical treatment for massive pulmonary embolism. Lancet 1994;343(8897):576–7.
110. Meneveau N, Seronde MF, Blonde MC, et al. Management of unsuccessful thrombolysis in acute massive pulmonary embolism. Chest 2006;129(4): 1043–50. http://dx.doi.org/10.1378/chest.129.4.1043.
111. Sukhija R, Aronow WS, Lee J, et al. Association of right ventricular dysfunction with in-hospital mortality in patients with acute pulmonary embolism and reduction in mortality in patients with right ventricular dysfunction by pulmonary embolectomy. Am J Cardiol 2005;95(5):695–6. http://dx.doi.org/10.1016/j.amjcard.2004.10.055.
112. Leacche M, Unic D, Goldhaber SZ, et al. Modern surgical treatment of massive pulmonary embolism: results in 47 consecutive patients after rapid diagnosis and aggressive surgical approach. J Thorac Cardiovasc Surg 2005;129(5): 1018–23. http://dx.doi.org/10.1016/j.jtcvs.2004.10.023.
113. Aklog L, Williams CS, Byrne JG, et al. Acute pulmonary embolectomy: a contemporary approach. Circulation 2002;105(12):1416–9.
114. Sareyyupoglu B, Greason KL, Suri RM, et al. A more aggressive approach to emergency embolectomy for acute pulmonary embolism. Mayo Clin Proc 2010;85(9):785–90. http://dx.doi.org/10.4065/mcp.2010.0250.
115. Goldhaber SZ. Advanced treatment strategies for acute pulmonary embolism, including thrombolysis and embolectomy. J Thromb Haemost 2009;7(Suppl 1):322–7. http://dx.doi.org/10.1111/j.1538-7836.2009.03415.x.
116. Kucher N, Rossi E, De Rosa M, et al. Massive pulmonary embolism. Circulation 2006;113(4):577–82. http://dx.doi.org/10.1161/CIRCULATIONAHA.105.592592.
117. Decousus H, Leizorovicz A, Parent F, et al. A clinical trial of vena caval filters in the prevention of pulmonary embolism in patients with proximal deep-vein thrombosis. Prevention du risque d'embolie pulmonaire par interruption cave study group. N Engl J Med 1998;338(7):409–15. http://dx.doi.org/10.1056/NEJM199802123380701.
118. Mismetti P, Rivron-Guillot K, Quenet S, et al. A prospective long-term study of 220 patients with a retrievable vena cava filter for secondary prevention of venous thromboembolism. Chest 2007;131(1):223–9. http://dx.doi.org/10.1378/chest.06-0631.
119. Tschoe M, Kim HS, Brotman DJ, et al. Retrievable vena cava filters: a clinical review. J Hosp Med 2009;4(7):441–8. http://dx.doi.org/10.1002/jhm.439.
120. Kuo WT, Gould MK, Louie JD, et al. Catheter-directed therapy for the treatment of massive pulmonary embolism: systematic review and meta-analysis of modern techniques. J Vasc Interv Radiol 2009;20(11):1431–40. http://dx.doi.org/10.1016/j.jvir.2009.08.002.
121. Kucher N. Catheter embolectomy for acute pulmonary embolism. Chest 2007; 132(2):657–63. http://dx.doi.org/10.1378/chest.07-0665.
122. US Food and Drug Administration. MAUDE adverse event report: Medrad Interventional/Possis Possis Angiojet Rheolytic Thrombectomy System Angiojet System. Available at: http://www.accessdata.fda.gov/scripts/cdrh/cfdocs/cfmaude/detail.cfm?mdrfoi__id=1397902. Accessed April 28, 2014.
123. Verstraete M, Miller GA, Bounameaux H, et al. Intravenous and intrapulmonary recombinant tissue-type plasminogen activator in the treatment of acute massive pulmonary embolism. Circulation 1988;77(2):353–60.

124. Greenfield LJ, Proctor MC, Williams DM, et al. Long-term experience with transvenous catheter pulmonary embolectomy. J Vasc Surg 1993;18(3): 450–7 [discussion: 457–8].
125. Chauhan MS, Kawamura A. Percutaneous rheolytic thrombectomy for large pulmonary embolism: a promising treatment option. Catheter Cardiovasc Interv 2007;70(1):121–8. http://dx.doi.org/10.1002/ccd.20997.
126. Ferrigno L, Bloch R, Threlkeld J, et al. Management of pulmonary embolism with rheolytic thrombectomy. Can Respir J 2011;18(4):e52–8.
127. Krichavsky MZ, Rybicki FJ, Resnic FS. Catheter directed lysis and thrombectomy of submassive pulmonary embolism. Catheter Cardiovasc Interv 2011; 77(1):144–7. http://dx.doi.org/10.1002/ccd.22696.
128. Mohan B, Chhabra ST, Aslam N, et al. Mechanical breakdown and thrombolysis in subacute massive pulmonary embolism: a prospective trial. World J Cardiol 2013;5(5):141–7. http://dx.doi.org/10.4330/wjc.v5.i5.141.
129. Kucher N, Goldhaber SZ. Cardiac biomarkers for risk stratification of patients with acute pulmonary embolism. Circulation 2003;108(18):2191–4. http://dx. doi.org/10.1161/01.CIR.0000100687.99687.CE.

Management of Right Heart Failure in the Critically Ill

Christopher King, MD[a,*], Christopher W. May, MD[b], Jeffrey Williams, MD[c], Oksana A. Shlobin, MD[d]

KEYWORDS

- Right ventricular failure • Right ventricular dysfunction • Pulmonary hypertension
- Acute respiratory distress syndrome

KEY POINTS

- Right ventricular failure complicates a number of commonly encountered conditions in the critically ill and is generally associated with worsened outcomes.
- An understanding of the pathophysiologic changes seen in the failing right ventricle is essential for developing an appropriate treatment strategy.
- Echocardiography is the screening test of choice for right ventricular failure. Focused critical care echocardiography can facilitate timely diagnosis by the bedside clinician.
- Timely diagnosis and treatment of the cause of right ventricular failure is essential.
- Reduction of right ventricular afterload and optimization of right ventricular preload and contractility form the principles of management. Oftentimes this requires combined use of vasopressors, inotropes, and pulmonary vasodilators.

INTRODUCTION

The critical importance of the right ventricle (RV) has long been underestimated, as classic teaching of cardiac physiology has emphasized left ventricular (LV) structure and function. Once thought a relatively unimportant conduit facilitating the flow of blood to the pulmonary vasculature, the RV is now recognized as a dynamic structure intricately linked to LV systolic and diastolic function. Likewise, research and clinical experience continue to demonstrate the importance of RV function in a variety of clinical conditions, including heart failure, myocardial infarction, congenital heart

Disclosures: The authors have no financial conflicts to disclose.
[a] Medical Critical Care Service, Inova Fairfax Hospital, 618 South Royal Street, Alexandria, VA 22314, USA; [b] Advanced Heart Failure and Cardiac Transplant Program, Inova Fairfax Hospital, 3300 Gallows Road, Falls Church, VA 22042, USA; [c] Medical Critical Care Service, Inova Fairfax Hospital, 3300 Gallows Road, Falls Church, VA 22042, USA; [d] Advanced Lung Disease and Transplant Program, Inova Fairfax Hospital, 3300 Gallows Road, Falls Church, VA 22042, USA
* Corresponding author.
E-mail address: Csking123@hotmail.com

disease, pulmonary embolism, and pulmonary hypertension. Critically ill patients in the intensive care unit (ICU) with RV failure have increased morbidity and mortality compared with those patients with preserved RV function, and clinical management of these patients remains a formidable challenge.[1] Despite advances in technology, support of the failing RV, whether acute or chronic, has lagged behind that of the failing LV.

In this review, we describe the anatomy and physiology of the healthy RV and contrast it with the maladaptive responses of the failing one. We provide a conceptual framework for the etiology of RV failure, discuss basic techniques for diagnosing RV dysfunction, and provide general management strategies for the critically ill patient with RV failure. Finally, the article focuses on the treatment of conditions frequently seen in the critically ill patients in the ICU, including decompensated severe pulmonary arterial hypertension (PAH), massive pulmonary embolism (PE), and RV infarction.

ANATOMY AND PHYSIOLOGY ON THE HEALTHY RV

The healthy RV serves 2 roles: to pump venous blood to the lungs and to fill the systemic LV. In the normal heart, the RV fills with blood from the inferior and superior vena cava and pumps it into the pulmonary arteries. During LV diastole, oxygenated blood returns from the lungs by the pulmonary veins. The RV and LV are pumps in series, with roughly equivalent cardiac outputs, although each is characterized by the vasculature they are connected to. The pulmonary vasculature is composed of thin-walled and large-diameter vessels, contrasting sharply with the high-resistance, muscular arteries of the systemic vasculature. Under normal conditions, the pulmonary vasculature is a low-impedance, high-capacitance system, with lower vascular resistance and greater distensibility than the systemic vasculature.[2] Accordingly, the myocardium of the RV is thin, approximately one-third the thickness of the LV, and is more compliant, allowing the RV to accommodate large variations in venous return without significantly altering end-diastolic pressures.[3] Compared with the LV, the RV has increased sensitivity to changes in afterload. Under normal conditions, the systolic pressure of the RV is approximately 25 mm Hg, less than one-fifth the systolic pressure generated by the LV.[2]

The RV appears triangular on longitudinal section and crescent-shaped in cross section.[4] The RV relies primarily on longitudinal shortening during systole whereas the LV uses circumferential constrictor fibers for contraction.[5] This results in a "peristaltic" contraction that moves in a wave from the RV apex to the outflow tract.[3,5] Under normal circumstances, the RV follows the Frank-Starling mechanism by which increases in preload improve myocardial contractility. Factors that influence RV filling include intravascular volume, RV compliance, heart rate and rhythm, LV filling, and abnormalities of the pericardium. Excessive RV volume loading can result in constraint by the pericardium, compression of the LV, and an increase in ventricular interdependence.

The RV has increased resistance to ischemic injury compared with the LV. Besides a lower rate of oxygen consumption, the RV has a more extensive system of collateral vessels. In most individuals, the right coronary artery (RCA) perfuses the RV free wall and the posterior third of the interventricular septum, whereas the anterior two-thirds of the interventricular septum and apex of the RV are supplied by the left anterior descending artery (LAD).[3] Because the RV tissue pressure is lower than aortic root pressure under normal conditions, the RV receives continuous perfusion throughout both systole and diastole.[5] Although patients with acute RV ischemic injury tend to be hemodynamically challenging to manage, those who recover typically do well because of the absence of permanent RV ischemic injury.

Ventricular interdependence acknowledges the relationship between the 2 ventricles. The size, shape, and compliance of one ventricle affects the size, shape, and compliance of the other ventricle through the direct mechanical interactions of sharing the ventricular septum and pericardial space. Systolic ventricular interdependence is characterized by the contribution of LV septal contraction on RV emptying; up to 40% of RV systolic function may be attributable to this mechanism.[6] Diastolic ventricular interdependence is characterized by acute RV pressure or volume overload states, where a shift of the interventricular septum toward the left results in decreased distensibility, potentially resulting in decreased preload and cardiac output.

PATHOPHYSIOLOGY OF THE FAILING RV

Right ventricular failure (RVF) is defined as low cardiac output and systemic hypoperfusion due to the inability of the RV to provide adequate circulation through the pulmonary vasculature despite normal central venous pressures.[7] RVF may occur secondary to increases in RV afterload, decreases in RV contractility, or alterations in RV preload.[8] (**Fig. 1**) understanding the underlying pathophysiological alterations is essential for the treatment of RVF. Of the 3 scenarios, the most common is that of increased afterload. Given the RV is a compliant structure well suited to changes in end diastolic volume, these same features leave the RV with little contractile reserve and vulnerable to increases in afterload. When a patient with previously normal pulmonary artery pressures is presented with an acute increase in pulmonary vascular resistance (PVR), the ability of the RV to compensate is quickly exceeded. A previously healthy RV can acutely increase peak systolic pressures to approximately 60 mm Hg before contractile failure and systemic hypotension ensue, resulting in decreased cardiac output and potential cardiovascular collapse.[9]

When faced with less abrupt increases in PVR, the RV undergoes changes in an effort to maintain adequate cardiac output. To maintain sufficient stroke volume, the

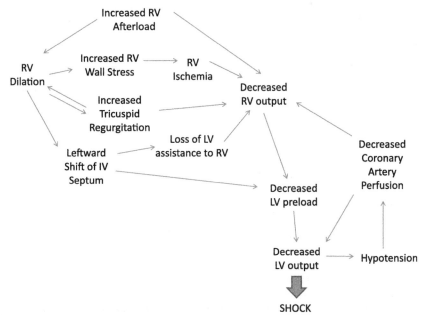

Fig. 1. Pathophysiologic changes in RVF.

RV initially dilates, thereby increasing preload.[1] However, if RV dilation progresses, a number of deleterious effects may occur. Alterations in the RV geometry will cause dilation of the tricuspid annulus and inadequate coaptation of the valve leaflets, resulting in regurgitation.[1] Further RV dilation and volume overload cause a leftward shift of the interventricular septum, reducing LV diastolic filling. LV systolic function decreases and the normal contribution of LV systolic function to RV emptying is impaired due to this geometric distortion.[3,5] Eventually, volume overload surpasses the compliance of the RV and pressure overload develops. RV pressure overload increases wall stress, leading to increased myocardial oxygen consumption.[5] If RV pressures are sufficiently elevated, myocardial blood supply from the RCA may occur only during diastole, leading to myocardial ischemia and further decreases in RV contractility.[5] Collectively, these maladaptive, inter-related physiologic derangements reduce cardiac output and result in significant hemodynamic compromise.

CAUSES OF RVF IN THE CRITICALLY ILL

Physicians caring for patients in the ICU must be well-versed in the management of RVF, as it complicates a number of commonly encountered disorders in the critically ill. RVF may develop de novo, as a direct result of critical illness (eg, massive PE, acute respiratory distress syndrome [ARDS]), or it may complicate the care of a patient with preexisting RV dysfunction (eg, sepsis in a patient with PAH). A simple method of categorizing causes of RVF is by the primary pathophysiologic disturbance responsible for the particular cause. Causes can be organized into 1 of 4 categories: increased RV afterload, decreased RV contractility, increased RV preload, or decreased RV preload. It should be emphasized that such categorization oversimplifies the underlying pathophysiology of RVF, as most causes of RVF are characterized by some degree of overlap of these pathophysiologic conditions. The most common causes of RVF encountered in the ICU are LV failure, acute PE, decompensated PAH, sepsis, ARDS, RV ischemia, cardiac tamponade, and post–cardiothoracic surgery, although several less common causes exist.[8] **Table 1** summarizes the causes of RVF.

EPIDEMIOLOGY AND IMPACT OF RVF

The prevalence of RVF and its impact on outcomes in the critically ill remain poorly defined. Multiple reasons exist for the gaps in our understanding of this process, including the relatively recent recognition of its importance, variable definitions of RVF, heterogeneity among ICU populations, and the myriad of etiologies leading to RVF. Examining the available data on individual diagnoses provides some insight.

RV dysfunction is a powerful predictor of mortality in patients with left heart failure.[10–13] Ghio and colleagues[10] examined right heart catheterization (RHC) data in 377 patients with chronic systolic heart failure and found that 75% of patients had a depressed RV ejection fraction, an independent predictor of death even after controlling for pulmonary hypertension. Isolated RVF or RVF in association with concurrent LVF is associated with mortality rates of approximately 40%.[14–16] Postoperative RVF also is well-described as a complication of cardiac surgery, including cardiac transplantation and left ventricular assist device (LVAD) implantation, and carries a similar mortality rate of nearly 40%.[17–20]

Of patients presenting with PE, 30% to 50% have "RV strain" either by elevated levels of biomarkers or echocardiographic evidence of RV dysfunction,[21] and 4.5% of patients with PE meet criteria for "massive PE," defined as systemic hypotension, cardiac arrest, syncope, or a decrease in systolic blood pressure by greater than 40 mm Hg for at least 15 minutes. Massive PE is associated with 90-day mortality rates

Table 1
Causes of RV failure

Primary Physiologic Disturbance	Etiology
Increased RV afterload	• Pulmonary arterial hypertension • Secondary causes of pulmonary hypertension • Pulmonary venous hypertension (owing to left heart failure) • Pulmonary embolism • Hypoxic pulmonary vasoconstriction • Mechanical ventilation • Post–cardiothoracic surgery • Acute chest syndrome in sickle cell disease • Pulmonary stenosis • Tumor emboli
Impaired RV contractility	• RV infarction • Cardiomyopathy • Sepsis (cytokine-mediated myocardial depression) • Arrhythmogenic RV dysplasia
Increased RV preload	• Tricuspid regurgitation • Pulmonary regurgitation • Post–left ventricular assist device • Atrial/ventricular septal defects
Decreased RV preload	• Superior vena cava syndrome • Tricuspid stenosis • Cardiac tamponade • Hypovolemia/Capillary leak

Abbreviation: RV, right ventricular.

of up to 50%.[21] The reported prevalence of RV dysfunction in sepsis ranges from 30% to 100% and is associated with decreased survival in some studies, although a recent meta-analysis failed to demonstrate a difference in RV ejection fraction or RV dimension between survivors and nonsurvivors.[22–28]

RV dysfunction in ARDS has been reported in multiple studies, with prevalence ranging from 14% to 73%.[29–38] This wide range is likely due to variability in the diagnostic techniques and patient populations examined. Early studies demonstrated poor outcomes in ARDS complicated by RV dysfunction.[38,39] Studies using a lung protective ventilatory strategy generally report a lower incidence of RV dysfunction and have failed to demonstrate an association between RV dysfunction in ARDS and mortality.[29,32] This suggests that mortality benefit associated with lung protective ventilation may be in part because of minimization of the impact of mechanical ventilation on the RV.[40,41]

Based on the available data, it appears that RVF commonly complicates the course of patients in the ICU, and when it occurs, is associated with poor outcomes. It comes as no surprise then that patients with chronic RV dysfunction fare poorly when acutely ill. Mortality rates of 32% to 41% have been reported in patients with PAH or inoperable chronic thromboembolic pulmonary hypertension when admitted to the ICU.[5]

DIAGNOSIS OF RV DYSFUNCTION IN THE CRITICALLY ILL

RVF in the critically ill patient may be difficult to detect, and requires a high degree of clinical suspicion. Physical examination findings of chronic right heart failure, such as peripheral edema, hepatomegaly, ascites, elevated jugular venous pressure with prominent *v* waves, and the blowing holosystolic murmur of tricuspid regurgitation may be absent in patients with acute RVF.[42] Hypotension and evidence of end-organ hypoperfusion due to low cardiac output may be the only clinically evident findings of RVF and should lead to further diagnostic investigation. Likewise, many of the diagnostic tests readily available in the ICU may lack sensitivity and specificity for RVF.

Clinically available biomarkers include brain natriuretic peptide (BNP), troponins, and creatininie phosphokinase-MB (CPK/MB), although each have limited utility in the diagnosis of RV dysfunction because of a lack of specificity. Released by the walls of the atria in response to increases in wall tension, plasma levels of BNP have been demonstrated to increase proportionally with increasing degrees of RV dysfunction. However, elevated levels of BNP alone do not constitute RVF. A number of commonly found conditions in patients in the ICU confound interpretation of BNP, including renal failure, which decreases clearance of BNP, and acute lung injury and chronic obstructive lung disease, both of which chronically elevate right atrial pressure.[43,44] Although BNP is nonspecific, the test has high negative predictive value, making RVF unlikely if BNP levels are normal.[45]

Standard 12-lead surface electrocardiography (ECG) lacks sensitivity for the diagnosis of RVF, although it may provide information in specific instances. The combination of right axis deviation, P pulmonale, and R/S wave >1 mm in V_1 with R wave >0.5 mV have greater than 90% specificity for RV hypertrophy.[46] Normotensive patients with PE and evidence of "RV strain," defined as complete or incomplete right bundle branch block, "S1Q3T3" pattern, and inverted T-waves in V_1 through V_4, were 8 times more likely to die or decompensate than those without these findings.[47]

Chest radiography or computed tomography (CT) cannot diagnose RV dysfunction, but may reveal evidence of parenchymal disease causing RV dysfunction or signs of chronic pulmonary hypertension, including RV hypertrophy, right atrial enlargement, or pulmonary artery enlargement.[8,46]

Transthoracic echocardiography remains the diagnostic test of choice for diagnosing structural and functional abnormalities of the RV. It is noninvasive, inexpensive, well-validated, and is easily obtained at the bedside. A complete study includes 2-dimensional imaging of the 4 cardiac chambers and valves in multiple planes, color flow and Doppler interrogation of the cardiac valves, interatrial and interventricular septums, and assessment of the great vessels and pericardium. Besides assessing RV and LV size and function, echocardiography allows assessment of valvular pathology, presence of a pericardial effusion, determination of tamponade physiology, detection of shunts, visualization of congenital abnormalities, and estimation of pulmonary arterial pressures.[42]

Echocardiographic signs of acute RVF include RV dilation and paradoxic septal motion.[48] Assessment of RV dilation is performed by comparing the size of the RV to that of the LV in an apical 4-chamber view. RV dilation is present when the RV is greater than two-thirds the size of the LV. If the RV is equal to or larger than the LV, then severe dilation exists (**Fig. 2**).[49] The absence of RV dilation on echocardiography in a patient with shock makes RVF unlikely to be the cause of shock.[50] RV dilation is also suggested by the appearance of a "D-shaped" septum on the parasternal short-axis view (**Fig. 3**). Paradoxic septal motion during systole is a specific sign of RV pressure overload.[40] More advanced techniques, such as the tricuspid annular plane systolic excursion (TAPSE) and Tei index, can provide assessments of RV systolic function.[51] In mechanically ventilated patients with poor acoustic windows precluding adequate transthoracic echocardiographic (TTE) assessment, transesophageal echocardiography can be used.[52]

Typically performed by dedicated echocardiography technicians and later interpreted by cardiologists once the study has been downloaded to a dedicated work

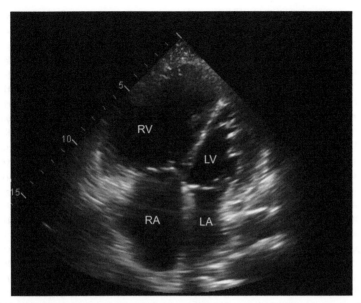

Fig. 2. Apical 4-chamber view from a TTE demonstrating severe RV dilation in a patient with severe PAH and RVF. LA, left atrium; RA, left atrium.

station, transthoracic studies are limited by the availability of resources, which can lead to substantial delays. More recently, focused critical care echocardiography (CCE) has allowed clinicians to rapidly diagnose a variety of cardiac conditions, including RVF, in a timely manner by using nondedicated, portable ultrasound machines.[53] In addition, serial CCE examinations allow assessment of response to interventions. With appropriate training, competence in basic CCE can be readily achieved

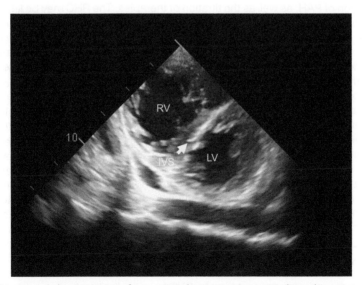

Fig. 3. Parasternal short-axis view from a TTE demonstrating a "D-shaped" septum in a patient with severe PAH and RVF. IVS, intraventricular septum.

by the noncardiologist clinician.[48] Although a substantial amount of information can be derived from a focused CCE study, CCE is not a substitute for a complete transthoracic echocardiography study.

RHC provides a wealth of hemodynamic data by allowing direct measurement of central venous pressure, right atrial pressure (RAP), RV pressure, pulmonary arterial pressure, and pulmonary artery occlusion pressure (PAOP). In patients without pulmonary arterial hypertension, PWP is a surrogate for left atrial pressure, and in the absence of mitral stenosis, reflects LV diastolic pressure. Both PVR and systemic vascular resistance (SVR) may be calculated. Cardiac output may be calculated by 2 different methods, although each have inherent flaws that require results to be carefully scrutinized. The assumed Fick method, which uses direct measurement of mixed venous oxygen saturation, assumes oxygen consumption of the patient, which is difficult in the critically ill patient. The thermodilution technique, in which a fixed quantity of a substance (typically room temperature saline) is injected and measured by a thermistor sensor, is unreliable in patients with moderate to severe tricuspid regurgitation and is vulnerable to operator error. The role of RHC in the management of patients in the ICU remains controversial.[54–57] The PAC-MAN trial randomized more than 1000 critically ill patients to management with versus without RHC. No difference in outcomes was detected.[54] The Fluid and Catheter Treatment Trial (FACTT) randomized 1000 patients with acute lung injury to treatment directed by pulmonary artery catheter versus care without one. No difference in mortality or end organ dysfunction was detected, but pulmonary artery catheters were associated with increased risk of complications.[56] Based on the negative outcomes of these trials, routine use of RHC in the ICU has declined in recent years. It should be noted that utility of RHC has never been studied specifically in the setting of RVF.

Understanding a critically ill patient's hemodynamics is important in a variety of settings, and RHC should be considered when a patient with RVF continues to decline despite attempted optimization of surrogate end points (central venous pressure [CVP], lactate, cardiac output) or when RVF is of unclear etiology. In patients with suspected decompensated PAH, RHC remains the gold standard for the diagnosis and classification of PAH, as well as the titration of therapies. The RHC may be left in place for a period of time, allowing for continuous hemodynamic monitoring and tailoring of therapies. As with any in-dwelling catheter, there are risks of complications, including infection, which limits its utility. The rate of serious complications from RHC is reported to be 1.1% when performed by experienced operators, although many of the procedures in this trial were not done in an ICU setting.[58]

A number of "minimally invasive" cardiac output monitors have been developed in recent years. These devices rely on pulse pressure analysis, pulse-Doppler technology, the applied Fick principles, or bioimpedance.[59] These devices have not been specifically validated in the setting of RVF but in the future may provide a less invasive means of continuously monitoring cardiac output in this population. Cardiac magnetic resonance (CMR) is the gold standard for assessment of RV size and function.[51] Cine images of the cardiac cycle can be obtained and allowing assessment of septal and regional wall motion. Dobutamine-stress CMR can be used to investigate contractile reserve.[51] The logistics of obtaining CMR limit its utility in the critically ill.

MANAGEMENT STRATEGIES IN ACUTE RVF

Despite increased recognition of acute RVF in critically ill patients and substantial progress in understanding the pathophysiologic changes of the failing RV, few experimental or clinical data exist to guide treatment. The goal of therapy is to maintain adequate end-organ perfusion until targeted therapies address the underlying etiology or until the initial insult responsible for decompensation resolves.[1] This is achieved through optimization of RV preload with volume management and rhythm control, afterload reduction by minimizing the harms of mechanical ventilation and the use of pulmonary vasodilator therapy, and augmentation of RV perfusion and contractility with pressors and inotropes. Although this article provides a general framework for treatment of RVF, optimal therapeutic strategies must be individualized to the patient's hemodynamics and underlying cause of RVF.

GENERAL MEASURES

Early diagnosis of RVF is essential, and an exhaustive search for possible precipitating factors should be undertaken immediately, with prompt institution of appropriate therapies so as to optimize outcomes. Supplemental oxygen should be administered to maintain oxygen saturations greater than 92% to avoid hypoxemic pulmonary vasoconstriction and increases in RV afterload.[8,60,61] Likewise, metabolic and respiratory acidosis should be corrected, as both can increase pulmonary vascular resistance.[62] Recent guidelines regarding the treatment of anemia and transfusion practice in the critically ill favor a conservative strategy. Although the optimal hemoglobin level in RVF is not known, correction of anemia causing inadequate end-organ perfusion should be corrected.[63]

OPTIMIZATION OF RV PRELOAD: VOLUME STATUS

Optimization of RV preload is crucial for maintenance of adequate cardiac output, and inadequate RV preload requires correction; however, clinicians should be cognizant of the deleterious effects of volume overload in these patients. Although some patients with acute RVF may be volume responsive, such as those with RV infarction or massive PE, the most patients in the ICU will be volume overloaded.[64–66] Inappropriate fluid administration in patients with RVF and volume overload can further hemodynamic deterioration by furthering RV dilation, increasing tricuspid regurgitation, causing RV ischemia, and impair LV filling by shifting the interventricular septum leftward.[1] If fluid administration is deemed appropriate, it should be done cautiously. Patients should receive small boluses of 250 to 500 mL with assessment of response after administration. The total volume administered should generally not exceed 2 L.[1] Fluid administration in patients with an elevated CVP should be done with caution.

Determining the volume status of a critically ill patient may be difficult. Tracking CVP in patients may be helpful, although filling pressures are poorly predictive of fluid responsiveness and low filling pressures do not predict which patients will benefit from volume administration.[67] Echocardiography may be helpful in assessing RV preload. Severe RV dilation, leftward shift of the interventricular septum in systole and diastole, or a decreased TAPSE all indicate elevation of RV preload, and further volume administration should be avoided.[50] Passive leg raising, by transiently increasing RV preload, simulates volume administration. This is an easy bedside test to assess whether a patient will respond to intravenous fluids without the harms of fluid administration in those who demonstrate no improvement in cardiac output.[68] Patients who are volume overloaded should be treated with intravenous (IV) diuretics, either by bolus administration or continuous infusion to achieve a negative fluid balance. Patients who are refractory to diuretic therapy may require hemofiltration, although this technique has not been shown to offer any mortality benefit.[5]

OPTIMIZATION OF RV PRELOAD: RHYTHM CONTROL

Atrial dysrhythmias are commonly encountered in critically ill patients. In RVF, augmentation of atrial contractility is an important compensatory mechanism.[69] Given the dependence of the failing RV on atrial contraction, atrial arrhythmias can lead to severe hemodynamic compromise.[4] Rate control alone is generally inadequate to restore hemodynamic stability, as these patients have increased reliance on atrial-ventricular synchrony.[65] Treatment with beta-blockers and calcium channel blockers may be harmful due to negative inotropic effects and can further impairment of RV function.[65] Prompt electrical cardioversion should be performed in the hemodynamically unstable patient. Antiarrhythmic therapy may be necessary to maintain sinus rhythm; IV amiodarone is typically well tolerated in patients with RVF, although it has a high volume of distribution. Sotalol should be avoided in patients with structural heart disease and digoxin should be used with caution in patients with impaired renal function.[4,65] Sequential atrioventricular pacing, either by the patient's indwelling device (if present) or by placement of a transcutaneous pacing wire, is another therapeutic consideration.[4] Ventricular dysrhythmias are typically poorly tolerated and require urgent cardioversion.

REDUCTION OF RV AFTERLOAD: MINIMIZING HARMS OF MECHANICAL VENTILATION

Intubation and mechanical ventilatory support of patients with RVF should be avoided if possible. Application of positive-pressure ventilation in combination with induction agents can result in systemic hypotension leading to RV ischemia and ultimate cardiovascular collapse.[65] If intubation is required, etomidate or ketamine are thought to be the induction agents of choice, as they provide adequate anesthesia while minimizing postinduction hypotension.[3] Vasopressors should be readily available or initiated preemptively to combat postintubation hypotension.[5] The optimal sedation regimen in mechanically ventilated patients with RVF is not known. A reasonable strategy in keeping with current sedation and analgesia guidelines is to first optimize analgesia with a fentanyl infusion, which has less propensity for hypotension than benzodiazepines or propofol. In addition, opiates do not adversely affect RV function.[70,71] If additional sedation is required, this can be achieved with incremental increases of propofol or a benzodiazepine.[65]

Mechanical ventilation exposes the RV to a number of detrimental physiologic effects. Positive intrathoracic pressure decreases RV preload and stroke volume and increases RV afterload. The optimal ventilatory strategy in RVF aims to minimize the impact of these effects by avoiding high lung volumes and pressures by using a combination of increased respiratory rate and small tidal volumes.[52] The minute ventilation must remain adequate to prevent hypercapnia, which can increase PVR.[46] Clinicians must also monitor for development of "auto-PEEP (positive end-expiratory pressure)," as it will adversely affect the RV. Plateau pressures should be maintained at less than 27 cm H_2O.[52] PEEP should be titrated to optimize lung recruitment, thus minimizing the adverse effects of atelectasis, while avoiding the harms of overdistention. Patients with severe ARDS may be difficult to oxygenate with this ventilatory strategy and may derive benefit in both gas exchange and hemodynamics with prone positioning.[31,52,72]

REDUCTION OF RV AFTERLOAD: PULMONARY VASODILATORS

Because of its thin-walled, highly compliant design, the RV is exquisitely sensitive to increased afterload and may fail with even minimal increases in PVR.[1] The primary pathophysiologic disturbance in many of the most commonly encountered causes of RVF in the ICU is increased RV afterload, including ARDS, massive PE, and decompensated PAH. Additionally, many of the physiologic derangements found in the critically ill (hypoxemia, hypercarbia, and acidosis) acutely raise PVR. Consequently, reducing RV afterload by pharmacologic means is a cornerstone of therapy in RVF. Pulmonary vasodilators can be delivered either locally by inhalation or systemically by IV infusion or oral delivery.

Inhaled nitric oxide (iNO) is a selective pulmonary vasodilator frequently used in the critical care setting. Following inhalation, nitric oxide is delivered to ventilated areas of the lungs, where it causes selective pulmonary vasodilation by increasing cyclic guanosine monophosphate, improving ventilation/perfusion matching and reducing PVR.[8,73] iNO is rapidly inactivated by hemoglobin in pulmonary capillaries, so SVR is not affected.[5] It may be delivered continuously by face mask or nasal cannula, but is most commonly used in mechanically ventilated patients.[5] iNO has been demonstrated to decrease PVR in heart transplant recipients and patients with pulmonary hypertension (PH) undergoing mitral valve replacement.[74,75] A small study of critically ill patients with RVF of varying etiologies found iNO improved cardiac output and decreased PVR in 14 (54%) of 26 patients.[76] Studies of iNO in ARDS demonstrate improved oxygenation, but no improvement in clinical end points, including duration of mechanical ventilation or mortality.[77–79] Caution should be exercised when weaning iNO, as rebound pulmonary hypertension may occur.[80] Other potential adverse effects associated with iNO are methemoglobinemia, renal failure, and worsened pulmonary edema in patients with biventricular failure.[46,81,82] iNO requires a specialized delivery system and the cost can be substantial.[45]

Inhaled prostanoids offer a cost-effective alternative to iNO therapy. Prostanoids promote vasodilation through activation of cyclic adenosine monophosphate.[1] Like iNO, inhaled prostanoids improve ventilation/perfusion matching and do not cause systemic hypotension.[8,83] Unlike iNO, they do not require specialized equipment for delivery. Inhaled epoprostenol (iEPO) performed as well as iNO in reducing PVR and improving cardiac output in a randomized, crossover study of 25 transplant recipients.[84] A retrospective study comparing iNO with iEPO found similar improvements in oxygenation in 105 critically ill patients with refractory hypoxemia.[85] Beneficial effects on hemodynamics and/or oxygenation have been demonstrated with inhaled iloprost in patients with ARDS, after cardiac surgery, and after heart transplantation.[86–89]

The role of IV prostanoid therapy in chronic pulmonary hypertension is well-established, but data to guide the use of these agents for RVF in the critically ill are extremely limited. When IV pulmonary vasodilators are used, epoprostenol is the drug of choice given its short half-life (3–6 minutes).[8] IV prostanoids have several side effects, including hypotension, nausea, vomiting, headache, rebound pulmonary hypertension following abrupt discontinuation, and the potential to worsen hypoxemia due to nonselective pulmonary vasodilation.[5] These agents should be avoided in patients with respiratory failure or LV dysfunction.[8] Limited data exist supporting the use of these agents for treatment of pulmonary hypertension following cardiac surgery or heart transplantation.[90,91] Given the paucity of studies supporting their use and the side-effect profile of these medications, we feel the utility of IV prostanoids in the care of acute RVF is limited. The primary role of IV pulmonary vasodilator therapy in the ICU is in the treatment of acutely decompensated PAH and should be done so in consultation with a pulmonary hypertension specialist.[46]

Endothelin receptor antagonists, phosphodiesterase-5 inhibitors, and soluble guanylate cyclase stimulators are oral agents used in the chronic care of pulmonary arterial hypertension. Lack of data and long half-lives limit their utility in the care of acute RVF. Small, nonrandomized studies suggest sildenafil may have a role in weaning inhaled or IV pulmonary vasodilators following cardiac surgery or LVAD implantation.[92,93]

IMPROVE RV CONTRACTILITY: AVOID ISCHEMIA BY ADDRESSING SYSTEMIC HYPOTENSION

Hypotension in RVF may lead to RV ischemia and should be rapidly corrected to prevent cardiovascular collapse. RV dilation leads to increased wall stress, leaving the RV myocardium susceptible to inadequate perfusion. The ratio of PVR to SVR is critical for RV perfusion. If PVR increases beyond SVR, RV perfusion will occur only during diastole, leading to RV myocardial ischemia.[5] This condition can occur through elevations in PVR, decreases in SVR, or some combination of the two. Systemic vasopressor therapy increases SVR and improves coronary perfusion, thereby offsetting RV ischemia.[94] The ideal vasopressor in RVF increases SVR maintaining or decreasing PVR. At a minimum, vasopressors should increase SVR to a greater extent than PVR, thus maintaining a favorable PVR-to-SVR ratio.

Norepinephrine is an $\alpha 1$-adrenergic receptor agonist and $\beta 1$-adrenergic receptor agonist with potent vasoconstrictor and limited inotropic properties.[5,46] A study of patients with chronic PH with anesthesia-induced hypotension found norepinephrine improved systemic blood pressure and decreased the ratio of pulmonary artery pressure–to–systemic blood pressure without altering cardiac index.[95] Another study of 10 patients with septic shock and RV dysfunction found low to moderate doses of norepinephrine improved the RV oxygen supply/demand ratio, and improved the ratio of PVR to SVR without altering cardiac index.[96] However, high doses of norepinephrine may negatively affect the PVR-to-SVR ratio, leading to worsening of RVF.[97]

Vasopressin is a systemic vasoconstrictor with direct effects on vascular smooth muscle at the vasopressinergic (V1) receptor and increases vascular responsiveness to catecholamines.[5,98] At low doses (0.03–0.067 U/min), vasopressin may reduce PVR and the PVR-SVR ratio through a nitric oxide–mediated mechanism.[99–101] Vasopressin induces fewer tachyarrhythmias than norepinephrine, although it can lead to bradycardia at high doses.[98] Unlike norepinephrine, vasopressin does not augment cardiac contractility.

Phenylephrine is a direct $\alpha 1$ agonist with no $\beta 1$ effects.[5] It is a potent vasoconstrictor that increases SVR; however, phenylephrine may worsen RV function by increasing PVR.[98] Epinephrine has both α-receptor and β-receptor activity, thus leading to vasoconstriction and increased inotropy.[5] A study of 14 patients with septic shock and RVF found epinephrine improved RV contractility despite increasing mean pulmonary artery pressure.[102] Tachycardia and tachyarrhythmias are common side effects of epinephrine and may be detrimental in RVF.

Based on the limited available data, norepinephrine is generally used as first-line therapy in the hypotensive patient with RVF.[98] Low-dose vasopressin may be a reasonable alternative, particularly in patients with tachycardia, although this recommendation is based on the limited available data.[98] In a patient requiring high-dose norepinephrine to maintain adequate mean arterial pressures, the combination of low-dose vasopressin and norepinephrine is reasonable, although no experimental data confirm this approach.

IMPROVE RV CONTRACTILITY: USE OF INOTROPES

Positive inotropic agents increase the force of myocardial contraction by increasing the force-velocity relationship of cardiac myocytes. Positive inotropes alter SVR,

PVR, and cardiac output. There are 2 primary classes of positive inotropes: the sympathomimetic inotropes, which include dopamine, epinephrine, and dobutamine, and the inodilators, which include phosphodiesterase (PDE) 3 inhibitors and levosimendan. Although commonly used in the critically ill patient, none of these agents has been shown to improve outcomes, and data exist suggesting increased mortality.

Dopamine is a dopaminergic and adrenergic agonist that increases both SVR and cardiac output.[46] Studies demonstrate variable effects of dopamine on the PVR-to-SVR ratio.[96,103,104] Dopamine typically produces significant tachycardia, which may adversely affect LV preload and precipitate RV ischemia.[46] A recent randomized control trial comparing dopamine with norepinephrine found dopamine increased the risk for arrhythmia and worsened mortality in the subgroup of patients with cardiogenic shock.[105]

Dobutamine exerts inotropic effects via the β1 receptor, and variable vasodilatory effects through β2 receptor stimulation.[5] At doses up to 5 μg/kg per minute, dobutamine increases cardiac contractility and reduces PVR and SVR.[98] Higher doses increase myocardial oxygen demand due to tachycardia, and fail to reduce PVR.[8] Use of dobutamine may cause hypotension requiring use of vasopressors, due to β2-mediated systemic vasodilation.[98]

Milrinone, a PDE-3 inhibitor, increases inotropy and causes vasodilation of both the systemic and pulmonary vasculature. Milrinone has been demonstrated to reduce pulmonary pressures and improve RV function in LV systolic heart failure, after cardiac transplantation, and after ventricular assist device implantation.[106–108] Like dobutamine, milrinone often induces systemic hypotension, necessitating the use of vasopressors. The combination of milrinone with vasopressin may be superior to norepinephrine in reducing the PVR-to-SVR ratio.[101]

Levosimendan sensitizes troponin-c to intracellular calcium, increasing contractility without affecting oxygen consumption.[8] The drug also acts as a vasodilator through calcium desensitization and PDE-3 inhibition.[98] Levosimendan reduces PVR and increases cardiac output.[8] Studies have demonstrated clinical improvement in the setting of RV infarction, ARDS, and after cardiac surgery.[109–111] This medication is not currently available for use in the United States.

In the absence of systemic hypotension, milrinone is the inotrope of choice in patients with RVF requiring inotropic support. If dobutamine is used, low-dose therapy is preferred so as to avoid tachycardia and increased myocardial oxygen demand.[98] Use of dopamine should generally be avoided in RVF because of the risk of tachycardia and data demonstrating increased mortality in cardiogenic shock.[98] Clinicians should anticipate the need to use concurrent vasopressor therapy with either milrinone or dobutamine.

MECHANICAL SUPPORT

In cases in which cardiogenic shock persists despite maximal medical therapy, mechanical support of the RV should be entertained. Mechanical support includes intra-aortic balloon pump counterpulsation (IABP), venoarterial extracorporeal membrane oxygenation (VA-ECMO), and RV assist devices (RVADs), and should only be used in carefully selected patients. Each of these therapies provides hemodynamic support in the acute setting, allowing for resolution of a potentially reversible process, definitive treatment of the underlying etiology, or bridging to a more permanent form of support.

IABP, while not directly unloading the RV, augments coronary artery blood flow, decreases myocardial oxygen demand, reduces LV afterload, and increases cardiac output.[112] Although these effects may benefit patients with RVF due to LV failure, the amount of support is limited.[112] IABP is considered the first line of mechanical support, as it is readily available and may be inserted either at bedside or in a cardiac catheterization laboratory.

In patients requiring full cardiac support, VA-ECMO and RVADs may be considered. VA-ECMO removes blood from the venous system, passes it through a pump head and oxygenator, and returns it to the arterial system, thus providing support of both the cardiac and respiratory systems.[42] Cannulation can be either via the femoral vessels or by direct cannulation of the right atrium and pulmonary artery. VA-ECMO does not fully offload the LV and, depending on the cannulation configuration, may reduce circulation to the pulmonary vessels. VA-ECMO is temporary support only, allowing for either resolution of the underlying process or determination of more permanent mechanical support. VA-ECMO is the mechanical support mode of choice in conditions resulting in severely elevated PVR, such as PAH and massive PE.[1]

Patients with refractory cardiogenic shock or end-stage heart failure may be supported by ventricular assist devices (VADs). Current-generation VADs are continuous-flow axial or centrifugal pumps designed for long-term support of the LV. Most patients require isolated LVAD support, although RVF after LVAD implantation is frequent and a leading cause of morbidity and mortality in this population. RVAD support may be temporary or long-term, although currently there is not a continuous-flow VAD that is approved by the Food and Drug Administration for RV support. There is increasing experience with the Heart Ware ventricular assist system (VAS) (Heart-Ware Inc, Framingham, MA, USA) in a biventricular configuration in patients awaiting cardiac transplantation. For patients ineligible for transplantation, permanent mechanical support of the RV should not be considered. RVADs should be avoided in the setting of significantly elevated PVR, as the increased flow of blood from the RVAD into the pulmonary circulation will lead to severely elevated pulmonary pressures and lung injury without effectively increasing cardiac output.[113]

TARGETED MANAGEMENT FOR SPECIFIC ETIOLOGIES OF RV FAILURE

We have described general management considerations for critically ill patients with RVF. **Table 2** provides a management "checklist" for providers caring for patients with RVF. In the next section, we briefly review specifics of targeted therapy for 3 specific causes of RVF: decompensated PAH, massive PE, and RV infarction.

DECOMPENSATED PAH

RVF secondary to decompensated PAH is a challenging disorder to manage with high associated mortality.[5] In the past 2 decades, significant progress has been made in treatment of PAH, including the development of 4 new classes of medications providing targeted treatment of PAH. Registry data indicate that patients affected with PAH live longer than before, likely due to improved management strategies.[114] Given an expanding population of patients actively treated with pulmonary vasodilator therapy, intensivists are increasingly likely to encounter patients with PAH in the ICU. Understanding of the nuances of management of this population is important, for many of the typical strategies used in a patient presenting with shock will be detrimental when applied to a decompensated patient with PAH.

Management of decompensated PAH is complex. Likely precipitating factors, such as PE, infection, or arrhythmia, should be actively sought out, as their presence will impact clinical management. Timely, aggressive therapy to restore adequate perfusion and prevent multiorgan system failure is required in decompensated PAH.

Table 2 Management of RVF checklist	
Management Consideration	**Comments**
Does this patient have RVF?	• TTE as initial screening test • TEE may be required if TTE is inadequate • Consider RHC to better define hemodynamics if echocardiography is suggestive
Has the cause of RVF been identified and appropriate treatment initiated?	• Anticoagulation and consideration of thrombolysis vs catheter-directed therapy vs surgical embolectomy for massive PE • Reperfusion if acute RV infarct • Appropriate treatment of left heart failure • Antibiotics and source control in sepsis • If decompensated chronic RVF, rule out PE, systemic infection, arrhythmia
Has RV preload been optimized?	• Avoid fluids if severe RV dilation on TTE • Judicious use of fluids if felt to be volume responsive • Most will be volume overloaded and require diuresis vs hemofiltration
Is the patient in sinus rhythm?	• Rate control is inadequate • Consider anti-arrhythmics (amiodarone) and cardioversion to restore sinus rhythm • Consider AV pacing if medications and cardioversion fail
Has RV afterload been minimized?	• Correct, hypoxia, hypercarbia, and acidosis • Minimize adverse effects of mechanical ventilation (plateau pressures <27; minimal PEEP; low tidal volumes) • Consider pulmonary vasodilators
Has RV contractility been optimized?	• Consider milrinone or low-dose dobutamine to augment contractility • Treat hypotension to maintain coronary perfusion • Norepinephrine is first-line vasopressor • Low-dose vasopressin is a reasonable choice as well
Has this patient failed medical therapy for RVF?	• Consider mechanical support

Abbreviations: AV, atrioventricular; PE, pulmonary embolism; PEEP, positive end-expiratory pressure; RHC, right heart catheterization; RV, right ventricular; RVF, RV failure; TEE, transesophageal echocardiography; TTE, transthoracic echocardiography.

Volume status is a key consideration in decompensated disease and is often assessed and managed incorrectly. In the setting of hypotension, the patients are generally volume overloaded. Fluid loading can be detrimental and precipitate cardiovascular collapse. Continuous IV diuretics and often continuous renal replacement therapy are required for fluid removal.[65] Prerenal acute kidney injury is common and often reversed with restoration of adequate perfusion achieved by diuresis and titration of pulmonary vasodilators. A combination of continuous IV diuretics and pressors is frequently necessary to restore adequate cardiac output. Focused TTE can rapidly confirm RV volume overload. RHC is used commonly to guide therapy and provides vital information, including cardiac output, filling pressures, and pulmonary artery pressures, thus allowing the clinicians to assess response to interventions.

Reduction of RV afterload with pulmonary vasodilator therapy is essential. IV prostanoids are the first-line therapy for treatment of decompensated PAH. Initial dosage and choice of prostanoid should take into consideration prior PAH therapy. Common dose-dependent side effects of prostanoid therapy are hypotension, headache, nausea, vomiting, and diarrhea.[46] Inhaled pulmonary vasodilators can be used in combination with IV therapy and will not worsen systemic hypotension.[65] New initiation of oral therapies is typically avoided in the critically ill patient with acute RVF, given their long half-life and ability to cause similar side effects to prostanoids. Titration of preexisting oral medications depends on a specific clinical situation. Patients with chronic PAH on IV vasodilator therapy who develop distributive shock may require dose adjustment to avoid high-output failure and systemic hypotension.[5] Consultation with a pulmonary hypertension specialist should be sought and interhospital transfer to an experienced center facilitated when appropriate.

MASSIVE PE

Ten percent of diagnosed cases of PE meet the definition of massive PE.[115] All patients with massive PE should be anticoagulated, barring contraindications. IV unfractionated heparin is typically used in massive PE, as this the preferred agent in patients receiving fibrinolytics or undergoing embolectomy.[116] In patients with suspected massive PE without prohibitive bleeding risk, heparin should be started immediately, rather than waiting for confirmatory testing.[117] Multidetector CT (MDCT) is the most commonly used diagnostic method. If PE is confirmed and the patient is hypotensive, current guidelines suggest thrombolytic therapy should be administered if bleeding risk is acceptable.[117] If hemodynamic instability precludes MDCT, TTE can be performed to assess for evidence of RV dilation.[115] If RV dilation is confirmed, European guidelines suggest consideration of thrombolysis.[118] Very limited randomized controlled trial data on the use of thrombolytic therapy in hypotensive patients exist. Jerjes-Sanchez and colleagues[119] compared heparin plus streptokinase to heparin alone in massive PE. The study was terminated after enrollment of only 4 patients to each arm for ethical reasons. All patients receiving streptokinase lived, whereas all patients in the heparin-only arm died. A meta-analysis of 5 studies that included patients with massive PE concluded that thrombolytic therapy reduces the risk of death or recurrent PE when compared with heparin alone.[120] Recent data suggest that "low-dose" recombinant tissue-type plasminogen activator, the recommended thrombolytic agent, may be as effective as standard doses with decreased risk of bleeding.[121] Supportive care with vasopressors, inhaled pulmonary vasodilators, inotropes, and optimization of volume status should be provided while awaiting hemodynamic improvement following thrombolytic therapy.

For patients with massive PE who have contraindications to thrombolysis, have failed thrombolysis, or who are expected to die from shock before thrombolysis can take effect, the American College of Chest Physicians guidelines recommend consideration of catheter-assisted thrombus removal or surgical embolectomy.[117] No large-scale studies validating catheter-based therapies have been performed, but available studies suggest hemodynamic stability can be restored in 86.5% of patients.[21] Surgical embolectomy was traditionally associated with high mortality rates, although recent studies using modern anesthesia and surgical techniques suggest in-hospital mortality rates as low as 5% to 6%.[122]

RV INFARCTION

The clinical presentation of RV infarction can vary widely, ranging from no hemodynamic effect to severe cardiogenic shock.[123] It is estimated that 25% to 50% of RV infarcts are hemodynamically significant.[123] Classic physical examination findings are hypotension, jugular venous distention, and clear lungs.[124] RV infarct should be entertained in all patients presenting with inferior ST-elevation myocardial infarction, the typical setting for RV infarction.[124] Larger ST elevations in lead III than in lead II are pathognomonic for RV infarct.[125] ST-elevations in right-sided precordial leads (RV1 through RV6) can be seen as well.[125] TTE reveals a dilated hypokinetic RV and preserved LV function.[123]

Restoration of coronary blood flow is critical when treating RV infarction. This is best accomplished with percutaneous coronary intervention.[126] Studies have demonstrated that successful revascularization is associated with RV recovery, decreased risk for ventricular arrhythmia, and excellent clinical outcomes.[123] Unsuccessful revascularization is associated with poor recovery of RV function and high mortality.[123] While awaiting revascularization, efforts focus on stabilization of hemodynamics. Diuretics and nitrates should be avoided, as they can precipitate significant hypotension. Traditionally, volume loading has been the initial therapy for correction of hypotension following RV infarction, as it was thought to improve RV preload, correct hypotension, and improve cardiac output.[126] Several studies have called this practice into question, reporting that volume loading did not improve cardiac output.[127–129] The disparate results seen in studies are likely due to variability in volume status of patients at the time of presentation. Invasive monitoring is recommended to aid clinicians in volume assessment. Exceeding a RAP or pulmonary capillary wedge pressure of 20 mm Hg is not recommended.[123] In patients with persistent shock after optimization of preload, inotropes are indicated. Dobutamine has been demonstrated to improve cardiac output and RV ejection fraction in RV infarction.[128] In patients with refractory shock despite maximal medical therapy, mechanical support with IABP or RVAD may be beneficial.[128]

SUMMARY

RVF is associated with a number of commonly encountered conditions in critically ill patients. Understanding the pathophysiology of the failing RV is essential to development of an appropriate treatment plan. Medical therapies focus on correction of the underlying cause, optimization of RV preload, and contractility and reduction of RV afterload. Mechanical support is an option for select patients who fail medical management. Given the prevalence of RVF and its association with poor outcomes, further study on optimal therapeutic strategies is warranted.

REFERENCES

1. Green EM, Givertz MM. Management of acute right ventricular failure in the intensive care unit. Curr Heart Fail Rep 2012;9:228–35.
2. Cecconi M, Johnston E, Rhodes A. What role does the right side of the heart play in circulation? Crit Care 2006;10(Suppl 3):S5.
3. Vandenheuvel MA, Bouchez S, Wouters PF, et al. A pathophysiological approach towards right ventricular function and failure. Eur J Anaesthesiol 2013;30:386–94.
4. Haddad F, Hunt SA, Rosenthal DN, et al. Right ventricular function in cardiovascular disease, part I: anatomy, physiology, aging, and functional assessment of the right ventricle. Circulation 2008;117:1436–48.
5. Poor HD, Ventetuolo CE. Pulmonary hypertension in the intensive care unit. Prog Cardiovasc Dis 2012;55:187–98.
6. Yamaguchi S, Harasawa H, Li KS, et al. Comparative significance in systolic ventricular interaction. Cardiovasc Res 1991;25:774–83.
7. McDonald MA, Ross HJ. Trying to succeed when the right ventricle fails. Curr Opin Cardiol 2009;24:239–45.

8. Lahm T, McCaslin CA, Wozniak TC, et al. Medical and surgical treatment of acute right ventricular failure. J Am Coll Cardiol 2010;56:1435–46.
9. Greyson C, Xu Y, Lu L, et al. Right ventricular pressure and dilation during pressure overload determine dysfunction after pressure overload. Am J Physiol Heart Circ Physiol 2000;278:H1414–20.
10. Ghio S, Gavazzi A, Campana C, et al. Independent and additive prognostic value of right ventricular systolic function and pulmonary artery pressure in patients with chronic heart failure. J Am Coll Cardiol 2001;37:183–8.
11. Polak JF, Holman BL, Wynne J, et al. Right ventricular ejection fraction: an indicator of increased mortality in patients with congestive heart failure associated with coronary artery disease. J Am Coll Cardiol 1983;2:217–24.
12. de Groote P, Millaire A, Foucher-Hossein C, et al. Right ventricular ejection fraction is an independent predictor of survival in patients with moderate heart failure. J Am Coll Cardiol 1998;32:948–54.
13. Juilliere Y, Barbier G, Feldmann L, et al. Additional predictive value of both left and right ventricular ejection fractions on long-term survival in idiopathic dilated cardiomyopathy. Eur Heart J 1997;18:276–80.
14. Davila-Roman VG, Waggoner AD, Hopkins WE, et al. Right ventricular dysfunction in low output syndrome after cardiac operations: assessment by transesophageal echocardiography. Ann Thorac Surg 1995;60:1081–6.
15. Haddad F, Fisher P, Pham M, et al. Right ventricular dysfunction predicts poor outcome following hemodynamically compromising rejection. J Heart Lung Transplant 2009;28:312–9.
16. Reichert CL, Visser CA, van den Brink RB, et al. Prognostic value of biventricular function in hypotensive patients after cardiac surgery as assessed by transesophageal echocardiography. J Cardiothorac Vasc Anesth 1992;6:429–32.
17. Matthews JC, Koelling TM, Pagani FD, et al. The right ventricular failure risk score: a pre-operative tool for assessing the risk of right ventricular failure in left ventricular assist device candidates. J Am Coll Cardiol 2008;51:2163–72.
18. Dang NC, Topkara VK, Mercando M, et al. Right heart failure after left ventricular assist device implantation in patients with chronic congestive heart failure. J Heart Lung Transplant 2006;25:1–6.
19. Kavarana MN, Pessin-Minsley MS, Urtecho J, et al. Right ventricular dysfunction and organ failure in left ventricular assist device recipients: a continuing problem. Ann Thorac Surg 2002;73:745–50.
20. Kaul TK, Fields BL. Postoperative acute refractory right ventricular failure: incidence, pathogenesis, management and prognosis. Cardiovasc Surg 2000;8:1–9.
21. Todoran TM, Sobieszczyk P. Catheter-based therapies for massive pulmonary embolism. Prog Cardiovasc Dis 2010;52:429–37.
22. Kimchi A, Ellrodt AG, Berman DS, et al. Right ventricular performance in septic shock: a combined radionuclide and hemodynamic study. J Am Coll Cardiol 1984;4:945–51.
23. Pulido JN, Afessa B, Masaki M, et al. Clinical spectrum, frequency, and significance of myocardial dysfunction in severe sepsis and septic shock. Mayo Clin Proc 2012;87:620–8.
24. Furian T, Aguiar C, Prado K, et al. Ventricular dysfunction and dilation in severe sepsis and septic shock: relation to endothelial function and mortality. J Crit Care 2012;27:319.e9–15.
25. Dhainaut JF, Lanore JJ, de Gournay JM, et al. Right ventricular dysfunction in patients with septic shock. Intensive Care Med 1988;14(Suppl 2):488–91.

26. Vincent JL, Reuse C, Frank N, et al. Right ventricular dysfunction in septic shock: assessment by measurements of right ventricular ejection fraction using the thermodilution technique. Acta Anaesthesiol Scand 1989;33:34–8.
27. Vieillard Baron A, Schmitt JM, Beauchet A, et al. Early preload adaptation in septic shock? A transesophageal echocardiographic study. Anesthesiology 2001;94:400–6.
28. Huang SJ, Nalos M, McLean AS. Is early ventricular dysfunction or dilatation associated with lower mortality rate in adult severe sepsis and septic shock? A meta-analysis. Crit Care 2013;17:R96.
29. Vieillard-Baron A, Schmitt JM, Augarde R, et al. Acute cor pulmonale in acute respiratory distress syndrome submitted to protective ventilation: incidence, clinical implications, and prognosis. Crit Care Med 2001;29:1551–5.
30. Page B, Vieillard-Baron A, Beauchet A, et al. Low stretch ventilation strategy in acute respiratory distress syndrome: eight years of clinical experience in a single center. Crit Care Med 2003;31:765–9.
31. Vieillard-Baron A, Charron C, Caille V, et al. Prone positioning unloads the right ventricle in severe ARDS. Chest 2007;132:1440–6.
32. Osman D, Monnet X, Castelain V, et al. Incidence and prognostic value of right ventricular failure in acute respiratory distress syndrome. Intensive Care Med 2009;35:69–76.
33. Mahjoub Y, Pila C, Friggeri A, et al. Assessing fluid responsiveness in critically ill patients: false-positive pulse pressure variation is detected by Doppler echocardiographic evaluation of the right ventricle. Crit Care Med 2009;37:2570–5.
34. Fougeres E, Teboul JL, Richard C, et al. Hemodynamic impact of a positive end-expiratory pressure setting in acute respiratory distress syndrome: importance of the volume status. Crit Care Med 2010;38:802–7.
35. Bull TM, Clark B, McFann K, et al. Pulmonary vascular dysfunction is associated with poor outcomes in patients with acute lung injury. Am J Respir Crit Care Med 2010;182:1123–8.
36. Brown SM, Pittman J, Miller Iii RR, et al. Right and left heart failure in severe H1N1 influenza A infection. Eur Respir J 2011;37:112–8.
37. Mekontso Dessap A, Boissier F, Leon R, et al. Prevalence and prognosis of shunting across patent foramen ovale during acute respiratory distress syndrome. Crit Care Med 2010;38:1786–92.
38. Jardin F, Gueret P, Dubourg O, et al. Two-dimensional echocardiographic evaluation of right ventricular size and contractility in acute respiratory failure. Crit Care Med 1985;13:952–6.
39. Monchi M, Bellenfant F, Cariou A, et al. Early predictive factors of survival in the acute respiratory distress syndrome. A multivariate analysis. Am J Respir Crit Care Med 1998;158:1076–81.
40. Gayat E, Mebazaa A. Pulmonary hypertension in critical care. Curr Opin Crit Care 2011;17:439–48.
41. Ventilation with lower tidal volumes as compared with traditional tidal volumes for acute lung injury and the acute respiratory distress syndrome. The Acute Respiratory Distress Syndrome Network. N Engl J Med 2000;342:1301–8.
42. Simon MA. Assessment and treatment of right ventricular failure. Nat Rev Cardiol 2013;10:204–18.
43. Christenson RH. What is the value of B-type natriuretic peptide testing for diagnosis, prognosis or monitoring of critically ill adult patients in intensive care? Clin Chem Lab Med 2008;46:1524–32.

44. Nagaya N, Nishikimi T, Okano Y, et al. Plasma brain natriuretic peptide levels increase in proportion to the extent of right ventricular dysfunction in pulmonary hypertension. J Am Coll Cardiol 1998;31:202–8.
45. Woods J, Monteiro P, Rhodes A. Right ventricular dysfunction. Curr Opin Crit Care 2007;13:532–40.
46. Zamanian RT, Haddad F, Doyle RL, et al. Management strategies for patients with pulmonary hypertension in the intensive care unit. Crit Care Med 2007; 35:2037–50.
47. Vanni S, Polidori G, Vergara R, et al. Prognostic value of ECG among patients with acute pulmonary embolism and normal blood pressure. Am J Med 2009; 122:257–64.
48. Mayo PH, Beaulieu Y, Doelken P, et al. American College of Chest Physicians/La Societe de Reanimation de Langue Francaise statement on competence in critical care ultrasonography. Chest 2009;135:1050–60.
49. Rudski LG, Lai WW, Afilalo J, et al. Guidelines for the echocardiographic assessment of the right heart in adults: a report from the American Society of Echocardiography endorsed by the European Association of Echocardiography, a registered branch of the European Society of Cardiology, and the Canadian Society of Echocardiography. J Am Soc Echocardiogr 2010;23:685–713 [quiz: 786–8].
50. Vieillard-Baron A. Assessment of right ventricular function. Curr Opin Crit Care 2009;15:254–60.
51. Mitoff PR, Beauchesne L, Dick AJ, et al. Imaging the failing right ventricle. Curr Opin Cardiol 2012;27:148–53.
52. Repesse X, Charron C, Vieillard-Baron A. Right ventricular failure in acute lung injury and acute respiratory distress syndrome. Minerva Anestesiol 2012;78: 941–8.
53. Laursen CB, Sloth E, Lambrechtsen J, et al. Focused sonography of the heart, lungs, and deep veins identifies missed life-threatening conditions in admitted patients with acute respiratory symptoms. Chest 2013;144:1868–75.
54. Harvey S, Harrison DA, Singer M, et al. Assessment of the clinical effectiveness of pulmonary artery catheters in management of patients in intensive care (PAC-Man): a randomised controlled trial. Lancet 2005;366:472–7.
55. Sandham JD, Hull RD, Brant RF, et al. A randomized, controlled trial of the use of pulmonary-artery catheters in high-risk surgical patients. N Engl J Med 2003; 348:5–14.
56. National Heart, Lung, and Blood Institute Acute Respiratory Distress Syndrome (ARDS) Clinical Trials Network, Wheeler AP, Bernard GR, et al. Pulmonary-artery versus central venous catheter to guide treatment of acute lung injury. N Engl J Med 2006;354:2213–24.
57. Binanay C, Califf RM, Hasselblad V, et al. Evaluation study of congestive heart failure and pulmonary artery catheterization effectiveness: the ESCAPE trial. JAMA 2005;294:1625–33.
58. Hoeper MM, Lee SH, Voswinckel R, et al. Complications of right heart catheterization procedures in patients with pulmonary hypertension in experienced centers. J Am Coll Cardiol 2006;48:2546–52.
59. Alhashemi JA, Cecconi M, Hofer CK. Cardiac output monitoring: an integrative perspective. Crit Care 2011;15:214.
60. Roberts DH, Lepore JJ, Maroo A, et al. Oxygen therapy improves cardiac index and pulmonary vascular resistance in patients with pulmonary hypertension. Chest 2001;120:1547–55.

61. Moloney ED, Evans TW. Pathophysiology and pharmacological treatment of pulmonary hypertension in acute respiratory distress syndrome. Eur Respir J 2003; 21:720–7.

62. Stengl M, Ledvinova L, Chvojka J, et al. Effects of clinically relevant acute hypercapnic and metabolic acidosis on the cardiovascular system: an experimental porcine study. Crit Care 2013;17:R303.

63. Retter A, Wyncoll D, Pearse R, et al. Guidelines on the management of anaemia and red cell transfusion in adult critically ill patients. Br J Haematol 2013;160:445–64.

64. Mercat A, Diehl JL, Meyer G, et al. Hemodynamic effects of fluid loading in acute massive pulmonary embolism. Crit Care Med 1999;27:540–4.

65. Hoeper MM, Granton J. Intensive care unit management of patients with severe pulmonary hypertension and right heart failure. Am J Respir Crit Care Med 2011; 184:1114–24.

66. Piazza G, Goldhaber SZ. The acutely decompensated right ventricle: pathways for diagnosis and management. Chest 2005;128:1836–52.

67. Marik PE, Cavallazzi R. Does the central venous pressure predict fluid responsiveness? An updated meta-analysis and a plea for some common sense. Crit Care Med 2013;41:1774–81.

68. Monnet X, Rienzo M, Osman D, et al. Passive leg raising predicts fluid responsiveness in the critically ill. Crit Care Med 2006;34:1402–7.

69. Goldstein JA, Tweddell JS, Barzilai B, et al. Right atrial ischemia exacerbates hemodynamic compromise associated with experimental right ventricular dysfunction. J Am Coll Cardiol 1991;18:1564–72.

70. Barr J, Fraser GL, Puntillo K, et al. Clinical practice guidelines for the management of pain, agitation, and delirium in adult patients in the intensive care unit. Crit Care Med 2013;41:263–306.

71. Forrest P. Anaesthesia and right ventricular failure. Anaesth Intensive Care 2009; 37:370–85.

72. Guerin C, Reignier J, Richard JC, et al. Prone positioning in severe acute respiratory distress syndrome. N Engl J Med 2013;368:2159–68.

73. Abman SH. Inhaled nitric oxide for the treatment of pulmonary arterial hypertension. Handb Exp Pharmacol 2013;218:257–76.

74. Ardehali A, Hughes K, Sadeghi A, et al. Inhaled nitric oxide for pulmonary hypertension after heart transplantation. Transplantation 2001;72:638–41.

75. Fattouch K, Sbraga F, Bianco G, et al. Inhaled prostacyclin, nitric oxide, and nitroprusside in pulmonary hypertension after mitral valve replacement. J Card Surg 2005;20:171–6.

76. Bhorade S, Christenson J, O'Connor M, et al. Response to inhaled nitric oxide in patients with acute right heart syndrome. Am J Respir Crit Care Med 1999;159:571–9.

77. Michael JR, Barton RG, Saffle JR, et al. Inhaled nitric oxide versus conventional therapy: effect on oxygenation in ARDS. Am J Respir Crit Care Med 1998;157: 1372–80.

78. Lundin S, Mang H, Smithies M, et al. Inhalation of nitric oxide in acute lung injury: results of a European multicentre study. The European Study Group of Inhaled Nitric Oxide. Intensive Care Med 1999;25:911–9.

79. Taylor RW, Zimmerman JL, Dellinger RP, et al. Low-dose inhaled nitric oxide in patients with acute lung injury: a randomized controlled trial. JAMA 2004;291: 1603–9.

80. Christenson J, Lavoie A, O'Connor M, et al. The incidence and pathogenesis of cardiopulmonary deterioration after abrupt withdrawal of inhaled nitric oxide. Am J Respir Crit Care Med 2000;161:1443–9.

81. Loh E, Stamler JS, Hare JM, et al. Cardiovascular effects of inhaled nitric oxide in patients with left ventricular dysfunction. Circulation 1994;90:2780–5.
82. Afshari A, Brok J, Moller AM, et al. Inhaled nitric oxide for acute respiratory distress syndrome and acute lung injury in adults and children: a systematic review with meta-analysis and trial sequential analysis. Anesth Analg 2011;112: 1411–21.
83. Walmrath D, Schermuly R, Pilch J, et al. Effects of inhaled versus intravenous vasodilators in experimental pulmonary hypertension. Eur Respir J 1997;10: 1084–92.
84. Khan TA, Schnickel G, Ross D, et al. A prospective, randomized, crossover pilot study of inhaled nitric oxide versus inhaled prostacyclin in heart transplant and lung transplant recipients. J Thorac Cardiovasc Surg 2009;138: 1417–24.
85. Torbic H, Szumita PM, Anger KE, et al. Inhaled epoprostenol vs inhaled nitric oxide for refractory hypoxemia in critically ill patients. J Crit Care 2013;28:844–8.
86. Sawheny E, Ellis AL, Kinasewitz GT. Iloprost improves gas exchange in patients with pulmonary hypertension and ARDS. Chest 2013;144:55–62.
87. Winterhalter M, Simon A, Fischer S, et al. Comparison of inhaled iloprost and nitric oxide in patients with pulmonary hypertension during weaning from cardiopulmonary bypass in cardiac surgery: a prospective randomized trial. J Cardiothorac Vasc Anesth 2008;22:406–13.
88. Rex S, Schaelte G, Metzelder S, et al. Inhaled iloprost to control pulmonary artery hypertension in patients undergoing mitral valve surgery: a prospective, randomized-controlled trial. Acta Anaesthesiol Scand 2008;52:65–72.
89. Theodoraki K, Tsiapras D, Tsourelis L, et al. Inhaled iloprost in eight heart transplant recipients presenting with post-bypass acute right ventricular dysfunction. Acta Anaesthesiol Scand 2006;50:1213–7.
90. Ocal A, Kiris I, Erdinc M, et al. Efficiency of prostacyclin in the treatment of protamine-mediated right ventricular failure and acute pulmonary hypertension. Tohoku J Exp Med 2005;207:51–8.
91. Schmid ER, Burki C, Engel MH, et al. Inhaled nitric oxide versus intravenous vasodilators in severe pulmonary hypertension after cardiac surgery. Anesth Analg 1999;89:1108–15.
92. Trachte AL, Lobato EB, Urdaneta F, et al. Oral sildenafil reduces pulmonary hypertension after cardiac surgery. Ann Thorac Surg 2005;79:194–7 [discussion: 194–7].
93. Klodell CT Jr, Morey TE, Lobato EB, et al. Effect of sildenafil on pulmonary artery pressure, systemic pressure, and nitric oxide utilization in patients with left ventricular assist devices. Ann Thorac Surg 2007;83:68–71 [discussion: 71].
94. Vlahakes GJ, Turley K, Hoffman JI. The pathophysiology of failure in acute right ventricular hypertension: hemodynamic and biochemical correlations. Circulation 1981;63:87–95.
95. Kwak YL, Lee CS, Park YH, et al. The effect of phenylephrine and norepinephrine in patients with chronic pulmonary hypertension*. Anaesthesia 2002;57: 9–14.
96. Schreuder WO, Schneider AJ, Groeneveld AB, et al. Effect of dopamine vs norepinephrine on hemodynamics in septic shock. Emphasis on right ventricular performance. Chest 1989;95:1282–8.
97. Morelli A, Ertmer C, Rehberg S, et al. Continuous terlipressin versus vasopressin infusion in septic shock (TERLIVAP): a randomized, controlled pilot study. Crit Care 2009;13:R130.

98. Price LC, Wort SJ, Finney SJ, et al. Pulmonary vascular and right ventricular dysfunction in adult critical care: current and emerging options for management: a systematic literature review. Crit Care 2010;14:R169.
99. Evora PR, Pearson PJ, Schaff HV. Arginine vasopressin induces endothelium-dependent vasodilatation of the pulmonary artery. V1-receptor-mediated production of nitric oxide. Chest 1993;103:1241–5.
100. Tayama E, Ueda T, Shojima T, et al. Arginine vasopressin is an ideal drug after cardiac surgery for the management of low systemic vascular resistant hypotension concomitant with pulmonary hypertension. Interact Cardiovasc Thorac Surg 2007;6:715–9.
101. Jeon Y, Ryu JH, Lim YJ, et al. Comparative hemodynamic effects of vasopressin and norepinephrine after milrinone-induced hypotension in off-pump coronary artery bypass surgical patients. Eur J Cardiothorac Surg 2006;29:952–6.
102. Le Tulzo Y, Seguin P, Gacouin A, et al. Effects of epinephrine on right ventricular function in patients with severe septic shock and right ventricular failure: a preliminary descriptive study. Intensive Care Med 1997;23:664–70.
103. Holloway EL, Polumbo RA, Harrison DC. Acute circulatory effects of dopamine in patients with pulmonary hypertension. Br Heart J 1975;37:482–5.
104. Leier CV, Heban PT, Huss P, et al. Comparative systemic and regional hemodynamic effects of dopamine and dobutamine in patients with cardiomyopathic heart failure. Circulation 1978;58:466–75.
105. De Backer D, Biston P, Devriendt J, et al. Comparison of dopamine and norepinephrine in the treatment of shock. N Engl J Med 2010;362:779–89.
106. Oztekin I, Yazici S, Oztekin DS, et al. Effects of low-dose milrinone on weaning from cardiopulmonary bypass and after in patients with mitral stenosis and pulmonary hypertension. Yakugaku Zasshi 2007;127:375–83.
107. Kihara S, Kawai A, Fukuda T, et al. Effects of milrinone for right ventricular failure after left ventricular assist device implantation. Heart Vessels 2002;16:69–71.
108. Eichhorn EJ, Konstam MA, Weiland DS, et al. Differential effects of milrinone and dobutamine on right ventricular preload, afterload and systolic performance in congestive heart failure secondary to ischemic or idiopathic dilated cardiomyopathy. Am J Cardiol 1987;60:1329–33.
109. Russ MA, Prondzinsky R, Carter JM, et al. Right ventricular function in myocardial infarction complicated by cardiogenic shock: improvement with levosimendan. Crit Care Med 2009;37:3017–23.
110. Morelli A, Teboul JL, Maggiore SM, et al. Effects of levosimendan on right ventricular afterload in patients with acute respiratory distress syndrome: a pilot study. Crit Care Med 2006;34:2287–93.
111. Cicekcioglu F, Parlar AI, Ersoy O, et al. Levosimendan and severe pulmonary hypertension during open heart surgery. Gen Thorac Cardiovasc Surg 2008; 56:563–5.
112. Boeken U, Feindt P, Litmathe J, et al. Intraaortic balloon pumping in patients with right ventricular insufficiency after cardiac surgery: parameters to predict failure of IABP Support. Thorac Cardiovasc Surg 2009;57:324–8.
113. Berman M, Tsui S, Vuylsteke A, et al. Life-threatening right ventricular failure in pulmonary hypertension: RVAD or ECMO? J Heart Lung Transplant 2008;27:1188–9.
114. Benza RL, Miller DP, Barst RJ, et al. An evaluation of long-term survival from time of diagnosis in pulmonary arterial hypertension from the REVEAL Registry. Chest 2012;142:448–56.
115. Vyas PA, Donato AA. Thrombolysis in acute pulmonary thromboembolism. South Med J 2012;105:560–70.

116. Piazza G, Goldhaber SZ. Fibrinolysis for acute pulmonary embolism. Vasc Med 2010;15:419–28.
117. Kearon C, Akl EA, Comerota AJ, et al. Antithrombotic therapy for VTE disease: antithrombotic therapy and prevention of thrombosis, 9th ed: American College of Chest Physicians evidence-based clinical practice guidelines. Chest 2012; 141:e419S–94S.
118. Torbicki A, Perrier A, Konstantinides S, et al. Guidelines on the diagnosis and management of acute pulmonary embolism: the Task Force for the Diagnosis and Management of Acute Pulmonary Embolism of the European Society of Cardiology (ESC). Eur Heart J 2008;29:2276–315.
119. Jerjes-Sanchez C, Ramirez-Rivera A, de Lourdes Garcia M, et al. Streptokinase and heparin versus heparin alone in massive pulmonary embolism: a randomized controlled trial. J Thromb Thrombolysis 1995;2:227–9.
120. Wan S, Quinlan DJ, Agnelli G, et al. Thrombolysis compared with heparin for the initial treatment of pulmonary embolism: a meta-analysis of the randomized controlled trials. Circulation 2004;110:744–9.
121. Zhang Z, Zhai ZG, Liang LR, et al. Lower dosage of recombinant tissue-type plasminogen activator (rt-PA) in the treatment of acute pulmonary embolism: a systematic review and meta-analysis. Thromb Res 2013;133(3):357–63.
122. He C, Von Segesser LK, Kappetein PA, et al. Acute pulmonary embolectomy. Eur J Cardiothorac Surg 2013;43:1087–95.
123. Ondrus T, Kanovsky J, Novotny T, et al. Right ventricular myocardial infarction: from pathophysiology to prognosis. Exp Clin Cardiol 2013;18:27–30.
124. Kinch JW, Ryan TJ. Right ventricular infarction. N Engl J Med 1994;330:1211–7.
125. Moye S, Carney MF, Holstege C, et al. The electrocardiogram in right ventricular myocardial infarction. Am J Emerg Med 2005;23:793–9.
126. Inohara T, Kohsaka S, Fukuda K, et al. The challenges in the management of right ventricular infarction. Eur Heart J Acute Cardiovasc Care 2013;2:226–34.
127. Shah PK, Maddahi J, Berman DS, et al. Scintigraphically detected predominant right ventricular dysfunction in acute myocardial infarction: clinical and hemodynamic correlates and implications for therapy and prognosis. J Am Coll Cardiol 1985;6:1264–72.
128. Dell'Italia LJ, Starling MR, Blumhardt R, et al. Comparative effects of volume loading, dobutamine, and nitroprusside in patients with predominant right ventricular infarction. Circulation 1985;72:1327–35.
129. Siniorakis EE, Nikolaou NI, Sarantopoulos CD, et al. Volume loading in predominant right ventricular infarction: bedside haemodynamics using rapid response thermistors. Eur Heart J 1994;15:1340–7.

Cardiothoracic Surgical Emergencies in the Intensive Care Unit

 CrossMark

Jessica Mitchell, MD[a],*, Linda Bogar, MD[b,c], Nelson Burton, MD[c]

KEYWORDS

- Cardiothoracic surgical emergencies • Operative intervention
- Collaborative team approach • ICU

KEY POINTS

- Patients with cardiothoracic surgical emergencies are frequently admitted to the ICU, either prior to operative intervention or after surgery.
- Recognition and appropriate timing of operative intervention are key factors in improving outcomes.
- A collaborative team approach with the cardiothoracic service is imperative in managing this patient population.

INTRODUCTION

Patients with cardiothoracic surgical emergencies are frequently admitted to the ICU, either prior to operative intervention or after surgery. Intensivists must be able to recognize and manage the medical aspects of cardiothoracic surgical emergencies, and know when to involve the cardiothoracic surgical team. This article covers common cardiothoracic surgical emergencies that require emergent intervention, the indications for surgery, and methods of acute stabilization of patients prior to operative intervention.

GREAT VESSEL PATHOLOGY
Thoracic Aortic Dissection

Acute aortic dissection, and the closely related entities of penetrating aortic ulcer and intramural hematoma, is a true life-threatening emergency. In the seminal work published by Hirst and colleagues[1] in 1958, they reported a 1% to 2% per hour mortality

[a] Department of Critical Care Medicine, Cooper University Hospital, 1 Cooper Plaza, Camden, NJ 08103, USA; [b] Inova Fairfax Hospital, 3300 Gallows Road, Falls Church, VA 22042, USA; [c] Cardiac Vascular & Thoracic Surgery Associates, Inova Fairfax Hospital, 2921 Telestar Court, Falls Church, VA 22042, USA
* Corresponding author.
E-mail address: mitchell-jessica@cooperhealth.edu

Crit Care Clin 30 (2014) 499–525
http://dx.doi.org/10.1016/j.ccc.2014.03.004
0749-0704/14/$ – see front matter © 2014 Elsevier Inc. All rights reserved.

rate early after symptom onset from an ascending aortic aneurysm. In the era prior to modern management of acute aortic dissection, it is estimated via autopsy series that 40% to 50% of patients with dissection of the proximal aorta died within 48 hours.[1] Death results from either frank exsanguination due to aortic rupture, pericardial tamponade, myocardial ischemia due to coronary dissection, or malperfusion to the brain, gut, kidney or spinal cord. In the modern era, patients with proximal ascending dissections who rapidly undergo surgery in experienced tertiary centers have a 30-day survival rate of 80% to 85%.[2] Patients with dissection of the descending aorta treated with aggressive antihypertensive therapy have a 30-day survival rate greater than 90%.[2]

The incidence of aortic dissection remains difficult to ascertain, because acute dissection often results in sudden death that may be attributed to another process. Population-based studies have estimated an incidence of 2 to 3.5 cases per 100,000 person-years, correlating with 6000 to 10,000 cases annually in the United States.[3] The International Registry of Acute Aortic Dissection (IRAD) was established in 1996 to help overcome small numbers in single-center registries and to promote further investigation of acute aortic dissection. It currently comprises 30 large referral centers in 11 different countries. Data from IRAD published in 2000 showed a mean age at presentation of 63 years, with a 65% male predominance.[4]

The aortic wall is composed of 3 tissue layers: the intima, which is continuous with the vessel lumen; the media; and the adventitia. Aortic dissection is defined as disruption of the media layer of the aorta with bleeding within and along the wall of the aorta, resulting in separation of the layers of the aorta. In a majority of patients, an intimal tear can be identified that results in pressurized blood cleaving a dissection plane within the media. The separation of the layers of the aorta results in the creation of 2 aortic lumens, the false lumen and the true lumen, with a septum, or intimal flap, separating the 2 lumens. The true lumen remains surrounded by intima, whereas the false lumen is surrounded by the intimal-medial dissection flap and a weak media-adventitial outer wall. The weakened false lumen may rupture externally or internally, may extend either anterograde down the aorta or retrograde back toward the aortic valve, or may thrombose over time.[2,5] Although on noninvasive imaging 15% of patients have an apparent intramural hematoma without evidence of an intimal tear, on autopsy only 4% are found to have no visible intimal tear (**Fig. 1**).[3]

Aortic dissection most commonly occurs in patients with a previously dilated or damaged aorta. Hypertension is the most common predisposing factor in 72% of patients, followed by atherosclerosis (31%), history of cardiac surgery (18%), Marfan syndrome (5%), and iatrogenic causes (4%).[4,6] Other predisposing factors are listed in **Box 1**.

Accurate classification of aortic dissection is important because it drives decisions regarding surgical versus nonsurgical management. The 2 most commonly used classification systems are the DeBakey and Stanford systems. For purposes of classification, ascending aorta is proximal to the brachiocephalic artery and descending aorta is distal to the left subclavian artery.

DeBakey Classification System
   Type I: Dissection originates in ascending aorta and propagates distally to include at least the aortic arch and typically the descending aorta.
   Type II: Dissection originates in and is confined to the ascending aorta.
   Type III: Dissection originates in the descending aorta and propagates most often distally.
      IIIa: Limited to the descending thoracic aorta

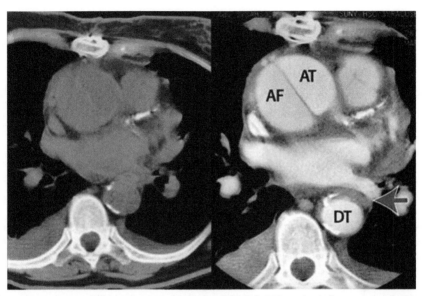

Fig. 1. Noncontrast (*left*) and contrast-enhanced (*right*) CT imaging of type A aortic dissection. *Arrow* points at descending false lumen. AF, ascending false lumen; AT, ascending true lumen; DT, descending true lumen. (*From* Tintinalli JE, Stapczynski JS, Ma OJ, et al, editors. Tintinalli's emergency medicine: a comprehensive study guide. 7th edition. New York: McGraw-Hill; 2011. p. 622–4; with permission.)

Box 1
Predisposing factors for aortic dissection
Hypertension
Atherosclerosis
History of cardiac surgery
Marfan syndrome
Trauma
Cocaine use
Pregnancy
Turner syndrome
Bicuspid aortic valve
Coarctation of the aorta
Tetralogy of Fallot
Syphilis
Aortitis
Behçet disease
Giant cell arteritis

IIIb: Extending below the diaphragm
Stanford Classification System
  Type A: All dissections involving the ascending aorta regardless of the site of
    origin
  Type B: All dissections that do not involve the ascending aorta (**Fig. 2**)

Surgery is usually recommended for DeBakey type I and type II dissections and in Stanford type A dissections. Regardless of classification system used, surgery is generally indicated for all dissections involving the ascending aorta, whereas dissections of the descending aorta are generally medically managed.[3]

Aortic dissection may also be classified as acute, subacute, or chronic depending on the amount of time from onset of symptoms to presentation. Acute dissection is defined as occurring within 2 weeks of onset of pain, subacute as between 2 and 6 weeks of onset, and chronic as more than 6 weeks from onset. This article focuses on acute presentations of aortic dissection.[3]

Acute aortic dissection remains a diagnostic dilemma for providers, because it is a rare cause of commonly encountered chief complaints of chest, abdominal, and back pain. It is estimated that coronary artery disease (CAD) is 100 to 200 times more common than aortic dissection and that there are an estimated 3 aortic dissections for every 100 patients presenting to an emergency department (ED) with chest pain and/or back pain.[7] Presentation often varies; chest pain is the most commonly

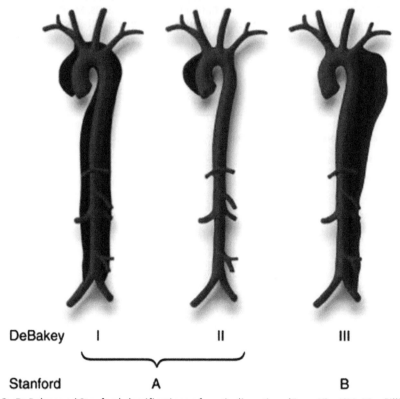

DeBakey   I   II   III

Stanford   A   B

Fig. 2. DeBakey and Stanford classifications of aortic dissection. (*From* Kim KM, MacGillivray TE. The management of acute aortic dissection. In: Cameron JL, Cameron AM. Current Surgical Therapy, Eleventh Edition. Philadelphia: Elsevier/Saunders, 2014; with permission.)

reported symptom but may be absent in up to 25% of presentations. For further signs and symptoms of acute aortic dissection, see **Table 1**.[4]

Due to the variation in presentation and diagnostic uncertainties, it is estimated that the diagnosis of aortic dissection may be missed, misdiagnosed, or substantially delayed in up to 40% of cases.[8] ECG may be normal (31.3%) or have nonspecific ST segment or T wave changes (41.4%). Chest radiography may show a widened mediastinum (61.6%) or may be entirely normal (12.4%).[4] Other diagnostic strategies are being explored, including the use of D-dimer assay to identify patients with acute aortic dissection. A recent meta-analysis shows that plasma D-dimer assay of less than 500 ng/mL has a good negative likelihood ratio (0.06; 95% CI, 0.03–0.12) for diagnosis of acute aortic dissection but limited positive likelihood ratio (2.43; 95% CI, 1.89–3.12). Plasma D-dimer assay may help rule out acute aortic dissection, but its use is limited currently and further studies are needed to confirm its utility.[9]

Due to its widespread availability, CT scanning (with and without contrast) is often the imaging modality used to diagnose acute aortic dissection. CT has been shown to have 92% accuracy for diagnosing abnormalities of the thoracic aorta.[3] MRI has been shown to have similar sensitivity to CT but is used less frequently due to access and timing limitations.[3] Echocardiography can also be used to visualize the thoracic aorta and its major branches. Transthoracic echocardiography (TTE) has a sensitivity of 77% to 80% and specificity of 93% to 96% for diagnosis of proximal aortic dissection. Transesophageal echocardiography has a superior sensitivity of 88% to 98% with a specificity of 90% to 95%. Advantages include portability, rapid imaging time, lack of IV contrast, and radiation.[3] The advantage of CT to cardiac surgeons is the availability to also view the anatomy of the axillary and femoral arteries for deciding on cannulation sites for cardiopulmonary bypass (CPB). Angiography was the historic gold standard for diagnosis of aortic dissection and provides accurate information about the site of dissection, branch artery involvement, and communication between true and false lumens. More recently, angiography is largely being replaced by CT,

Table 1	
Presenting signs and symptoms of acute aortic dissection (Hagan)	
Location of pain	
Chest	>75%
Back	53.2%
Abdomen	29.6%
Descriptors of pain	
Sudden onset	84.4%
Severe	90.6%
Sharp	64.4%
Ripping/tearing	50.6%
Blood pressure	
Hypertensive	49%
Normotensive	34.6%
Hypotensive	16.4%
Aortic insufficiency murmur	31.6%
Pulse deficit	15.1%
Stroke	4.7%
Heart failure	6.6%

MRI, and transesophogeal echocardiogram (TEE) as the first-line test for diagnosis of acute aortic syndrome. This is due to concerns regarding its availability, the invasiveness of the procedure, and exposure to dye. Another downside of angiography is the potential for false-negative results with intramural hematoma or a thrombosed false lumen, and reported sensitivities and specificities for angiography are slightly lower than those for the other less-invasive modalities.[3]

The 2010 guidelines on thoracic aortic disease published by the American Heart Association (AHA) and the American College of Cardiology (ACC) give the following level 1 recommendations:

- Urgent surgical consultation should be obtained for all patients diagnosed with thoracic aortic dissection regardless of the anatomic location (ascending vs descending) as soon as a diagnosis is made or highly suspected (level of evidence: C).
- Acute thoracic aortic dissection involving the ascending aorta should be urgently evaluated for emergent surgical repair because of the high risk of associated life-threatening complications, such as rupture (level of evidence: B).
- Acute thoracic aortic dissection involving the descending aorta should be managed medically unless life-threatening complications develop (eg, malperfusion syndrome, progression of dissection, enlarging aneurysm, and inability to control blood pressure or symptoms) (level of evidence: B).

Initial management strategies in the ICU should focus on prevention of propagation of the false lumen by controlling the amount of aortic shear stress. Aortic wall stress is affected by the velocity of ventricular contraction (dP/dt), the rate of contraction, and blood pressure. β-Blockade helps control these 3 parameters. Titratable IV agents are preferred. Labetalol, with both α- and β-receptor antagonism, may work as a single agent to control both heart rate and blood pressure. Esmolol, with an extremely short half-life, may be appropriate for patients in whom it is unsure if they can tolerate β-blockade. Vasodilators are frequently used as an adjunct agent for blood pressure control. IV sodium nitroprusside is the most established agent, with other alternatives, including nicardipine and nitroglycerin. Use of a vasodilator without β-blockade is not recommended because reflex tachycardia may result in greater aortic wall stress. Reasonable initial goal parameters are a heart rate less than 60 beats per minute and a systolic blood pressure between 100 and 120 mm Hg.[3] Therapy should be initiated while patients are evaluated for possible surgical or endovascular intervention.

Acute ascending aortic dissection has a mortality of 1% to 2% per hour during the first 24 to 48 hours of presentation. Medical management alone is associated with mortality of approximately 20% at 24 hours, 30% by 48 hours, and 50% at 1 week.[10] The main principles of acute ascending aortic dissection surgery are resection of the primary intimal tear with stabilization of the aortic wall. This prevents rupture, stopping end-organ malperfusion syndromes.[5] In patients who develop aortic valve incompetence, restoration of aortic valve competence should be attempted by either resuspension of the native aortic valve or by aortic valve replacement.[10] The aortic arch is dissected in more than 70% of acute ascending aortic dissections and dilatation or obstruction of supra-aortic vessels is common. Possible interventions include tissue adhesive, proximal arch or hemiarch procedure, total arch replacement, trifurcated graft procedure, or frozen elephant trunk procedure.[5] Endovascular repair of descending aortic dissection has been performed since the late 1990s and has increasingly become the standard of care for many types of descending aortic dissections.[5,11,12] Investigation is ongoing to see if endovascular techniques may have a role in ascending aortic dissection.[5]

Current estimates of in-hospital and early mortality in acute ascending aortic dissection range from 15% to 32% in surgically treated patients, whereas medically managed patients have an overall in-hospital mortality of 56% to 58%. Recent studies have demonstrated long-term survival in surgically treated patients ranging from 96% to 97.6% at 1 year to 88.3% to 90.5% at 3 years (**Fig. 3**).[13]

Controversy exists about surgical intervention on elderly patients. A recent registry trial showed that octogenarians (ages 80–89) with uncomplicated ascending thoracic aortic dissection treated with emergency surgery had early and midterm outcomes close to their younger counterparts. Acute ascending aortic dissection complicated by cerebrovascular accident (CVA), paraplegia, coma, visceral ischemia, and CPR, however, in the octogenarian group were associated with poor outcomes.[14] Similarly, there has been controversy over management strategy for patients who present with an acute ascending aortic dissection and major brain injury. A recent study published from the IRAD group showed that nearly 1 of 10 ascending thoracic aortic dissection cases are complicated by brain injury, resulting in 2- to 3-fold increase in mortality. Surgery, as opposed to medical therapy, seemed to be associated with better early and late outcomes, and brain injury reversal occurred in 84.3% of patients with CVA and 78.8% of patients with coma.[15]

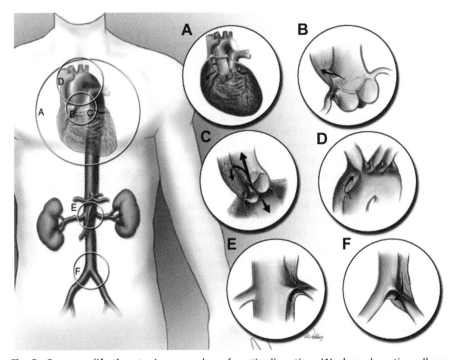

Fig. 3. Common life-threatening sequelae of aortic dissection. Weakened aortic wall can rupture at any location and often results in fatal exsanguination. Rupture of ascending aorta into pericardial space (*A*) causes cardiac tamponade. Aortic dissection can lead to acute cardiac failure via (*B*) extension into coronary ostia, causing myocardial ischemia, and (*C*) disruption of aortic valve commissures, causing valvular insufficiency. Complications of branch vessel malperfusion include (*D*) stroke or upper-extremity ischemia when brachio-cephalic branches are involved, paraplegia when segmental intercostal and lumbar arteries are compromised, (*E*) renal failure or mesenteric ischemia when visceral vessels are disrupted, and (*F*) lower-limb ischemia when iliac arteries are occluded. (*From* Creager MA, Beckman JA, Loscalzo J. Vascular medicine: a companion to Braunwald's Heart Disease. Second Edition. Philadelphia: Elsevier/Saunders, 2013; with permission.)

Brain protection strategies to prevent stroke and preserve cognitive function are a key element of the surgical, anesthetic, and perfusion techniques used to accomplish repairs of the ascending aorta and transverse aortic arch (class 1B recommendation).[3] Deep hypothermic circulatory arrest, selective antegrade brain perfusion, and retrograde brain perfusion are available techniques for brain protection. Monitoring of brain function and metabolic suppression by electroencephalography, evoked potentials, bispectral index, transcranial Doppler, noninvasive cerebral oximetry, and jugular bulb oxyhemoglobin saturation are additional methods used to guide extracorporeal circulation interruption during repair of the ascending aorta. Data are limited to suggest one strategy over another at this time.[3,16] Ideal management strategies for acute ascending aortic dissection remain an active area of research and practice is likely to change in the future.

Penetrating Aortic Ulcer and Intramural Hematoma

Acute aortic syndrome is a term that encompasses the related conditions of aortic dissection, intramural hematoma, and penetrating atherosclerotic ulcer. These disease processes have similar presentation, diagnostic testing, and management. Intramural hematoma is a contained hemorrhage within the aortic layers in the absence of a clearly detectable intimal tear. It originates from ruptured vasa vasorum followed by an aortic wall infarction. This may weaken and rupture and progress to a classic acute aortic dissection.[17] Penetrating aortic ulcer is a focal atherosclerotic lesion that ulcerates and disrupts the internal elastic lamina of the aortic wall. Complications can include progression to intramural hematoma, pseudoaneurysm formation, and progression to acute aortic dissection with a propensity to rupture. Although acute ascending aortic dissection has a 7% risk of rupture, penetrating aortic ulcer has an up to 40% risk of rupture.[18] In the absence of randomized clinical trials, the level of evidence in treatment of penetrating aortic ulcer is low.[10] General indications for urgent surgical intervention include rapid increase in aortic diameter, hemodynamic instability, recurrent or refractory pain, presence of a pleural effusion, presence of intramural hematoma, and maximum ulcer diameter of 2.1 cm or depth of 1.3 cm. Ulcerations of the descending thoracic aorta may be amenable to endograft repair with coverage of the ulceration, particularly in patients who are not good candidates for an open procedure.[17,18] Differentiation of penetrating aortic ulcer, intramural hematoma, and acute aortic dissection may be difficult. Regardless of which process is present, surgical evaluation is warranted and should be sought emergently, especially for intramural hematoma or penetrating aortic ulcer involving the ascending aorta (**Fig. 4**).[10,17,18]

VALVULAR PATHOLOGY
Acute Severe Mitral Regurgitation

In acute severe mitral regurgitation, sudden volume overload is imposed on the left atrium. This increase in left ventricular (LV) preload, in the absence of ventricular dilatation and remodeling, results in inadequate forward stroke volume and cardiac output.[19] This results in the clinical picture of pulmonary edema, hypotension, and, possibly, cardiogenic shock. A new pansystolic murmur is best auscultated at the apex with radiation to the axilla. This murmur may be absent due to poor LV systolic function and elevated left atrial pressure.[20] Pulmonary artery (PA) catheterization may reveal a prominent V wave, although these may also be seen in ventricular septal rupture or severe LV failure.[21]

When considering acute mitral regurgitation, it is important to remember the distinction between organic and functional causes of regurgitation. Organic causes include

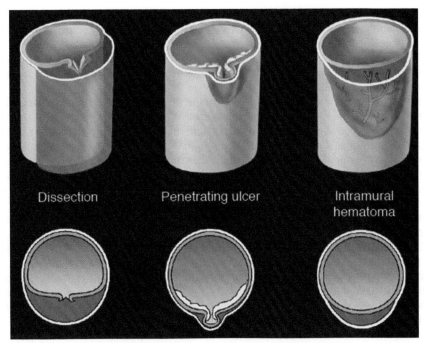

Fig. 4. Variants of aortic dissection: classic aortic dissection versus penetrating ulcer versus intramural hematoma. (*From* Elefteriades JA. Thoracic aortic aneurysm: reading the enemy's playbook. Curr Probl Cardiol 2008;33:203–77; with permission.)

leaflet perforation, chordal or papillary muscle rupture, and prosthetic valve dysfunction due to endocarditis or perivalvular leak. Functional causes of mitral regurgitation result from abnormalities of the LV and are generally chronic. Acute changes to the structure of the LV can occur with acute myocardial infarction (AMI), Takotsubo cardiomyopathy, and peripartum cardiomyopathy, which may result in functional mitral regurgitation. Organic causes of acute mitral regurgitation frequently require surgical repair or valve replacement, whereas a majority of functional causes improve after medical management of the underlying disease process.[22] This article focuses on an acute organic cause of mitral regurgitation, specifically mitral valve papillary rupture.

Acute Mitral Valve Papillary Muscle Rupture

The most common cause of mitral valve papillary muscle rupture is AMI. Rupture secondary to infarction is recognized as a life-threatening complication with a poor prognosis.[23,24] In the era of percutaneous coronary intervention (PCI) for AMI, papillary muscle rupture occurs in only 0.25% of patients after myocardial infarction (MI) and it represents the reason 7% of patients are in cardiogenic shock after an AMI.[25] Traditionally, it is thought to occur 2 to 7 days post-MI, but the SHOCK [Should we emergently revascularize occluded coronaries for cardiogenic shock trial] registry showed a median time of 12.8 hours to onset of shock in the setting of acute mitral regurgitation.[20,24,26] Patients presenting with inferior infarcts are at the highest risk of papillary muscle ischemia and subsequent rupture because the posteromedial papillary muscle receives its blood supply from the posterior descending artery, whereas the anterolateral papillary muscle receives dual blood supply from the left anterior descending (LAD) and the left circumflex coronary artery.[20]

Electrocardiogram and chest radiography should be obtained, although changes are generally nonspecific. The diagnostic test of choice is echocardiogram with color-flow Doppler. TTE should demonstrate severe mitral regurgitation; however, a TEE may be needed to for more definitive assessment of valve anatomy and pathology.[19,20] TTE initial diagnostic sensitivity is 65% to 85% compared with TEE's diagnostic sensitivity of 95% to 100% (**Fig. 5**).[27]

In acute papillary muscle rupture, medical therapy has a limited role and should be aimed at hemodynamic stabilization prior to surgery. The goal is to diminish the degree of regurgitant flow, augment forward output, and reduce pulmonary congestion. Nitroprusside provides afterload reduction, helps maintain forward cardiac output, and may partially restore MV competence as LV size diminishes. In patients whose hemodynamics do not tolerate a vasodilator, intra-aortic balloon counterpulsation (IABP) increases forward output and mean arterial pressure. IABP also decreases mechanical afterload, thereby decreasing regurgitant volume and LV filling pressure.[19] Medical management only of post-MI acute mitral regurgitation due to papillary muscle rupture is associated with 80% to 90% mortality.[24]

Both European Society of Cardiology (ESC) and AHA/ACC guidelines recommend urgent surgery in patients with papillary muscle rupture.[19,28] Mitral valve repair is preferred to replacement, but often papillary muscle rupture results in valve replacement due to technical considerations.[19,28] A recent study showed no statistically significant difference in mortality between MV repair and replacement.[29] This series of 54 patients with papillary muscle rupture post-MI showed an operative mortality of 18.5%. In patients who had operations after 1990 in conjunction with coronary artery bypass grafting (CABG), operative mortality decreased to 8.7%. Patients who need MV repair should have coronary resvascularization if it is needed. Overall 5-year survival was 65%, and survival free of congestive heart failure was 52%.[29] Other recent

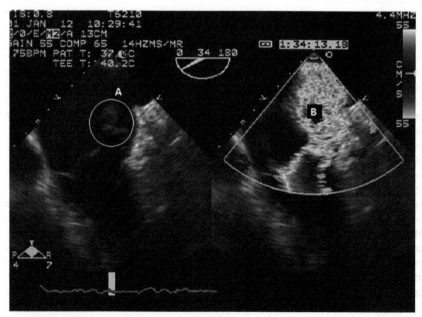

Fig. 5. Papillary muscle rupture with acute severe mitral regurgitation. TEE showing papillary muscle rupture (*A*) and resultant severe mitral valve regurgitation on color Doppler (*B*). (*Courtesy of* P. Peters, MD, Camden, New Jersey.)

studies have shown a 30-day mortality rate after mitral valve surgery due to ischemic papillary muscle rupture as high as 39.3%. In this trial, predictors of mortality included low cardiac output, renal failure, and implementation of extracorporeal membrane oxygenation therapy (ECMO).[30]

Severe Acute Aortic Regurgitation

Severe acute aortic regurgitation (AR) is a surgical emergency. Although medical management may provide temporizing measures, predicted mortality from pulmonary edema, ventricular arrhythmias, electromechanical dissociation, or circulatory collapse is upward of 75% without surgical intervention.[19,28,31–33] Acute severe AR is most commonly caused by infective endocarditis or ascending aortic dissection, although it may also be seen with traumatic rupture of the valve or rupture of a fenestrated aortic cusp in the setting of systemic hypertension[32] or in the setting of prosthetic valve with dehiscence.

With chronic AR, the LV responds to the increased end-diastolic volume with LV enlargement and hypertrophy, resulting in an increase in chamber compliance with little or no increase in LV end-diastolic pressure. In acute severe AR, the LV does not have time to compensate for the increase in LV end diastolic volume; LV end-diastolic pressure rises and the LV subsequently is shifted to a less compliant portion of the pressure-volume curve.

Echocardiography is the key to diagnosis of acute severe AR. It is used to confirm the presence and severity of valvular regurgitation and helps determine the cause of valvular dysfunction. It may also help determine the presence of rapid equilibration of aortic and LV diastolic pressure. This is supported by the echocardiographic findings of a short AR diastolic half time (less than 300 ms), a short mitral deceleration time (less than 150 ms), or premature closure of the mitral valve. TEE may help further demonstrate the mechanism of AR if not evident on the TTE.[19,34]

Both ESC and AHA guidelines recommend urgent/emergent surgical intervention for acute severe AR.[19,28] Patients with acute severe AR who are treated medically have a mortality rate of up to 75%, as opposed to surgical therapy, which reduces mortality to 25%.[33] Medical therapy should be used as a bridge to surgical therapy. Vasodilators, such as nitroprusside, are used to increase forward flow but also can worsen hypotension. Inotropic agents, such as dobutamine, are used to increase cardiac output and forward flow. IABP is contraindicated because it increases regurgitant flow through the incompetent valve. β-Blockers are contraindicated because they block compensatory tachycardia and could lead to cardiovascular collapse. In patients with severe acute AR due to endocarditis, surgery should not be delayed regardless of infection status and duration of antibiotic therapy.[19,34]

Aortic Root Abscess

Infective endocarditis is a common diagnosis in the ICU setting. Extension of infective endocarditis beyond the valve annulus with abscess formation predicts a higher mortality rate. Periannular extension is common and occurs in 10% to 40% of all native valve endocarditis and in 56% to 100% of prosthetic valve endocarditis. In aortic valve endocarditis, the weakest portion of the annulus is near the membranous septum and atrioventricular node and abscesses commonly form in this location (**Fig. 6**). Perivalvular abscesses are more common with prosthetic valves because the annulus is the usual primary site of infection. Under systemic intravascular pressures, abscesses may progress to form fistula tracts and create intracardiac or pericardial shunts.[35]

Patients at risk for perivalvular extension of infective endocarditis require prompt evaluation. Persistent bacteremia or fever, recurrent emboli, heart block, congestive

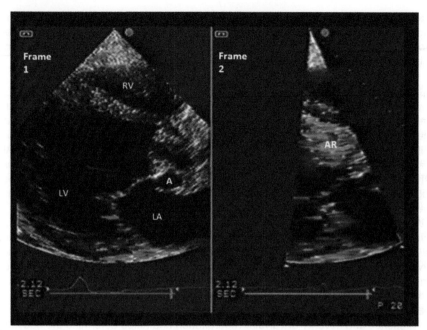

Fig. 6. Aortic root abscess. (*Frame 1*) Transthoracic parasternal long axis view of aortic root abscess (A) and surrounding inflammation. LA, left atrium; RV, right ventricle. (*Frame 2*) Color Doppler demonstrates severe AR. (*Courtesy of* P. Peters, MD, Camden, New Jersey.)

heart failure, or a new pathologic murmur in a patient on appropriate antibiotics suggest uncontrolled infection and the possible need for surgical therapy. A new atrioventricular block on ECG has a positive predictive value of 88% for abscess formation but a low sensitivity (45%).[35]

Evaluation of perivalvular extension of disease should be performed with echocardiography. The sensitivity of TTE for detecting perivalvular abscess is only 18% to 63% in prospective and retrospective studies. The use of TEE dramatically increases sensitivity (76%–100%) with excellent specificity (95%). With color Doppler techniques, the structural anatomy of the abscess and/or fistula may be assessed. TEE is the modality of choice to assess for perivalvular extension of infective endocarditis.[35]

Once an aortic root abscess is detected, urgent surgery is required, because antibiotic therapy alone is inadequate to control the infection. If an aortic root abscess is not treated, most patients progress to death due to heart failure or sepsis.[36] Both AHA and ESC guidelines give a 1B recommendation for surgical management of perivalvular abscess, fistula, or penetrating valvular lesions.[19,37] Delay in surgical intervention leads to greater destruction of the aortic root, resulting in LV-aortic discontinuity and more complicated surgical repair.[38] Depending on the extent of the abscess formation and the structures involved, these cases may be technically difficult to manage. Débridement of all infected and necrotic tissue is the mainstay of treatment. Reconstruction of the annulus involves patching the defect with either autologous or bovine pericardium followed by valve replacement or reconstruction of the entire annulus and valve with a cadaveric aortic homograft.

Reported operative mortality rates for infective endocarditis with paravalvular abscesses vary from 3.7% to 31%. Outcomes are worse in patients with prosthetic valve endocarditis as opposed to native valve endocarditis. Patients with sepsis or renal failure or requiring concomitant CABG are at higher risk of poor outcomes. Recent studies have suggested that early surgery in active endocarditis with complications, such as paravalvular abscess, leads to better outcomes.[39]

CORONARY ARTERY PATHOLOGY

The mortality rate due to CAD has declined steadily over the past half century.[40] Both a reduction in incidence and improvements in treatment seem responsible for this trend.[40] Since the introduction of CABG in 1968 and PCI in 1977 as treatment of revascularization in the setting of coronary CAD, there has been debate about the ideal method of revascularization. The goals of revascularization are both to improve overall survival and to relieve symptoms. As of 2011, there were 26 randomized controlled trials (RCTs) published comparing CABG and PCI, with further studies continuing to be published on both perioperative survival and long-term outcomes.[41]

A majority of recent interest has been focused on the areas of intervention for left main CAD, triple-vessel CAD, and CAD in diabetic patients. Large RCTs, such as SYNTAX, continue to show higher repeat revascularization rates with PCI than with CABG, even when drug-eluting stents are used. There was no significant difference between death or MI, and stroke was more likely to occur with CABG in the SYNTAX trial.[42] The FREEDOM trial addressed multivessel disease in patients with diabetes and showed a decrease in all-cause mortality and MI but again an increase in stroke with CABG.[43] Both trials looked at quality-of-life postintervention and found that CABG patients experienced greater relief of angina symptoms, albeit small.[44,45] This remains an active area of investigation and guidelines continue to change based on the best evidence available.

In certain populations, the indications for emergent CABG remain clear.

2011 American College of Cardiology Foundation (ACCF)/AHA guidelines class 1 recommendations for emergent CABG from the (level of evidence: B, unless otherwise stated):
- AMI with primary PCI failure or inability to perform PCI
- Coronary artery anatomy is suitable for CABG
- Persistent ischemia of a significant area of myocardium at rest
- Hemodynamic instability refractory to nonsurgical management
- Patients already undergoing surgical repair of a postinfarction mechanical complication of MI (ventricular septal rupture, papillary muscle rupture, or free wall rupture)
- Cardiogenic shock
- Life-threatening ventricular arrhythmias thought to be ischemic in origin in the presence of left main stenosis greater than or equal to 50% and/or 3-vessel CAD (level of evidence: C)[41]

Failed PCI of Culprit Lesion in AMI

Many technologic and pharmacologic advances have been made in PCI since its introduction in 1977. With the improvements in PCI, the need for emergency CABG in the setting of failure PCI has been decreasing. A review of prospective registry data from the Mayo Clinic defining indications for emergency CABG found that the need for emergency CABG decreased from 2.9% in the prestent era to 0.3% in the current era.[46] The indications for emergent CABG in that study include abrupt vessel closure, extensive coronary artery dissection, incomplete revascularization, coronary perforation, unsuccessful dilation, or other situations resulting in hemodynamic instability. A review at Cleveland Clinic showed a similar trend, with emergency CABG occurring in 1.5% of PCIs in 1992 to 0.14% in 2000.[47]

2011 ACCF/AHA guidelines for emergency CABG after failed PCI:
- Ongoing ischemia or threatened occlusion with substantial myocardium at risk (1B)
- Hemodynamic compromise after failed PCI in patients without impairment of the coagulation system and without a previous sternotomy (1B)
- Retrieval of foreign body (eg, fractured guide wire or stent, in a crucial anatomic location [class 2a level C])
- Hemodynamic compromise after failed PCI with impairment of the coagulation system and without previous sternotomy (class 2a level C)
- Hemodynamic compromise after failed PCI with previous sternotomy (class 2b level C)
- Emergency CABG should not be performed after failed PCI in the absence of ischemia or threatened occlusion (class 3 level C)
- Emergency CABG should not be performed after failed PCI if revascularization is impossible due to target anatomy or a no-reflow state (class 3 level C)[41]

Subjects most likely to require emergency CABG after failed PCI include those with evolving ST-segment elevation myocardial infarciton (STEMI), cardiogenic shock, 3-vessel CAD, or the presence of a type C coronary arterial lesion. A type C coronary lesion is defined as greater than 2 cm in length, an excessively tortuous proximal segment, an extremely angulated segment, a total occlusion greater than 3 months in duration, or a degenerated saphenous vein graft that appears to be friable. Variables that predict increased perioperative morbidity and mortality include depressed LV systolic function, recent acute coronary syndrome, multivessel CAD and complex lesion morphology, cardiogenic shock, advanced age, absence of angiographic collaterals, previous PCI, and a prolonged time of delay in transfer to an operating room (OR).[41]

Despite the reduction in need for emergency CABG in the setting of PCI, in-hospital mortality rates remain higher than patients undergoing a planned procedure at 10% to 15%.[46,47] If complete revascularization is achieved with minimal delay after failure of PCI, long-term prognosis is similar to that of patients undergoing elective CABG.[41]

Coronary Artery Dissection

Coronary artery dissection is a rare cause of acute coronary syndrome and possible sudden death. Coronary artery dissection may be spontaneous, the result of extension of an aortic root dissection, iatrogenic during coronary angiography, and the result of chest trauma. The dissection may be between the intima and media or media and adventitia and results in creation of a false lumen. Hemorrhage or thrombus in the false lumen may result in compression of the true lumen of the coronary artery, resulting in partial or full occlusion with subsequent myocardial ischemia.[48]

Spontaneous coronary artery dissection affects a young, often otherwise healthy, population. A recently published series of 87 patients showed an 82% female predominance with a mean age of onset of 42.6 years; 18% of women affected were postpartum. STEMI was the initial presentation in one-half of patients, whereas others presented with non-STEMI/unstable angina and 14% experienced a ventricular arrhythmia requiring emergent defibrillation. The LAD was the most commonly affected artery; however, multivessel coronary dissection was present in 23% of patients.[49] Past studies have shown a higher incidence of peripartum status. Other associations with spontaneous coronary artery dissection exist with cocaine abuse, hypertension, collagen disorders, vasculitis, mild coronary atherosclerosis, smoking, oral contraceptives, extreme exertion, and fibromuscular dysplasia,[48–50] although the true etiology remains unclear. Retrospective registry studies have shown an incidence of spontaneous coronary artery dissection in 0.07% to 1.1% of all coronary angiograms performed[48,49]; 1 in 5 women, but no men, experienced a recurrence in spontaneous coronary artery dissection during long-term follow-up.[49]

There are no specific guidelines for management of patients with spontaneous coronary artery dissection. Hemodynamically stable patients may have successful medical management, with therapy similar to the treatment of acute coronary syndrome.[48] PCI with stenting of the lesion can be therapeutic, although Tweet and colleagues[49] reported PCI complicated by technical failure in 35% of patients. CABG may be used, particularly in unstable patients, or in patients with dissections of the left main or with no obvious intimal tear, or in which tandem stenting is not possible. The goal of CABG for spontaneous coronary artery dissection should be to restore flow beyond the obstruction and minimize the chance for further dissection.[50] A recent study of 23 patients with spontaneous coronary artery dissection showed a 26% need for urgent CABG.[51] In cases of severe cardiac failure, heart transplantation has been used.[50]

Traumatic coronary artery dissection is a rare event but has been well described after blunt chest trauma, most commonly in motor-vehicle collision-related steering wheel injuries. Mechanism of injury is thought to be due to shearing of the vessel wall. The most commonly affected artery is the LAD, occurring in 76% of cases. A recently published literature review showed that of 24 reported cases, 33% were treated with CABG, 29% were treated with PCI, and 38% were treated conservatively with medical management.[52]

Iatrogenic coronary artery dissection during PCIs is a rare occurrence but accounts for a large proportion of emergency CABG procedures after failed PCI. As discussed previously, the number of patients with failed PCI requiring emergent CABG has been declining with improvements in technology and therapeutic interventions. In published series, however, dissection was the indication for emergent CABG in failed PCI in 14% to 54% of cases.[46,47,53]

Preoperative Hemodynamic Optimization

Prior to emergent revascularization in the OR, patients should undergo stabilization and hemodynamic optimization. Vasopressors and inotropes should be used as needed to stabilize patients for the OR. PA catheter placement and invasive hemodynamic monitoring may help guide supportive medical therapy in select patient populations: those with refractory shock or heart failure or those being worked up for possible cardiac transplantation.[54] Use of an IABP device may be considered. In current clinical practice, IABP is used preoperatively in several clinical settings, including unstable angina refractory to medical management, cardiogenic shock after PCI, poor LV function, left main stem disease, and diffuse CAD.[55] The use of IABP and LV assist devices is discussed in the article on cardiogenic shock and mechanical assist devices.

There are not a lot of data to help guide hemodynamic optimization. Some studies have looked at cardiac surgery–associated acute kidney injury (AKI), because AKI has been reported in up to 29.7% of cases, and an increase of greater than 0.5 mg/dL is associated with more than an 18-fold increase in 30-day mortality.[56] Proposed preoperative methods of optimization include ensuring adequate hydration, avoidance of loop diuretics, continuing aspirin use, optimization of anemia through erythropoietin or packed red blood cell transfusion, or even prophylactic hemodialysis for patients with elevated serum creatinine.[56] A recent RCT looked at the use of the calcium sensitizer, levosimendan, in patients with severe LV dysfunction and an ejection fraction less than 25%. A preoperative 23-hour infusion was shown to decrease mortality as well as use of inotropes, vasopressors, and intraaortic balloon pumps.[57] The preoperative optimization of the cardiac patient remains an active area of research and further developments should be expected.

PERICARDIAL/MYOCARDIAL PATHOLOGY
Cardiac Tamponade

Cardiac tamponade is a life-threatening emergency resulting from pericardial effusion causing increased pressure in the pericardial sac and on the heart, leading to cardiovascular collapse. Possible causes include malignancy, infectious processes (fungal, tuberculous, parasitic, bacterial, and viral), myxedema, autoimmune disease (systemic lupus erythematosus and rheumatoid arthritis), uremia, aortic dissection, trauma, and postsurgical or iatrogenic during invasive coronary procedures.[58–60]

Pathophysiology of cardiac tamponade

Understanding the pathophysiology of cardiac tamponade is key to recognizing the disease process and developing management strategies. The pericardium is a bilayered sac that contains an inner visceral layer made of thin elastic membrane and a stiff thick outer parietal layer consisting predominantly of collagen and elastic fibers. The pericardium envelops the cardiac chambers but does not connect directly to any of them. Between the 2 layers is the pericardial space, which generally contains a small (15–50 mL) amount of physiologic pericardial fluid.[61,62] The pressure-volume curve of the normal pericardium resembles a J-shaped curve; there is an initial shallow portion in which the pericardium may stretch to accommodate more fluid. Once this volume is exceeded, further small increases in volume lead to a dramatic rise in pressure, resulting in acute cardiac tamponade (**Fig. 7**). In acute effusions, such as hemopericardium due to traumatic etiology, an increase of even 100 to 200 mL can result in tamponade physiology. In slower accumulations of fluid, pericardial compliance may increase, resulting in 1 to 2 L effusion without hemodynamic compromise. Once the volume increases to the steep portion of the pressure-volume curve, further small increases in volume result in dramatic tamponade physiology.[60]

In cardiac tamponade, pericardial pressure is elevated. The true filling pressure of the heart is represented by myocardial transmural pressure, which is intracardiac minus pericardial pressure. The circulation adapts by increasing venous pressure to allow for cardiac filling and prevent collapse of cardiac chambers. As pericardial pressure continues to rise, the left and right ventricular diastolic, right atrial, and pulmonary wedge pressures all rise to equal pericardial pressure, one of the hallmarks of cardiac tamponade (**Fig. 8**). If the pericardial pressure rises above the capability of venous pressures to allow cardiac filling, stroke volume drops and hemodynamic collapse occurs. The elevation of pressure in the enclosed pericardial sac also results in ventricular interdependence, because any change in volume on one side of the heart results in the opposite change in volume on the other side. For example, as the right side of the heart receives increased venous return during inspiration, the volume of the left side of the heart decreases, resulting in the classic clinical finding of pulsus paradoxus.[63–66]

Diagnosis of cardiac tamponade

The pressure relationships in the pericardial sac are illustrated by echocardiography, the imaging modality of choice. It is crucial to detect the pericardial effusion, establish extent and location, assess hemodynamic significance, and guide therapeutic

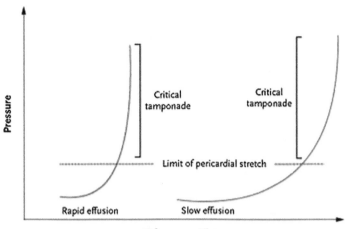

Volume over Time

Fig. 7. Cardiac Tamponade: Pericardial pressure–volume (or strain–stress) curves are shown in which the volume increases slowly or rapidly over time. In the left-hand panel, rapidly increasing pericardial fluid first reaches the limit of the pericardial reserve volume (the initial flat segment) and then quickly exceeds the limit of parietal pericardial stretch, causing a steep rise in pressure, which becomes even steeper as smaller increments in fluid cause a disproportionate increase in the pericardial pressure. In the right-hand panel, a slower rate of pericardial filling takes longer to exceed the limit of pericardial stretch, because there is more time for the pericardium to stretch and for compensatory mechanisms to become activated. (*From* Spodick DH. Acute cardiac tamponade. N Engl J Med 2003;349:684–90; with permission.)

pericardiocentesis. Cardiac tamponade remains, however, a clinical diagnosis, and the mere presence of a large effusion does not necessarily mandate intervention.[61] The expected findings on echocardiography in the setting of cardiac tamponade include collapse of the right atrium and right ventricle during diastole (**Fig. 9**). In some cases, the left atrium may collapse in diastole, but the LV rarely collapses due to its thick wall. Other possible findings on echocardiogram include signs of ventricular interdependence with respiration, an increase in mitral and tricuspid inflow E wave velocity with inspiration, and vena cava dilation without collapse with inspiration.[59]

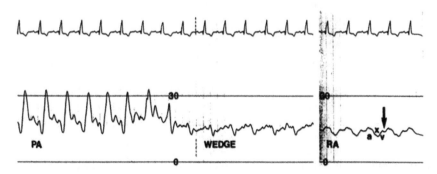

Fig. 8. PA catheter tracing in pericardial tamponade. Tracings show characteristic equalization of wedge and right atrial pressures and blunting of they descent (*arrow*). (*From* Hall JB, Schmidt GA, Wood LD. Principles of critical care. 3rd edition. New York: McGraw-Hill Professional; 2005; with permission.)

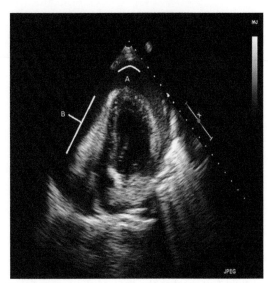

Fig. 9. Echocardiographic findings of cardiac tamponade. Transthoracic apical 4-chamber view demonstrating circumferential pericardial effusion (A) and right chamber collapse during diastole (B). (*Courtesy of* P. Peters, MD, Camden, New Jersey.)

Loculated effusions and regional cardiac tamponade may exist in postoperative cardiac surgery patients. These presentations may make diagnosis more difficult. TTE can be unrevealing and transesophogeal echocardiography may be needed to make the diagnosis.[58,66]

Treatment of cardiac tamponade

Treatment of cardiac tamponade is drainage of the pericardial space. Medical therapy may be attempted while preparing for intervention. Volume infusion may be helpful in patients with hypovolemia to help increase venous pressure and filling pressure but may be detrimental in other states and should be used cautiously. Positive pressure ventilation unless necessary should avoided, because it decreases venous return. The use of inotropes and vasopressors is controversial.[66,67] Cardiac tamponade may be drained via needle pericardiocentesis under echocardiographic or fluoroscopic guidance or in an OR by a cardiothoracic surgeon. In an emergency where imaging is not immediately available, a blind pericardiocentesis may be performed (**Fig. 10**). A pigtail catheter is often left in place for continued drainage. Surgical drainage is preferred in patients with intrapericardial bleeding, hemopericardium, and is required in aortic dissection resulting in cardiac tamponade.[66] Removal of small amounts of volume has a dramatic effect on hemodynamics as the pressure-volume curve returns to the compliant portion. Surgical approaches include a vertical subxiphoid incision, where the xiphoid is elevated or even cut to expose the pericardium, or a left anterolateral thoracotomy. In either approach, a small piece of pericardium is removed and sent to pathology (especially if the diagnosis is unknown) and at least one drainage tube is left in place. The choice of approach with surgical interventions depends on a patient's body habitus and prior chest surgery and if there is a concomitant left pleural effusion to be drained. Other interventions for pericardial effusion include sclerosing agents, chemotherapy or radiation therapy in the setting of malignancy, pericardiectomy, or a pericardial window allowing for continued drainage.[60,66]

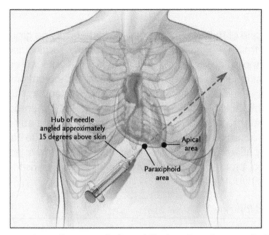

Fig. 10. Most common sites of approach for a blind pericardiocentesis. In the paraxiphoid approach, the needle should be aimed toward the left shoulder. In the apical approach, the needle is aimed internally. Bedside ultrasound may be used to visualize pericardial fluid. (*From* Spodick DH. Acute cardiac tamponade. N Engl J Med 2003;349:684–90; with permission.)

The ESC guidelines from 2004 recommend a surgical approach with pericardiectomy be reserved for patients with large chronic effusion in whom repeated pericardiocentesis and/or intrapericardial therapy was not successful.[68]

Ventricular Free Wall Rupture

Ventricular free wall rupture and ventricular septal rupture together constitute the second most common cause of in-hospital death in patients with AMI.[20] Based on the SHOCK registry, free wall rupture was the cause of 1.7% of cases of cardiogenic shock post-MI and had a 30-day mortality of 55%.[20] Since the introduction of PCI for revascularization for STEMI, the incidence of LV free wall rupture has been reported as 0.5% of patients after AMI.[21] Free wall rupture generally occurs within the first week after a transmural MI, and 90% of cases present within the first 2 weeks. Risk factors include age greater than 55, female gender, hypertension, large area of infarct, first-time infarct, and single-vessel involvement, which likely reflects a limited collateral coronary blood supply.[20,21]

There are different proposed classifications for ventricular free wall rupture, but the most common classifications seem to be early (<48 hours from infarct) versus late (>48 hours from infarct) and acute (cardiac tamponade, hemodynamic instability, and sudden death) versus subacute (moderate to severe effusion with or without tamponade physiology).[20,21,69] Clinical presentation are similar to the presentation of cardiac tamponade. Medical therapy with fluids and inotropes may be used a bridge to surgical intervention while the OR is prepared. Immediate pericardiocentesis may be required. Emergent surgical repair remains a patient's best chance for survival and surgical repair may be performed using resection and closure with Teflon or Dacron patches and/or biologic glue.[20]

In cases of LV free wall rupture, there is a subset of patients who have small areas of leak that become contained either by thrombus formation or pericardial adhesions and present more similarly to a pseudoaneurysm. There are reports of medical management in patients with small areas of rupture and contained hemorrhage, although these seem to be the exception rather than the rule.[69]

TRAUMA

Thoracic trauma is one of the leading causes of death in all age group, and represents 25% to 50% of all traumatic injuries.[70] There are many surgical indications for traumatic injury to the thoracic cavity, but a majority of patients with chest trauma may be managed with simple tube thoracostomy.[71] Classic indications for thoracotomy in the trauma setting include initial output after thoracostomy tube placement of greater than 1500 mL, output of 200 mL/h for 2 to 4 hours, or hemodynamic instability with suspected intrathoracic injury,[72] although there is debate as to whether specific numeric cutoffs are appropriate or if the decision should be made based on the clinical presentation of the patient.[71,73,74] This review focuses on a few specific indications for surgery: penetrating cardiac injuries, descending aortic transection due to blunt trauma, and severe hypothermia.

Penetrating Cardiac Injury

Penetrating injuries to the cardiac box (the area below the clavicles, above the costal margins, and between the nipple lines)[74] are of immediate concern for penetrating cardiac injury. Penetrating trauma with entry wounds outside of this area do not exclude cardiac injury. Due to the anatomy of the heart in the chest cavity, stab wounds to the chest most commonly involve the right ventricle (35%), LV (25%), or are dual chamber (30%). Other, less common, possible penetrating cardiac injuries due to a stab wound are coronary artery lacerations, valve injury, or ventricular septal defects. Missile injuries have the potential to affect any cardiac chamber.[75]

Patients with penetrating cardiac injuries present with clinical features of either hemorrhage or cardiac tamponade.[76] As discussed previously, small amounts of blood (as little as 50 mL), which accumulate in the pericardial sac acutely, may be sufficient to result in tamponade physiology. Up to 65% of patients with penetrating injuries to the chest arrive to an ED with no obtainable blood pressure.[76] ED thoracotomy (EDT) is a potential life-saving procedure for penetrating cardiac trauma, although its use has been debated. Generally accepted guidelines include the use of EDT for impending or witnessed cardiac arrest with cardiopulmonary resuscitation less than 15 minutes in the setting of penetrating trauma. The outcomes of EDT for blunt trauma are less favorable and are generally reserved for patients with witnessed cardiac arrest after arrival to the trauma center or with CPR less than 5 minutes.[71,74,76,77] Overall survival after EDT is reported at 7.4%, although the survival for patients surviving stab wounds was reported at 16.8% whereas the survival for gunshot wounds was reported at 4.3%.[78]

Hemodynamically stable patients with penetrating thoracic injuries should be monitored closely, because there is a high risk for decompensation. Work-up should be performed via focused assessment with sonography for trauma (FAST) or formal TTE/TEE as well as CT of the chest.[71,74] Identification of penetrating cardiac injury warrants surgical exploration. Most lacerations can be repaired with pledgeted sutures, although complex lacerations may require patch grafting with autologous or bovine pericardium. Most coronary artery injuries warrant bypass grafting.[75] Reported outcomes after penetrating cardiac injury remain variable, likely due to differences in transport systems, extent, and mechanism of the injury and the presence of other associated injuries.[75] It does remain clear that penetrating cardiac injury is a true life-threatening surgical emergency.

Descending Aortic Transection due to Blunt Trauma

Thoracic aortic injury is second only to brain injury as the leading cause of death in motor vehicle collisions.[75,79] The most commonly proposed mechanism of thoracic aortic transection in blunt trauma is rapid deceleration resulting in a shearing force on the aorta. In 65% of patients in an autopsy series, or 85% of patients who present to the hospital, the site of transection is at the isthmus, distal to the left subclavian artery and proximal to the third intercostal artery.[80] This is where the ligamentum arteriosum tethers the aorta, representing the junction between the more mobile aortic arch and the relatively fixed descending thoracic aorta. This supports the theory of shear forces in deceleration injury. Other proposed theories include the water-hammer theory, in which a sudden increase in the intravascular hydrostatic pressure at the time of impact results in a tear in the aorta at its weakest point. The osseous pinch theory suggests that a compressive mechanism from blunt trauma may result in the bony structures coming together and resulting in a tear of interposed vascular structures.[75,80] Regardless of the cause, thoracic aortic injuries should be suspected in patients who undergo rapid decelerations, such as high-speed motor vehicle collisions or falls from a great height.

The original study on thoracic aortic transection resulting from blunt trauma was published in 1958. This study estimated that 85% of patients with blunt aortic injury died on scene, whereas of those who survived at least 1 hour, 30% died within 6 hours, 49% with 24 hours, and 90% within 4 months.[81] Complete transection of the aorta, including the adventitia and the periadventitial connective tissue, leads to immediate death. A mediastinal hematoma contained within the adventitia may allow temporary survival.[79]

Rapid recognition of this injury is key, and it should be sought in patients who present with a mechanism of rapid deceleration injury. Chest radiograph is often used as an initial screening tool and may show a widened mediastinum or abnormal aortic contour; a left-sided apical pleural cap or hemothorax; depression of the left main stem bronchus; fractures of the sternum, clavicle, or first 2 ribs; and rightward displacement of the trachea or esophagus.[82] Angiography is the historic gold standard for diagnosis of thoracic aortic injury, but CT angiography (CTA) is the most commonly used diagnostic tool today, with a reported 100% sensitivity and 83% to 95% specificity.[80] Once an aortic injury is recognized, medical management should be initiated with short-acting vasodilators and β-blockers, hemodynamically tolerated, in order to reduce shear stress in the aorta, while decisions are made regarding other injuries and definitive management strategies. Hypertension and tachycardia should be avoided, as in aortic dissection.[80]

Due to the high incidence of other serious injuries complicating patients with thoracic aortic transection, delayed therapy to allow stabilization of other emergent injuries has been proposed. Heparinization may not be possible in the setting of serious abdominal or intracranial injuries for possible bypass procedures. Pulmonary contusion may also occur with blunt thoracic trauma and may make open surgical techniques difficult. Recent studies have shown that delayed open surgical management or endovascular management may be preferred in this patient population. With delayed definitive therapy, there must be strict attention to treatment of hypertension and reduction of shear forces on the aorta.[75,79,80]

Prospective multicenter studies conducted by the American Association for the Surgery of Trauma (AAST), the AAST1 and AAST2, were published in 1997 and 2007. The diagnosis and management of traumatic aortic transections underwent many significant changes over this 10-year period. Aortography and TEE were almost eliminated as diagnostic studies in favor of CTA. There was a shift from open surgical techniques (100%–35.2%) to endovascular repair (0%–64.8%). Mortality decreased from 22% to 13%, whereas the incidence of procedure-related paraplegia also decreased from 8.7% to 1.6%. Delayed intervention also became more common, with the time to intervention increasing from 16.5 hours to 54.6 hours.[83]

Thoracic aortic transection due to blunt trauma remains an injury with extremely high mortality rates, but recent changes in diagnostic technique and definitive management seem to be improving mortality. Long-term outcomes need to be assessed with the use of endovascular grafts in otherwise young, healthy adults, because studies have not yet been able to assess long term durability and complications of grafting.[75,79,82,83]

Severe Hypothermia

When exposed to cold, the initial reaction of the body is to maintain a normal core temperature through adaptive responses, such as physical exertion or involuntary shivering. Eventually these resources are overcome, and core body temperature drops. Hypothermia is defined as a core body temperature below 35°C (95°F). Hypothermia may be further classified as mild (32°–35°C or 89.6°–95°F), moderate (30°–32°C or 86°–89.6°F), or severe (below 30°C or 86°F). Primary hypothermia refers to otherwise healthy individuals who are overcome by excessive cold, whereas secondary hypothermia refers to patients with an underlying illness leading to their hypothermic state. At temperatures less than 28°C (82.4°F) the risk of cardiac arrest increases substantially.[84] This section focuses on primary severe hypothermia. CPB and ECMO are therapeutic options for patients with severe hypothermia and hemodynamic instability or cardiac arrest.[72,84–86]

Patients with mild and moderate hypothermia who are hemodynamically stable are generally managed in a warm environment with surface rewarming as well as warm IV fluid resuscitation. If intubated, warm humidified air may be used. If a patient is in cardiac arrest due to severe hypothermia, CPB or ECMO is indicated.[72,84,86] CPR should be instituted for pulseless patients until rewarmed. The optimal timing of vasopressors and attempted defibrillation is unclear.[86] In a setting where CPB or ECMO is not available, other invasive strategies, including thoracic lavage, peritoneal lavage, and dialysis, may be tried.[84,86] Increased serum potassium level has a strong association with nonsurvival in studies looking at CPB and ECMO for severe hypothermia, and proposed protocols suggest a cutoff of either 12 or 10 mmol/L, at which point further CPR and resuscitative measures would be considered futile.[84,87]

In 1997 Walpoth and colleagues[85] published a report of patients who survived deep hypothermia with circulatory arrest with rewarming via CPB; 15 of 32 (46%) patients treated with CPB survived to discharge. Mean time of discovery of patient to rewarming with CPB was 141 ± 50 minutes in survivors. At follow-up, all patients had resumed their former activities and lifestyles with minimal to no residual neurologic affects from hypothermia. Importantly, no patients were thought to have asphyxia prior to hypothermia and circulatory arrest, which has been associated with worse outcomes. In 2001, Farstad and colleagues[87] published a series of patients with severe hypothermia who underwent extracorporeal circulation for rewarming. The found that patients with nonasphyxiated deep accidental hypothermia have a reasonable prognosis (63% survival) in sharp contrast to the cases where asphyxia was believed to have preceded hypothermia (5% survival). Studies are limited due to the small sample sizes, but the surprisingly high survival rates with good neurologic outcomes favorably reflect aggressive resuscitation of severe hypothermia with CPB and ECMO.

SUMMARY

Cardiothoracic surgical emergencies are frequently admitted to the ICU and it is important that intensivists are prepared to recognize the situation and provide medical stabilization as well as work collaboratively with the cardiothoracic surgeons to provide optimal care for this patient population. Several cardiothoracic surgical emergencies are discussed. Recognition and appropriate timing of operative intervention are key factors in improving outcomes. A collaborative team approach with the cardiothoracic service is imperative in managing this patient population.

REFERENCES

1. Hirst AE Jr, Johns VJ Jr, Kime SW Jr. Dissecting aneurysm of the aorta: a review of 505 cases. Medicine (Baltimore) 1958;37(3):217–79.
2. Klompas M. Does this patient have an acute thoracic aortic dissection? JAMA 2002;287(17):2262–72.
3. Hiratzka LF, Bakris GL, Beckman JA, et al. 2010 ACCF/AHA/AATS/ACR/ASA/SCA/SCAI/SIR/STS/SVM guidelines for the diagnosis and management of patients with thoracic aortic disease: a report of the American College of Cardiology Foundation/American Heart Association Task Force on Practice Guidelines, American Association for Thoracic Surgery, American College of Radiology, American Stroke Association, Society of Cardiovascular Anesthesiologists, Society for Cardiovascular Angiography and Interventions, Society of Interventional Radiology, Society of Thoracic Surgeons, and Society for Vascular Medicine. Circulation 2010;121(13):e266–369.
4. Hagan PG, Nienaber CA, Isselbacher EM, et al. The International Registry of Acute Aortic Dissection (IRAD): new insights into an old disease. JAMA 2000; 283(7):897–903.
5. Kruger T, Conzelmann LO, Bonser RS, et al. Acute aortic dissection type A. Br J Surg 2012;99(10):1331–44.
6. Braverman AC. Acute aortic dissection: clinician update. Circulation 2010; 122(2):184–8.
7. Tsai TT, Trimarchi S, Nienaber CA. Acute aortic dissection: perspectives from the International Registry of Acute Aortic Dissection (IRAD). Eur J Vasc Endovasc Surg 2009;37(2):149–59.
8. Bonser RS, Ranasinghe AM, Loubani M, et al. Evidence, lack of evidence, controversy, and debate in the provision and performance of the surgery of acute type A aortic dissection. J Am Coll Cardiol 2011;58(24):2455–74.
9. Shimony A, Filion KB, Mottillo S, et al. Meta-analysis of usefulness of d-dimer to diagnose acute aortic dissection. Am J Cardiol 2011;107(8):1227–34.
10. Nienaber CA, Powell JT. Management of acute aortic syndromes. Eur Heart J 2012;33(1):26–35b.
11. Nienaber CA, Fattori R, Lund G, et al. Nonsurgical reconstruction of thoracic aortic dissection by stent-graft placement. N Engl J Med 1999;340(20): 1539–45.
12. Dake MD, Kato N, Mitchell RS, et al. Endovascular stent-graft placement for the treatment of acute aortic dissection. N Engl J Med 1999;340(20):1546–52.
13. Booher AM, Isselbacher EM, Nienaber CA, et al. The IRAD classification system for characterizing survival after aortic dissection. Am J Med 2013;126(8): 730.e19–24.
14. Piccardo A, Le Guyader A, Regesta T, et al. Octogenarians with uncomplicated acute type a aortic dissection benefit from emergency operation. Ann Thorac Surg 2013;96(3):851–6.
15. Di Eusanio M, Patel HJ, Nienaber CA, et al. Patients with type A acute aortic dissection presenting with major brain injury: should we operate on them? J Thorac Cardiovasc Surg 2013;145(Suppl 3):213–21.e1.

16. Harrington DK, Fragomeni F, Bonser RS. Cerebral perfusion. Ann Thorac Surg 2007;83(2):S799–804 [discussion: S824–31].

17. Akin I, Kische S, Ince H, et al. Penetrating aortic ulcer, intramural hematoma, acute aortic syndrome: when to do what. J Cardiovasc Surg (Torino) 2012; 53(1 Suppl 1):83–90.

18. Bischoff MS, Geisbusch P, Peters AS, et al. Penetrating aortic ulcer: defining risks and therapeutic strategies. Herz 2011;36(6):498–504.

19. Bonow RO, Carabello BA, Chatterjee K, et al. 2008 Focused update incorporated into the ACC/AHA 2006 guidelines for the management of patients with valvular heart disease: a report of the American College of Cardiology/American Heart Association Task Force on Practice Guidelines (Writing Committee to Revise the 1998 Guidelines for the Management of Patients with Valvular Heart Disease): endorsed by the Society of Cardiovascular Anesthesiologists, Society for Cardiovascular Angiography and Interventions, and Society of Thoracic Surgeons. Circulation 2008;118(15):e523–661.

20. Ng R, Yeghiazarians Y. Post myocardial infarction cardiogenic shock: a review of current therapies. J Intensive Care Med 2013;28(3):151–65.

21. Kutty RS, Jones N, Moorjani N. Mechanical complications of acute myocardial infarction. Cardiol Clin 2013;31(4):519–31, vii–viii.

22. Mokadam NA, Stout KK, Verrier ED. Management of acute regurgitation in left-sided cardiac valves. Tex Heart Inst J 2011;38(1):9–19.

23. Bizzarri F, Mattia C, Ricci M, et al. Cardiogenic shock as a complication of acute mitral valve regurgitation following posteromedial papillary muscle infarction in the absence of coronary artery disease. J Cardiothorac Surg 2008;3:61.

24. Wei JY, Hutchins GM, Bulkley BH. Papillary muscle rupture in fatal acute myocardial infarction: a potentially treatable form of cardiogenic shock. Ann Intern Med 1979;90(2):149–52.

25. French JK, Hellkamp AS, Armstrong PW, et al. Mechanical complications after percutaneous coronary intervention in ST-elevation myocardial infarction (from APEX-AMI). Am J Cardiol 2010;105(1):59–63.

26. Thompson CR, Buller CE, Sleeper LA, et al. Cardiogenic shock due to acute severe mitral regurgitation complicating acute myocardial infarction: a report from the SHOCK Trial Registry. Should we use emergently revascularize Occluded Coronaries in cardiogenic shocK? J Am Coll Cardiol 2000;36(3 Suppl A):1104–9.

27. Czarnecki A, Thakrar A, Fang T, et al. Acute severe mitral regurgitation: consideration of papillary muscle architecture. Cardiovasc Ultrasound 2008;6:5.

28. Joint Task Force on the Management of Valvular Heart Disease of the European Society of Cardiology, et al. Guidelines on the management of valvular heart disease (version 2012). Eur Heart J 2012;33(19):2451–96.

29. Russo A, Suri RM, Grigioni F, et al. Clinical outcome after surgical correction of mitral regurgitation due to papillary muscle rupture. Circulation 2008;118(15): 1528–34.

30. Schroeter T, Lehmann S, Misfeld M, et al. Clinical outcome after mitral valve surgery due to ischemic papillary muscle rupture. Ann Thorac Surg 2013;95(3): 820–4.

31. Nkomo VT. Indications for surgery for aortic regurgitation. Curr Cardiol Rep 2003;5(2):105–9.

32. Morganroth J, Perloff JK, Zeldis SM, et al. Acute severe aortic regurgitation. Pathophysiology, clinical recognition, and management. Ann Intern Med 1977; 87(2):223–32.

33. Carabello BA. Progress in mitral and aortic regurgitation. Prog Cardiovasc Dis 2001;43(6):457–75.
34. Hamirani YS, Dietl CA, Voyles W, et al. Acute aortic regurgitation. Circulation 2012;126(9):1121–6.
35. Baddour LM, Wilson WR, Bayer AS, et al. Infective endocarditis: diagnosis, antimicrobial therapy, and management of complications: a statement for healthcare professionals from the Committee on Rheumatic Fever, Endocarditis, and Kawasaki Disease, Council on Cardiovascular Disease in the Young, and the Councils on Clinical Cardiology, Stroke, and Cardiovascular Surgery and Anesthesia, American Heart Association: endorsed by the Infectious Diseases Society of America. Circulation 2005;111(23):e394–434.
36. David TE, Komeda M, Brofman PR. Surgical treatment of aortic root abscess. Circulation 1989;80(3 Pt 1):I269–74.
37. Thuny F, Grisoli D, Collart F, et al. Management of infective endocarditis: challenges and perspectives. Lancet 2012;379(9819):965–75.
38. Okada K, Okita Y. Surgical treatment for aortic periannular abscess/pseudoaneurysm caused by infective endocarditis. Gen Thorac Cardiovasc Surg 2013;61(4):175–81.
39. Leontyev S, Borger MA, Modi P, et al. Surgical management of aortic root abscess: a 13-year experience in 172 patients with 100% follow-up. J Thorac Cardiovasc Surg 2012;143(2):332–7.
40. Fang J, Centers for Disease Control and Prevention. Prevalence of coronary heart disease – United States, 2006-2010. MMWR Morb Mortal Wkly Rep 2011;60:1377–81.
41. Hillis LD, Smith PK, Anderson JL, et al. 2011 ACCF/AHA guideline for coronary artery bypass graft surgery: a report of the American College of Cardiology Foundation/American Heart Association Task Force on Practice Guidelines. Circulation 2011;124(23):e652–735.
42. Serruys PW, Morice MC, Kappetein AP, et al. Percutaneous coronary intervention versus coronary-artery bypass grafting for severe coronary artery disease. N Engl J Med 2009;360(10):961–72.
43. Farkouh ME, Domanski M, Sleeper LA, et al. Strategies for multivessel revascularization in patients with diabetes. N Engl J Med 2012;367(25):2375–84.
44. Abdallah MS, Wang K, Magnuson EA, et al. Quality of life after PCI vs CABG among patients with diabetes and multivessel coronary artery disease: a randomized clinical trial. JAMA 2013;310(15):1581–90.
45. Cohen DJ, Van Hout B, Serruys PW, et al. Quality of life after PCI with drug-eluting stents or coronary-artery bypass surgery. N Engl J Med 2011;364(11):1016–26.
46. Yang EH, Gumina RJ, Lennon RJ, et al. Emergency coronary artery bypass surgery for percutaneous coronary interventions: changes in the incidence, clinical characteristics, and indications from 1979 to 2003. J Am Coll Cardiol 2005;46(11):2004–9.
47. Seshadri N, Whitlow PL, Acharya N, et al. Emergency coronary artery bypass surgery in the contemporary percutaneous coronary intervention era. Circulation 2002;106(18):2346–50.
48. Vrints CJ. Spontaneous coronary artery dissection. Heart 2010;96(10):801–8.
49. Tweet MS, Hayes SN, Pitta SR, et al. Clinical features, management, and prognosis of spontaneous coronary artery dissection. Circulation 2012;126(5):579–88.
50. Glamore MJ, Garcia-Covarrubias L, Harrison LH Jr, et al. Spontaneous coronary artery dissection. J Card Surg 2012;27(1):56–9.

51. Ito H, Taylor L, Bowman M, et al. Presentation and therapy of spontaneous coronary artery dissection and comparisons of postpartum versus nonpostpartum cases. Am J Cardiol 2011;107(11):1590–6.
52. Lobay KW, MacGougan CK. Traumatic coronary artery dissection: a case report and literature review. J Emerg Med 2012;43(4):e239–43.
53. Lotfi M, Mackie K, Dzavik V, et al. Impact of delays to cardiac surgery after failed angioplasty and stenting. J Am Coll Cardiol 2004;43(3):337–42.
54. McMurray JJ, Adamopoulos S, Anker SD, et al. ESC Guidelines for the diagnosis and treatment of acute and chronic heart failure 2012: The Task Force for the Diagnosis and Treatment of Acute and Chronic Heart Failure 2012 of the European Society of Cardiology. Developed in collaboration with the Heart Failure Association (HFA) of the ESC. Eur Heart J 2012;33(14): 1787–847.
55. Theologou T, Bashir M, Rengarajan A, et al. Preoperative intra aortic balloon pumps in patients undergoing coronary artery bypass grafting. Cochrane Database Syst Rev 2011;(1):CD004472.
56. Vives M, Wijeysundera D, Rao V. Cardiac surgery-associated acute kidney injury. Interact Cardiovasc Thorac Surg 2014. [Epub ahead of print].
57. Levin R, Degrange M, Del Mazo C, et al. Preoperative levosimendan decreases mortality and the development of low cardiac output in high-risk patients with severe left ventricular dysfunction undergoing coronary artery bypass grafting with cardiopulmonary bypass. Exp Clin Cardiol 2012;17(3):125–30.
58. Bodson L, Bouferrache K, Vieillard-Baron A. Cardiac tamponade. Curr Opin Crit Care 2011;17(5):416–24.
59. Saito Y, Donohue A, Attai S, et al. The syndrome of cardiac tamponade with "small" pericardial effusion. Echocardiography 2008;25(3):321–7.
60. Imazio M, Adler Y. Management of pericardial effusion. Eur Heart J 2013;34(16): 1186–97.
61. Goldstein JA. Cardiac tamponade, constrictive pericarditis, and restrictive cardiomyopathy. Curr Probl Cardiol 2004;29(9):503–67.
62. Khandaker MH, Espinosa RE, Nishimura RA, et al. Pericardial disease: diagnosis and management. Mayo Clin Proc 2010;85(6):572–93.
63. Shabetai R. Pericardial effusion: haemodynamic spectrum. Heart 2004;90(3): 255–6.
64. Reddy PS, Curtiss EI, O'Toole JD, et al. Cardiac tamponade: hemodynamic observations in man. Circulation 1978;58(2):265–72.
65. Hoit BD. Pericardial disease and pericardial tamponade. Crit Care Med 2007; 35(Suppl 8):S355–64.
66. Spodick DH. Acute cardiac tamponade. N Engl J Med 2003;349(7):684–90.
67. Seferovic PM, Ristic AD, Imazio M, et al. Management strategies in pericardial emergencies. Herz 2006;31(9):891–900.
68. Maisch B, Seferovic PM, Ristic AD, et al. Guidelines on the diagnosis and management of pericardial diseases executive summary; the Task force on the diagnosis and management of pericardial diseases of the European society of cardiology. Eur Heart J 2004;25(7):587–610.
69. Figueras J, Cortadellas J, Soler-Soler J. Left ventricular free wall rupture: clinical presentation and management. Heart 2000;83(5):499–504.
70. Hunt PA, Greaves I, Owens WA. Emergency thoracotomy in thoracic trauma-a review. Injury 2006;37(1):1–19.
71. Demetriades D, Velmahos GC. Penetrating injuries of the chest: indications for operation. Scand J Surg 2002;91(1):41–5.

72. Advanced trauma life support for doctors: ATLS student course manual. 8th edition. Chicago: American College of Surgeons; 2008.
73. Bernardin B, Troquet JM. Initial management and resuscitation of severe chest trauma. Emerg Med Clin North Am 2012;30(2):377–400, viii–ix.
74. Bastos R, Baisden CE, Harker L, et al. Penetrating thoracic trauma. Semin Thorac Cardiovasc Surg 2008;20(1):19–25.
75. Cook CC, Gleason TG. Great vessel and cardiac trauma. Surg Clin North Am 2009;89(4):797–820, viii.
76. Embrey R. Cardiac trauma. Thorac Surg Clin 2007;17(1):87–93, vii.
77. Mejia JC, Stewart RM, Cohn SM. Emergency department thoracotomy. Semin Thorac Cardiovasc Surg 2008;20(1):13–8.
78. Rhee PM, Acosta J, Bridgeman A, et al. Survival after emergency department thoracotomy: review of published data from the past 25 years. J Am Coll Surg 2000;190(3):288–98.
79. Fattori R, Russo V, Lovato L, et al. Optimal management of traumatic aortic injury. Eur J Vasc Endovasc Surg 2009;37(1):8–14.
80. Nzewi O, Slight RD, Zamvar V. Management of blunt thoracic aortic injury. Eur J Vasc Endovasc Surg 2006;31(1):18–27.
81. Parmley LF, Mattingly TW, Manion WC, et al. Nonpenetrating traumatic injury of the aorta. Circulation 1958;17(6):1086–101.
82. Vrancken Peeters MP, Muhs BE, Van Der Linden E, et al. Endovascular treatment of traumatic ruptures of the thoracic aorta. J Cardiovasc Surg (Torino) 2007;48(5):557–65.
83. Demetriades D, Velmahos GC, Scalea TM, et al. Diagnosis and treatment of blunt thoracic aortic injuries: changing perspectives. J Trauma 2008;64(6):1415–8 [discussion: 1418–9].
84. Brown DJ, Brugger H, Boyd J, et al. Accidental hypothermia. N Engl J Med 2012;367(20):1930–8.
85. Walpoth BH, Walpoth-Aslan BN, Mattle HP, et al. Outcome of survivors of accidental deep hypothermia and circulatory arrest treated with extracorporeal blood warming. N Engl J Med 1997;337(21):1500–5.
86. Vanden Hoek TL, Morrison LJ, Shuster M, et al. Part 12: cardiac arrest in special situations: 2010 American Heart Association Guidelines for Cardiopulmonary Resuscitation and Emergency Cardiovascular Care. Circulation 2010;122(18 Suppl 3):S829–61.
87. Farstad M, Andersen KS, Koller ME, et al. Rewarming from accidental hypothermia by extracorporeal circulation. A retrospective study. Eur J Cardiothorac Surg 2001;20(1):58–64.

Perioperative Complications of Cardiac Surgery and Postoperative Care

CrossMark

Howard Nearman, MD, MBA*, John C. Klick, MD,
Paul Eisenberg, MD, Nicholas Pesa, MD

KEYWORDS

- Cardiac complications • Vasoplegia • Pulmonary complications
- Gastrointestinal complications • Acute kidney injury • Hematologic complications
- Infections • Neurological problems

KEY POINTS

- Caring for the postoperative cardiac surgical patient is challenging because of the number and severity of potential complications.
- By definition, the patient presents postoperatively with some degree of cardiac dysfunction, and the procedure itself may cause (at least transiently) further deterioration.
- Diagnostic, therapeutic and preventative measures are discussed.

CARDIAC COMPLICATIONS
Surgical and Physiologic Complications

Cardiac complications of open heart surgery can be divided into 2 distinct categories, surgical and physiologic. Mechanical complications are addressed by surgical intervention, whereas physiologic complications may be attributed to changes in preload, afterload, heart rate, and the inotropic or lusitropic state of the heart. Dysrhythmias are not uncommon after cardiac surgery, and have direct effects on myocardial performance. The use of cardiopulmonary bypass (CPB) is also associated with its own set of complications.

Proper monitoring is essential in the intensive care unit (ICU) to determine the etiology of changes in cardiac performance. Continuous telemetry, a central venous and/or pulmonary artery catheter, and direct arterial blood pressure monitoring are frequently used for both intraoperative and postoperative monitoring. These

The authors have no financial interests to disclose.
Department of Anesthesiology and Perioperative Medicine, University Hospitals Case Medical Center, Case Western Reserve University School of Medicine, 11100 Euclid Avenue, Cleveland, OH 44106, USA
* Corresponding author.
E-mail address: Howard.Nearman@UHhospitals.org

Crit Care Clin 30 (2014) 527–555
http://dx.doi.org/10.1016/j.ccc.2014.03.008
0749-0704/14/$ – see front matter © 2014 Elsevier Inc. All rights reserved.

criticalcare.theclinics.com

monitoring devices, along with the selective use of bedside echocardiography (particularly transesophageal echocardiography [TEE]), enable the critical care clinician to determine the cause of and appropriate response to most hemodynamic disturbances. The use of intraoperative TEE has had a significant impact on surgical decision making during cardiac surgery. One large case series of more than 12,000 patients found that intraoperative use of TEE altered the surgical plan in more than 9% of patients, particularly in those undergoing combined coronary artery bypass grafting (CABG) and valve procedures.[1] Both the American Society of Anesthesiologists and the Society of Cardiovascular Anesthesiologists recommend the use of intraoperative TEE in all open heart and thoracic aortic procedures in the adult population.[2]

Mechanical complications may be detected by echocardiography or with hemodynamic monitoring. Spasm or acute occlusion of a coronary graft can lead to acute myocardial ischemia and decrements in myocardial contractility. After the surgical placement of a prosthetic valve, perivalvular leak may lead to hemodynamic compromise and hemolysis. Failure of any surgical repair of a valvular defect must also be ruled out.

Myocardial dysfunction after cardiac surgery is often multifactorial, and frequently involves perioperative myocardial ischemia. Underlying coronary artery disease (CAD), hemodynamic instability, coronary artery embolization, and poor myocardial protection during cardiopulmonary bypass may all play a role in impaired myocardial contractility in the early postoperative period. Restoration of blood flow to the chronically ischemic myocardium may result in the phenomenon of myocardial ischemia reperfusion injury and further temporary compromise in myocardial contractility.[3] CPB is known to initiate a systemic inflammatory response. These inflammatory mediators may lead to not only myocardial injury but also injury in multiple other organ systems.[4]

The incidence of perioperative myocardial infarction is around 3% to 15% in all patients undergoing open heart surgery.[5] Several factors are known contributors to myocardial injury, as outlined in **Box 1**.

Owing to their underlying disease, patients undergoing CABG are at particularly high risk for the development of myocardial ischemia. A multitude of factors are known to trigger myocardial ischemia in these patients in the immediate postoperative period (**Box 2**).[6]

Pericardial Tamponade

Acute cardiac tamponade caused by hemopericardium may occur in up to 5.8% of patients after open heart surgery,[7] and may be suspected by acute tachycardia, rising central venous pressures, and poor response to fluid challenges. Bedside echocardiography can expeditiously provide the diagnosis and allow early operative intervention

---

Box 1
Causes of perioperative myocardial injury after cardiac surgery

Incomplete myocardial protection during aortic cross-clamping

Incomplete revascularization

Coronary vasospasm

Air embolism

Thrombosis of a graft or native vessel

Atheromatous emboli from a previous bypass graft or from the aorta

---

Box 2
Risk factors for perioperative myocardial ischemia in patients undergoing coronary artery bypass grafting

Increased plasma catecholamines

Increased heart rate

Increased pain

Increased temperature variation

Impaired gas exchange

Coagulation abnormalities

Decreased fibrinolysis

Mechanical graft damage

Intimal flap due to probing of graft

Size mismatch of anastomosed vessels

Internal mammary occlusion

Left ventricular dysfunction

Narrowing distal to graft insertion

Increased fibrointimal hyperplasia

Suboptimal anastomotic technique

---

to restore hemodynamic stability. Risk factors include advanced age, complex surgery, aortic surgery, and the use of anticoagulants in the perioperative period.[7] Common sites of direct surgical bleeding are small arterial vessels behind the sternum, vein side graft branches, and graft suture lines. Tamponade can also result from the removal of epicardial pacing wires. Delayed cardiac tamponade by as long as 1 to 3 weeks can be seen with anticoagulation for prosthetic heart valves, atrial fibrillation, or deep venous thrombosis (DVT).[7] Tamponade leads to hemodynamic instability by the impairment of diastolic cardiac filling. The hemodynamic impact depends on the rate of fluid accumulation in the pericardium. A large volume of fluid may be well tolerated if it accumulates slowly. Bleeding in the early postoperative period leads to rapid fluid accumulation, and as little as 100 mL of fluid may lead to hemodynamic decompensation. Physical examination often reveals significant tachycardia, a narrow pulse pressure, elevated neck veins, and constriction of the peripheries. Elevated left ventricular end-diastolic pressure (LVEDP) and decreased diastolic perfusion pressure lead to myocardial ischemia and worsening of hemodynamics. Aggressive volume resuscitation to raise intracardiac pressure while maintaining an elevated heart rate to increase cardiac output can be temporizing measures, but definitive treatment can only be accomplished by relief of the fluid accumulation.[8]

Systolic Anterior Motion of the Mitral Valve

Systolic anterior motion of the mitral valve (SAM) occurs when the anterior mitral leaflet is pulled into the left ventricular outflow tract (LVOT) during systole, limiting blood outflow through the LVOT. It should be suspected in the setting of worsening hypotension during escalating inotropic support. SAM occurs in approximately 2% to 7% of patients after operative repair of the mitral valve. Several underlying anatomic features put the patient at higher risk of developing SAM, as outlined in **Box 3**. When the correct physiologic conditions arise in the anatomically prone heart, SAM will occur.

Box 3
Anatomic factors predisposing to systolic anterior motion of the mitral valve

Small left ventricle

Mitral chordal anomaly

Bulging interventricular septum

Papillary muscle displacement

Redundant posterior mitral leaflet

Redundant anterior mitral leaflet

Hypovolemia, tachycardia, reduced afterload, and hypercontractility of the left ventricle can all bring out the manifestations of SAM in the anatomically prone heart. The diagnosis can be made by TEE (**Fig. 1**), and immediate treatment consists of volume loading while decreasing inotropic and chronotropic support. Increasing afterload and the judicious use of β-blocking medications may also help to restore normal cardiac geometry and relieve SAM. SAM is typically seen in the setting of hypertrophic obstructive cardiomyopathy or surgical repair of the mitral valve. It may also be seen after replacement of a stenotic aortic valve whereby increased blood velocity in the LVOT causes drag on the anterior mitral leaflet. This situation is exacerbated by the hypertrophic, smaller left ventricular (LV) cavity frequently found in these patients. SAM has also been described as a manifestation of cardiac allograft rejection. For reasons that are not understood, diabetic patients seem to be exceptionally prone to develop SAM when β-agonist medications are used. If SAM cannot be reliably managed medically, further surgical intervention may be necessary.[9]

The astute clinician must keep in mind that not all mechanical complications of cardiac surgery involve the heart. Acute pneumothorax, hemothorax, or acute respiratory changes may also lead to hemodynamic compromise, and must be ruled out.[10]

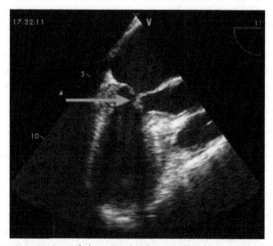

Fig. 1. Systolic anterior motion of the mitral valve. *Arrow* shows the anterior mitral leaflet obstructing the left ventricular outflow tract transesophageal echocardiography view of systolic anterior motion of the mitral valve. (*From* Chandrasegaram MD, Celermajer DS, Wilson MK. Apical ballooning syndrome complicated by acute severe mitral regurgitation with left ventricular outflow obstruction—case report. J Cardiothorac Surg 2007;2:18.)

Physiologic complications can be addressed immediately by the intensivist, but require rapid assessment, diagnosis, and intervention to prevent major morbidity. Low cardiac output may be due to low stroke volume from inadequate preload. This deficiency should respond to volume challenges, although causes of decreased stroke volume, including bleeding, need to be evaluated for. Increasing the heart rate via direct epicardial pacing will increase the cardiac output, but again this is a temporizing measure. Transthoracic echocardiography or TEE can rapidly determine if there has been a significant change in myocardial contractility. Regional wall motion changes in a bypassed coronary distribution may indicate early compromise of a graft and necessitate an immediate return to the operating. Patients with globally poor LV contractility may require additional inotropic support.[11] Hypotension in the setting of an adequate cardiac output and stroke volume is most likely due to a state of low systemic vascular resistance, and may require additional vasopressor support. By contrast, postoperative hypertension in the setting of low cardiac output may require selective afterload reduction with short-acting agents such as clevidipine or nicardipine.[12] A pulmonary artery catheter may prove useful in these settings.

Acute heart failure in the postoperative period may occur in patients with preexistent congestive heart failure, or may be the direct result of acute events that occur in the operating room. Despite the use of cardioplegia, aortic cross-clamping on cardiopulmonary bypass results in acute intraoperative ischemia and reperfusion injury. These events may result in a period of stunned myocardium, leading to an acute impairment in ventricular function that may recover with time.[13]

Patients with chronic cardiomyopathy live in a state of sustained endogenous catecholamine release, leading to progressive downregulation of β1 receptors.[14,15] Inotropic response in these patients becomes progressively mediated by β2 receptors, with clear implications for inotropic choices during the postoperative period.[16] Phosphodiesterase inhibitors such as milrinone are effective inotropic agents in this setting.

Postoperative diastolic dysfunction must also be taken into consideration. Impaired relaxation of the left ventricle is particularly common in the elderly and in patients with significant LV hypertrophy. Postischemic injury and myocardial stunning related to cardiopulmonary bypass may exacerbate the problem. These patients will require a higher LVEDP to maintain an adequate postoperative preload. Progressive impairment in diastolic function is a hallmark of aging, even in patients with apparently normal systolic function and without hypertrophy of the left ventricle. On a structural level, aging results in a decreased number of ventricular myocytes and an increase in the amount of connective tissue matrix. The result is a stiffer, less compliant ventricle. The degree of diastolic dysfunction in a given patient may be demonstrated through the use of various echocardiographic techniques. Patients with diastolic dysfunction may demonstrate increased sensitivity to changes in loading conditions, making them less able to tolerate rapid volume shifts. Nevertheless, their ventricle will be intensely dependent on preload to maintain filling. Positive lusitropic agents such as milrinone may be of benefit in the immediate postbypass period.[17]

Failure to improve cardiac output through medical means may occasionally necessitate the use of circulatory support devices such as the intra-aortic balloon pump, the Impella pump (Abiomed USA, Inc, Danvers, MA), venoarterial extracorporeal membrane oxygenation, or even implantable ventricular assist devices in extreme cases.

Acute exacerbations of postoperative pulmonary hypertension can be mitigated through the avoidance of hypoxemia, hypercarbia, acidosis, or excessive sympathetic tone.[18] Patients with chronic pulmonary arterial hypertension or pulmonary venous hypertension secondary to left-sided cardiac lesions are at high risk for acute right ventricular (RV) failure in the immediate postoperative period. Management of severe pulmonary hypertension and RV failure mandates the maintenance of systemic blood pressure to maintain coronary perfusion against a high intracavitary RV pressure. Vasopressin permits systemic vasoconstriction without causing pulmonary vasoconstriction. Inhaled nitric oxide and prostacyclin analogues allow selective vasodilation of the pulmonary vasculature to decrease RV afterload, and inodilators such as milrinone and dobutamine augment RV contractility while helping to decrease pulmonary vasculature resistance.[18]

Dysrhythmias are not uncommon in the postoperative period after cardiac surgery. Supraventricular tachyarrhythmias, particularly atrial fibrillation and atrial flutter, occur frequently after cardiac surgery. Atrial fibrillation occurs in 10% to 65% of patients after open heart surgery requiring cardiopulmonary bypass.[19] The decreased diastolic time impairs ventricular filling time and causes loss of atrial kick during ventricular filling. This combination may lead to hemodynamic compromise. The ensuing decreased diastole time decreases myocardial perfusion and may lead to ischemia.[20] Atrial fibrillation disrupts atrioventricular synchrony and can result in a 15% to 25% reduction in cardiac output. Pharmacologic rate control is the first line in management, with a goal ventricular rate of 80 to 100 beats per minute. If the patient is hemodynamically unstable, electrical or pharmacologic cardioversion should be performed.[20] A randomized trial demonstrated the efficacy of atorvastatin, 40 mg/d initiated 7 days before surgery, in the reduction of postoperative atrial fibrillation in patients undergoing cardiac surgery with cardiopulmonary bypass.[19] Preoperative oral amiodarone has also been shown to significantly reduce the incidence of postoperative atrial fibrillation.[21] β-Blockers have the most evidence to support their use in the prevention of postoperative atrial fibrillation in patients undergoing cardiac surgery, and should be used routinely in the absence of a contraindication.[22]

Ventricular arrhythmias frequently result in hemodynamic instability, and need to be converted promptly either chemically or electrically. Ischemia and electrolyte abnormalities must be ruled out in this setting. Age older than 65 years, peripheral vascular disease, LV ejection fraction (LVEF) less than 45%, and emergent surgery are all associated with a higher incidence of postoperative ventricular arrhythmias.[23]

Bradyarrhythmias and atrioventricular (AV) blocks are common after valvular surgery as a consequence of direct surgical injury and edema affecting the conduction system. Temporary epicardial pacing can be used to adjust the heart rate and rhythm. If the bradyarrhythmia or AV block does not resolve with time, a permanent pacemaker may be necessary. Approximately 1.5% of patients undergoing cardiac surgery develop conduction disturbances that will require the placement of a permanent pacemaker. Those undergoing aortic valve replacement are at exceptionally high risk because of the proximity of the valve to the conduction tissue. Up to 8.5% of patients may require a permanent pacemaker after aortic valve replacement. The presence of proximal disease of the left anterior descending coronary artery also seems to increase the risk.[24]

The postcardiotomy or postpericardiotomy syndrome occurs in approximately 18% of adult patients after open heart surgery, but the incidence decreases with advancing age.[25] The syndrome appears to be an autoimmune phenomenon, attributable to high titers of heart-reactive antibodies that develop in all patients who undergo open heart surgery. Viruses have also been implicated. The syndrome may eventually progress to pericardial effusion and, rarely, to constrictive pericarditis. The most common presentation includes fever, pleuritic pain, malaise, and a pericardial friction rub. Patients may occasionally develop pleural or pericardial effusions or experience pain with swallowing. The symptoms usually appear within the first month postoperatively, and usually within the first week. Mild leukocytosis may be present along with nonspecific ST changes on the electrocardiogram. In general the syndrome is self-limited, usually lasting about 1 month. Nonsteroidal anti-inflammatory agents are often prescribed, and patients with severe symptoms may benefit from a tapered dose of corticosteroids. The syndrome is not associated with any increase in perioperative mortality.[26]

Constrictive pericarditis is a rare occurrence after cardiac surgery, although the actual incidence may be as high as 2% to 3%. The disease starts with pericardial hemorrhage and inflammation, and progresses to organization into a fibrotic pericardial shell that may or may not contain calcium. The etiology is unclear, but nearly half of these patients will have experienced the postcardiotomy syndrome. Patients may present 2 weeks to 17 years after an operation with exertional dyspnea, fatigue, and peripheral edema. Echocardiography, magnetic resonance imaging, and computed tomography (CT) scan all demonstrate pericardial thickening, effusions, and occasional pericardial calcium. Most commonly, echocardiography will demonstrate biatrial dilation, small to normal ventricular size, and a rigid shell of pericardium. Surgical decortication remains the only effective treatment, and usually results in an immediate improvement in cardiac performance.[27] Late pericardial stripping is associated with a mortality rate of up to 12%.[28]

VASOPLEGIA

Vasoplegic syndrome occurring in the immediate postoperative period may be defined as low mean arterial pressure (<60 mm Hg), a high cardiac index (>3.5 L/min/m^2), and adequate cardiac chamber filling pressures. This syndrome was first described in 1994 by Gomes and colleagues,[29] who observed 6 patients in the early postoperative period with this syndrome. The investigators noted that restoration of volume was not sufficient to restore hemodynamic parameters back to normal, and that high doses of pressor agents were required for anywhere up to 48 to 72 hours. This suspected inflammatory response occurring after cardiopulmonary bypass was further quantified several years later by Carrel and colleagues,[30] who described a mean arterial pressure (MAP) of less than 60 mm Hg with normal LV contractility and normal filling pressures. In these patients, MAP responded immediately to norepinephrine infusion.

Vasoplegia may occur in up to 25% of postoperative cardiac surgical patients, but the exact etiology of this syndrome is not clear. It is likely a combination of multiple different vasodilatory mechanisms coupled with a resistance to the actions of vasopressor agents. Initially it was thought that vasoplegia resulted from an inflammatory response to synthetic surfaces of the cardiopulmonary bypass circuit, perhaps mediated by C3a, tumor necrosis factor, and/or interleukin-6. Other hypotheses over the years have implicated vasodilators such as bradykinin that are released and/or altered during cardiopulmonary bypass. Linking the changes seen in the peripheral vasculature to cardiopulmonary bypass may be too simplistic, however. The syndrome occurs in off-pump cases, although at decreased incidence (6.9% vs 2.8%).[31] Whatever the initiating factor(s) may be that produce the dysregulation of endothelial homeostasis, the final effector mechanism most likely involves activation of nitric oxide synthase, with the resultant production of cyclic guanosine monophosphate signaling smooth muscle relaxation.

Preoperative risk factors for the development of vasoplegia include the use of the angiotensin-converting enzyme (ACE) inhibitors, angiotensin-receptor blockers (ARBs), and calcium-channel blockers (CCBs). ACE inhibitors decrease angiotensin II levels and increase plasma levels of bradykinin. The lungs, which are the major site of bradykinin metabolism, are excluded during CPB and therefore potentiate the vasodilating effect of this polypeptide. Other drugs that have been associated with an increased risk of vasoplegia are amiodarone, β-blockers, and heparin. Patient-independent risk factors include valvular surgery, surgery for treatment of heart failure, red blood cell transfusion, and LVEF less than 35%.[32]

Once the diagnosis of vasoplegia is made and adequate volume resuscitation obtained, the use of vasopressors is usually effective. Vascular tone can be resistant and high-dose vasopressor therapy can have adverse consequences. The catechol-amines phenylephrine and norepinephrine, primarily α-agonists, are often used as first-line agents (**Table 1**). Vasopressin may be a better initial choice, as vasoplegia patients have been associated with a reduction in circulating endogenous vasopressin levels. In patients already receiving catecholamines, the addition of vasopressin may allow a reduction in these agents.[33] Methylene blue, which inhibits nitric oxide synthase, has been successfully used in the treatment of refractory hypotension caused by vasoplegia. A recent study has questioned this practice, linking the use of methylene blue in postoperative cardiac surgical patients with poor outcomes.[34] More studies are needed to better define the role of this agent in the treatment of vasoplegia.

Because of the clinical circumstances whereby vasoplegia develops, it is difficult to define the potential increase in morbidity and mortality associated with this syndrome. In one study, cardiac surgery patients who developed postoperative vasoplegia had 2 to 3 times the incidence of mortality or a prolonged hospital stay (>10 days). Catecholamine-refractory vasogenic shock that lasts longer than 48 hours may have mortality as high as 25%.[34]

Prevention of vasoplegia is important because of its associated comorbidities. Reducing controllable risk factors may be helpful, but questions remain regarding this strategy. ACE inhibitors, ARBs, and CCBs are associated with an increased incidence of vasoplegia, but it is unclear as to whether stopping their administration preoperatively will prevent its development. Preoperative methylene blue and intraoperative vasopressin have been shown to decrease the incidence of postoperative vasoplegia and improve mortality, and may be considered for use in those patients deemed to be at high risk.[35,36]

PULMONARY COMPLICATIONS

Pulmonary dysfunction is a leading cause of postoperative morbidity in the cardiac surgical population. A thorough history and physical examination, along with preoperative pulmonary function tests, may help predict those patients at high risk for postoperative pulmonary complications. In one large study, moderate or severe airway

Table 1			
Pressor agents for the treatment of vasoplegia			
Agent	Receptor/Action	Dosage	Comments
Phenylephrine	α1 agonist	40–60 μg/min	
Norepinephrine	α1, α2, and β1 agonist	0.01–0.3 μg/kg/min	
Vasopressin	V1a agonist	0.01–0.04 U/min	Potential for mesenteric ischemia
Methylene blue	Inhibits nitric oxide synthase	2 mg/kg over 20 minutes	Should not be used in patients using SSRI or those with G6PD deficiency

Abbreviations: G6PD, glucose-6-phosphate dehydrogenase; SSRI, selective serotonin reuptake inhibitor.

obstruction (forced expiratory volume in 1 second [FEV_1] to forced vital capacity [FVC] ratio<0.7 and FEV_1 <80% predicted) and diffusion capacity of carbon monoxide of less than 50% were independent predictors of operative mortality, prolonged mechanical ventilation, and longer stay in hospital.[37]

Sternotomy and thoracotomy incisions produce pain, leading to altered pulmonary mechanics and a decreased ability to cough, breathe deeply, or clear secretions. After surgery, there are decreases in the FVC, FEV_1, forced expiratory flow at 50% of vital capacity, peak expiratory flow rate, and maximum voluntary ventilation. The FVC and FEV_1 may decrease by more than 50% compared with preoperative values. The changes are attributed to uncoordinated rib-cage expansion from the median sternotomy, along with pain and pleural effusions. Use of internal mammary artery grafts is associated with lower FVC and FEV_1 in CABG patients because of violation of the pleural cavity and the more extensive dissection. Use of partial sternotomies and other minimally invasive approaches may speed the recovery of postoperative respiratory function.[38]

Oxygenation may be impaired for a week or more after cardiac surgery with CPB. Potential mechanisms include poor preoperative oxygenation, leukocyte activation, atelectasis, and pulmonary edema of both cardiogenic and noncardiogenic origin.[39]

CPB leads to increases in expiratory airway resistance caused by inhomogeneous constriction in peripheral airways, perhaps due to the release of bronchoconstricting mediators during cardiopulmonary bypass. However, this is not observed in patients undergoing off-pump surgery.[38]

Atelectasis and pleural effusions are extremely common after cardiac surgery, and may be seen in up to 63% of patients on postoperative chest radiographs. Atelectasis is multifactorial in origin. Induction of general anesthesia, manual compression of the lungs, and apnea during CPB are all contributing factors. Poor postoperative coughing, pleural effusions, increased interstitial lung water, gastric distension, and poor inspiratory effort may all contribute to atelectasis in the postoperative setting. Longer operative and bypass times, entrance into the pleural space, and lower body temperature during bypass have also all been associated with an increase in postoperative atelectasis.[38]

Various ventilator strategies in the immediate postoperative period may help to reduce the degree of atelectasis. Lung-recruitment maneuvers and the use of positive end-expiratory pressure (PEEP) may improve both lung volumes and the degree of oxygenation. Avoidance of 100% fraction of inspired oxygen may also help limit the degree of reabsorption atelectasis.[38]

Pleural effusions are extremely common in the immediate postoperative period. Up to 6.6% of patients may require drainage of a pleural effusion after CABG. A history of heart failure, more advanced peripheral arterial disease, and atrial fibrillation are more common among patients who develop significant postoperative pleural effusions. Valve replacement and prolonged operative times are associated with a higher incidence of pleural effusions.[39] Postoperative bleeding, atelectasis, pneumonia, disruption of pleural lymphatic drainage from internal mammary harvesting, and leakage of fluid from the mediastinum may all contribute. Pulmonary edema of cardiogenic and noncardiogenic origins may also contribute to the formation of effusions. Most effusions do resolve within a year.[38]

Pulmonary edema can be of both cardiogenic and noncardiogenic origin. Cardiogenic pulmonary edema resulting from reduced LV function is one of the leading causes of prolonged mechanical ventilation after cardiac surgery. Treatment of cardiogenic pulmonary edema is aimed at improvement of the underlying cardiac function using inotropic agents, afterload reduction, and diuretics. Mechanical circulatory support may be considered in medically refractory situations.[38]

Pneumothoraces may occur after cardiac surgery, as a result of direct injury to the lung during surgery, spontaneous rupture of blebs, or barotrauma secondary to mechanical ventilation. The overall incidence is reported as 0.7% to 1.7%. Pleural and mediastinal tubes are routinely placed at the time of surgery in an effort to evacuate residual air.[38]

The reported incidence of pneumonia after cardiac surgery varies widely from 2% to 22%, owing to differences in study designs. Many patients undergoing cardiac surgery have a history of cigarette smoking and associated chronic obstructive pulmonary disease (COPD). In general, postoperative pulmonary complications are significantly higher in smokers than in nonsmokers. Silent aspiration secondary to pharyngeal dysfunction or cognitive impairment may contribute to postoperative pneumonia, along with poor clearance of secretions due to poor coughing from pain. Prolonged postoperative intubation and ventilation leaves the patient prone to ventilator-associated pneumonia (VAP). Pneumonia after cardiac surgery is associated with high morbidity and mortality, up to 27% in one series. Reintubation, the presence of a nasogastric tube, use of broad-spectrum antibiotics, and transfusion of blood products are all risk factors for the development of pneumonia. Other risk factors for VAP include diabetes mellitus, COPD, previous myocardial infarction, prior cerebrovascular accident, and age older than 75 years. The supine position, presence of a nasogastric tube, and the use of H2-receptor blocking drugs have also been implicated in changing the colonization of gastric fluid with gram-negative bacteria, which may in turn be aspirated and lead to VAP.[38]

Diaphragmatic dysfunction secondary to intraoperative phrenic nerve injury has been described in about 2% of patients after cardiac surgery. Direct phrenic injury during harvest of the internal mammary artery, cold injury from pericardial ice slush, and inadvertent stretch injury during intrapericardial manipulation of the heart are all documented causes. The postoperative chest radiograph may show a high hemidiaphragm or lower-lobe atelectasis of the affected lung, but nerve conduction, fluoroscopic, or ultrasonographic studies are required to definitively make the diagnosis. Most phrenic nerve palsies resolve within 18 months, but permanent paralysis of the hemidiaphragm has been described.[40]

The acute respiratory distress syndrome (ARDS) is a rare event after the use of cardiopulmonary bypass, complicating fewer than 2% of cardiac surgical procedures. The mortality of patients with ARDS may be as high as 50% after the use of cardiopulmonary bypass.[41] Care remains supportive, with the use of low-tidal-volume ventilation to prevent further iatrogenic injury to the lungs. A less severe degree of lung injury is much more common, and may affect up to 20% of patients who undergo cardiopulmonary bypass.[42,43]

ARDS in the postoperative cardiac surgical patient leads to prolonged mechanical ventilation, prolonged stay in the ICU and hospital, and leads to increased morbidity from renal, neurologic, and infectious complications.[42]

Most evidence points to the pathogenesis of ARDS after cardiopulmonary bypass as being from the acute inflammatory response to CPB.[44] The additional use of cardiopulmonary bypass with aortic cross-clamping subject patients' lungs to ischemia/reperfusion injury.[45] During rewarming on CPB, half of all circulating neutrophils are sequestered in the pulmonary capillaries. The subsequent degranulation of these neutrophils damages pulmonary endothelial cells.[43] Complement activation from CPB worsens postoperative pulmonary dysfunction.[45]

Transfusion-related acute lung injury (TRALI) is another important cause of pulmonary dysfunction after cardiac surgery, emphasizing the need to be judicious with the administration of blood products.[46] The onset of TRALI is due to the presence of leukocyte antibodies in an implicated donor product. TRALI is initiated during or within 6 hours of blood-product transfusion.[47,48] In general, the clinical course of TRALI is not as severe as with other causes of ARDS. Mortality is much lower, on the order of 5% to 8%, and complete recovery occurs in up to 80% of cases.[48]

Pulmonary embolism occurs in roughly 1% of patients following cardiac surgery, most commonly the result of DVT occurring in the lower extremities. Whereas symptomatic DVT occurs in only 1% to 2% of patients after cardiac surgery, noninvasive screening studies have documented an incidence of up to 20%, half occurring in the nonharvest leg. There are no data to suggest that patients after cardiac surgery are at any lower risk for the development of DVT and pulmonary embolism than are general surgical patients. The use of venous compressions devices, early mobilization, and selective use of pharmacologic prophylaxis can help mitigate the incidence.[49]

The need for prolonged mechanical ventilation beyond 24 hours in modern cardiac surgery is uncommon, less than 5% in some studies. However, it is associated with a very high mortality rate. Predictors of the need for prolonged postoperative mechanical ventilation include preoperative renal failure, emphysema, low LVEF (<30%), urgent operation, preoperative critical illness, prolonged CPB time, prolonged cross-clamp time, and perioperative myocardial infarction.[50]

GASTROINTESTINAL COMPLICATIONS

Following cardiac surgery, gastrointestinal (GI) complications are infrequent, with a recent prospective study finding an incidence of 0.35%.[51] Although on the lower end, this is consistent with prior data showing the incidence over the past 15 years to be between 0.5% and 1.5%.[51–53] The most common GI complications following cardiac surgery include upper and lower GI bleeding, acute pancreatitis, acute cholecystitis, perforation of the GI tract, paralytic ileus, visceral ischemia, and liver failure.[54] The pathophysiology of these complications is complex, with hypoperfusion of the viscera as the underlying cause, often as a result of the low flow state during the intraoperative and postoperative period and potential embolic events.[55] The most frequent of these complications is upper GI bleeding, while mesenteric ischemia requires the highest frequency of surgical intervention.[51–53] The mortality from these associated complications ranges from 11% to 67%.[51,52] The combination of a low incidence, significant mortality, and often insidious presentation make the need for perioperative vigilance of these complications very important.[56]

The practice of classifying patients into risk categories based on perioperative factors could be beneficial. **Box 4** lists factors in the perioperative period that have been associated with an increased risk of GI complications.[51–54,56] Studies have not been consistent regarding the threshold at which certain variables lead to increased risk (age, creatinine level in chronic renal insufficiency). Both CPB and prolonged CPB times have been associated with an increased risk of GI complications, but not consistently.[52,57] Despite this potential association, the use of off-pump cardiac surgery has not consistently led to a decrease in the incidence of complications.[57–59] A recent prospective analysis showed a reduction in GI complications when comparing off-pump with on-pump cardiac surgeries.[51] Of note, certain variables have not been associated with an increased risk of GI complications: patient gender, diabetes, preoperative use of anticoagulants or antiplatelet agents, and postoperative utilization of these agents.[53]

A prospective, multivariate analysis study found that after New York Heart Association Class III and IV, and smoking were the strongest independent predictors of death after a GI complication.[52] The same study found that intraoperative variables such as

---

Box 4
Risk factors for gastrointestinal complications following cardiac surgery

Age older than 65 years[a]

Chronic obstructive pulmonary disease

Steroid use

History of cerebrovascular accident

Low cardiac output

Peripheral vascular disease

Reoperative surgery

History of peptic ulcers

Chronic renal insufficiency[b]

Blood transfusion

Prolonged cardiopulmonary bypass time[c,d]

Arrhythmias

Intra-aortic balloon pumping

Combined bypass/valve[d]

Heparin-induced thrombocytopenia type II

Prolonged mechanical ventilation (>24 hours)

Sepsis

   [a] Analysis by a study cited age older than 70 leading to increased risk.[56]
   [b] Lowest value cited as increased risk is 1.4 mg/dL.[52]
   [c] Longer than 98 minutes.[57]
   [d] Studies disagree over associated increased risk.[52]
   Data from Refs.[51–54,56]

CPB time, type of operation, off-pump procedure, and degree of hemorrhage did not influence the probability of death after a GI event.[52]

The most important overall decision is early and aggressive workup, especially in the setting of mesenteric ischemia where survival depends on early recognition.[60] Difficulty in diagnosing mesenteric ischemia is also due to its timing in relation to cardiac surgery, whereby it usually occurs within the first few days postoperatively. During this period the patient's status of mechanical ventilation, sedation, and analgesia remove the signs and symptoms associated with a physical examination consistent with mesenteric ischemia. Other GI pathologic processes such as pancreatitis, peptic ulcer disease, and upper GI bleeds may occur further out from the surgical event, but can still occur in a shorter time frame.[52]

The management of the GI complications depends on the specific complication and the patient's clinical status.[61] One retrospective study found that 21 of 22 cases of GI hemorrhage were medically managed, with no significant difference in mortality between the 2 groups. In the same study, all 3 cases of mesenteric ischemia required surgical intervention.[53]

Prevention of GI complications is difficult because many of the risk factors cannot be modified (age, history of cerebrovascular accident), and those that one can potentially optimize (COPD, chronic respiratory infection, steroid use, blood transfusion, cardiac output) have not been proved to reduce the incidence of GI complications. One area of potential prevention could be in the use of stress ulcer prophylaxis. The overall incidence of stress ulcers following cardiac surgery is low (0.45%) according to a literature review, and this decreased to 0.35% when using histamine receptor–2 antagonists (H2As).[62] Concerns exist about the benefit of stress ulcer prophylaxis in the cardiac population and whether it outweighs the risks associated with it, including increased pneumonia.[63] If stress ulcer prophylaxis is used, the choice between proton-pump inhibitors (PPIs) and H2As is also unclear. A recent meta-analysis supports the utilization of PPIs over H2As in the critically ill, though not specifically the postoperative cardiac surgery population.[64] The difference between the quality of trials, sparse data, and possible publication bias make the results of this meta-analysis questionable. The investigators did conclude that no differences were noted between the 2 classes of drugs regarding increased incidence of pneumonia, death, or length of stay in the ICU.[64] Meta-analysis does not clearly support one of either sucralfate or H2As over the other. However, these data are not specific to postoperative cardiac surgery patients.[65] Both the decision to use stress ulcer prophylaxis in cardiac surgery patients and the choice of drug remain unclear.

ACUTE KIDNEY INJURY

The incidence of acute kidney injury (AKI) in the postoperative period following cardiac surgery occurs in 5% to 30% of patients.[66–71] This wide range of reported incidence is partly due to the lack of specificity in defining AKI. The Acute Dialysis Quality Initiative Group helped establish the RIFLE criteria (Risk, Injury, Failure, Loss, and End-stage renal disease) in 2004 to help define and identify AKI.[72] Moreover, the Acute Kidney Injury Network (AKIN) published a modification of the RIFLE criteria to improve its reliability in identifying AKI.[73] These criteria have been used in large populations of significant variation, including cardiac surgery patients.[68,74,75] Two studies that did use these criteria in cardiac surgery patients found no significant difference between the 2 systems (**Table 2**).[74,75]

Table 2
Criteria of each system in defining acute kidney injury

RIFLE Criteria		
Class	**Glomerular Filtration Rate**	**Urine Output**
Risk	Inc. SCr × 1.5 or GFR dec. >25%	<0.5 mL/kg/h for >6 h
Injury	Inc. SCr × 2 or GFR dec. >50%	<0.5 mL/kg/h for >12 h
Failure	Inc. SCr × 3 or GFR dec. >75% or SCr >4 mg/dL with acute increase of 0.5	<0.5 mL/kg/h for >24 h or anuria >12 h
Loss	Complete loss of renal function >4 wk	
ESRD	Complete loss of renal function >3 mo	
AKIN Criteria		
Stage	**SCr**	**Urine Output**
1	Inc. SCr >0.3 mg/dL or inc. SCr × 1.5	<0.5 mL/kg/h for >6 h
2	Inc. SCr × 2	<0.5 mL/kg/h for >12 h
3	Inc. SCr × 3 or SCr >4 mg/dL (acute inc. SCr >0.5 mg/dL)	<0.5 mL/kg/h for >24 h or anuria >12 h

Abbreviations: dec., decrease; ESRD, end-stage renal disease; GFR, Glomerular filtration rate; Inc., increase; SCr, serum creatinine.

Patients who experience AKI after cardiac surgery have associated increases in their morbidity, mortality, and health care costs. Mortality associated with AKI has been cited as high as 60% in those who require dialysis.[76] Mild elevations in serum creatinine that remain within the normal limit have been associated with increased mortality in cardiac surgery patients.[77] The mortality and morbidity associated with AKI has not significantly changed over the past 2 decades.

Numerous investigators have analyzed patient-related and procedure-related factors in the perioperative period, and their association with the risk of AKI. Consistent risk factors have been noted to be present across multiple studies (**Box 5**).

Procedure-related risk factors that might lead to a decrease in the risk of AKI (while not as consistent across studies) include length of CPB, cross-clamp time, off-pump versus on-pump, nonpulsatile flow, hemolysis, and hemodilution.[69] The importance of recognizing risk factors is important, as patients who are exposed to nephrotoxins (intravenous contrast) might benefit from a delay of nonurgent surgery.

The presumed cause of most incidents of AKI following cardiac surgery is acute tubular necrosis.[78] Owing to the high incidence of AKI in addition to the associated morbidity and mortality, significant research has attempted to reduce the risk. The overall goal has been to maintain adequate renal perfusion while avoiding toxic insults. Euvolemia has been established as reducing the risk of AKI, but cardiac surgery patients postoperatively frequently deal with fluid overload as opposed to hypovolemia. Hydration has been established as reducing the risk of contrast-induced AKI that many cardiac surgery patients are exposed to in the days before surgery secondary to cardiac catherization.[79,80] Hydration has not been established to prevent postoperative AKI in cardiac surgery patients. Limited data seem to suggest that conservative fluid management does not increase the incidence of AKI and that positive fluid balance in the postoperative period is associated with an increased incidence of AKI.[81,82] These data, along with failed attempts at goal-directed fluid resuscitation before cardiac surgery, imply that hydration of cardiac surgery patients does not lead to a decrease in the incidence of AKI.[83] Worsening renal function has been associated with synthetic colloids based on starches, including third generations developed with lower molecular weights.[84–86] Although this evidence is not solely derived from the cardiac surgery population, it is the authors' practice to avoid this class of colloids for their patients. The data concerning prevention of AKI with the use of this frequently used class of drugs in cardiac surgery patients has not been encouraging. Although in theory this drug class decreases oxygen utilization and prevents tubule

---

Box 5
Consistent risk factors for acute kidney injury

Female gender

Chronic obstructive pulmonary disease

Diabetes

Peripheral vascular disease

Renal insufficiency

Congestive heart failure

Left ventricular ejection fraction less than 35%

Emergent surgery

Cardiogenic shock[69]

obstruction, its use has not decreased the incidence of AKI. Prophylactic use of diuretics has led to either an increased incidence or no effect on the incidence of AKI.[78,87] Diuretics are not recommended for prevention of AKI, but continue to play a primary role in treating patients with volume overload.

Despite hopes that alkalization of the urine would reduce the incidence of AKI following cardiac surgery, trials of perioperative alkalization of blood and urine using infusions of sodium bicarbonate have not reduced the incidence of AKI and, in fact, might increase mortality.[88,89] Based on the current evidence, this is not recommended as a preventive measure to reduce AKI.

Both anemia and transfusion of stored blood are risk factors for AKI.[90] The risk of AKI with transfusion is not negligible, and transfusions of blood products should only be used in the proper clinical context.

Research into the potential role of antioxidants (N-acetylcysteine) and vasodilators (dopamine and fenoldopam) in reducing the incidence of AKI has shown their clinical ineffectiveness. N-Acetylcysteine as an oxygen free radical scavenger has failed to demonstrate any benefit in cardiac surgery patients, both those without prior renal injury and those with chronic renal insufficiency.[91] Dopamine has failed to prove benefit in the prevention of AKI and should not be used in this setting.[87] Fenoldopam has mixed evidence to support its use in the setting of AKI prevention, and its use can lead to systemic hypotension.[92–94] A large randomized trial would be most beneficial before fenoldopam can be recommended for prevention of AKI in cardiac surgery patients.

Evidence does show a decrease in the incidence of AKI in off-pump CABG versus on-pump bypass; however, the 30-day rates of death, myocardial infarction, stroke, or need for dialysis were not different between the 2 groups. Based on this information, reduced AKI incidence alone would not be a reason to use off-pump bypass.[95]

Renal replacement therapy (RRT) is often needed in the setting of kidney injury after cardiac surgery for the management of severe acidemia, electrolyte abnormalities refractory to medical management, fluid overload, and significant uremia. Evidence remains inconclusive regarding whether early intervention with RRT before blood urea nitrogen and creatinine are markedly elevated can improve outcomes.[96–98] The specific modality of therapy depends on the underlying need for treatment and on the urgency of the treatment, but otherwise does not have significant influence on outcome.[99]

Despite significant research into the pathophysiology of AKI and attempts to reduce risk and shorten the clinical course, most attempts have not met with clinical success. Future research into other biomarkers might help identify AKI at an earlier stage than the current biomarkers, and thus lead to therapies that can improve outcomes.

CONTROL OF BLOOD GLUCOSE

Hyperglycemia is a common occurrence in cardiac surgical patients even without the preoperative diagnosis of diabetes. Exposure to extracorporeal circulation, hypothermia, and the release of endogenous catecholamines, cortisol, and glucagon all combine to decrease insulin secretion and increase peripheral resistance to the effects of insulin. It has been long known that elevated blood glucose levels are associated with increasing morbidity and mortality in critically ill patients of all types. Postoperative cardiac surgical patients are no exception, as hyperglycemia also leads to higher rates of infection and, potentially, the vasoplegic syndrome.[100]

Whereas there is no doubt that blood glucose control in the perioperative period is important, there exists significant controversy regarding what level should be targeted, and even if intensive insulin therapy does more good than harm. Although the classic intensive insulin therapy study published in 2001 demonstrated improved general clinical outcome,[85] subsequent studies have not consistently demonstrated this beneficial effect. In fact, an alarmingly high rate of hypoglycemia in patients on intensive insulin therapy was seen in one, and a significantly increased risk of stroke noted in another.[101,102] Clinicians need to be cognizant of the prevalence and risk of hyperglycemia in the perioperative period. The question becomes one of how tight control needs to be, and how best to accomplish this. In its 2009 guidelines, The Society of Thoracic Surgeons recommended maintaining serum glucose levels at less than 180 mg/dL.[103] The Surgical Care Improvement Project (SCIP) has recently changed its benchmark to have blood glucose levels less than or equal to 180 mg/dL in the time frame between 18 and 24 hours after the end-anesthesia time.[104]

INFECTIOUS DISEASE

Infections in the postoperative period are not uncommon, with one prospective study reporting an incidence of almost 14%.[105] Infections may arise from multiple sites including the operative field, indwelling catheters and devices, the lungs, and urine. The presentation may vary from local inflammation in a superficial wound infection all the way up to bacteremia and sepsis. Nosocomial infection after cardiac surgery may occur in up to 20% of patients, with VAP the most common (4%–10%), followed by catheter-associated urinary tract infection (1%–3%) and central line–associated bloodstream infections (1%).[106]

Sepsis

Sepsis is fortunately a rare event, occurring in fewer than 2% of postoperative cardiac surgical patients, but causes significant morbidity and mortality. Increases in ventilator dependence, and length of stay in ICU and hospital are seen, with each episode of sepsis estimated to add US$25,000 to $30,000 to the cost of care. Mortality is also significantly increased, with studies demonstrating an increase of 6- to 10-fold. Risk factors for the development of sepsis include increasing patient age, duration of procedure, increased blood loss requiring reoperation, or significantly more blood transfused and low cardiac output syndrome.[107,108]

Sternal Wound Infection and Mediastinitis

Deep sternal wound infection and mediastinitis is a serious complication of cardiac surgery, and has been reported in approximately 1.1% of patients undergoing CABG. It is associated with a higher risk of mortality, with one study showing a mortality of 14% in those with diagnosed sternal wound infections.[109] Rates for infection may be higher in specific subsets of patients such as heart transplant recipients or in the setting of cardiac assist devices, where infection rates have been reported to be 2.5% and higher.[110,111]

The pathogenesis of sternal wound infection is multifactorial and complex, involving wound contamination with subsequent inability to clear the infectious inoculum. Although poorly understood, there do appear to be identifiable associated risk factors (**Box 6**).[16,109–118]

There is a lack of data and consensus regarding the contribution of each of these factors to the risk of sternal wound infection, but it is thought that any underlying process that impairs vascular supply, nutrition, or immunologic status can contribute to the risk of sternal wound infection.

Box 6
Risk factors associated with sternal wound infections

Obesity

Diabetes mellitus or perioperative hyperglycemia

Mobilization of bilateral internal mammary artery for grafting

Prolonged duration of surgery (>5 hours)

Staple use for skin closure

Obstructive airway disease

Dual antiplatelet therapy within 5 days of surgery

Tobacco use

Prior cardiac surgery

Blood transfusion

End-stage renal failure on dialysis

Practically any pathogenic organism can cause mediastinitis, although it has been reported that in up to 83% of cases a single pathogen is isolated, thus indicating monomicrobial infection.[110,111] **Fig. 2** illustrates the distribution of pathogens.

The time course of postoperative sternal wound infection is usually subacute, with one study showing a range of 3 to 416 (time frame) days and a median onset of 7 days.[112] The typical presentation includes fever, leukocytosis, and sternal instability/wound drainage, with sternal wound drainage/cellulitis being present in 85% of patients.[119,120] This characteristic presentation should raise suspicion, with diagnosis confirmed with prompt surgical reexploration. During surgical reexploration the presence of pus in the mediastinum establishes the definitive diagnosis.

In the absence of superficial findings (sternal wound instability, drainage, cellulitis), diagnosis may be more difficult. Signs of systemic infection should still be present, and imaging and/or culture data may help elucidate the diagnosis. CT scanning has

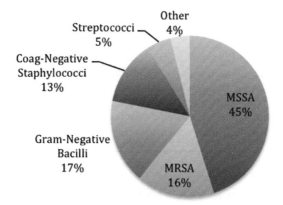

Fig. 2. Pie chart demonstrating the microbiology of mediastinal infections. Coag, coagulase; MRSA, methicillin-resistant *Staphylococcus aureus*; MSSA, methicillin-sensitive *Staphylococcus aureus*. (*Adapted from* Trouillet JL, Vuagnat A, Combes A, et al. Acute poststernotomy mediastinitis managed with debridement and closed-drainage aspiration: factors associated with death in the intensive care unit. J Thorac Cardiovasc Surg 2005;129:518; with permission.)

been found to have high sensitivity (100%) but can have low specificity (33%) if performed before postoperative day 14. The specificity increases as time goes on, and thus a delayed CT scan can greatly aid in diagnosis.[121] Culture data are helpful because the detection of bacteremia, especially *Staphylococcus aureus*, has a strong association with mediastinitis.[122]

Treatment of mediastinitis requires both surgical debridement and antimicrobial therapy. Surgical debridement should be performed urgently in an operating room equipped for complex cardiac surgical procedures. All nonviable tissue and foreign material need to be removed, as they serve as a nidus for infection. Sharp bone edges need to be filed down to minimize risk to underlying structures such as the heart. Total sternectomy was previously advocated, but the increased morbidity associated with chest-wall instability has caused this technique to lose favor.[123] After surgical debridement immediate or delayed closure may take place, although robust evidence supporting either technique is absent.

Initial antimicrobial therapy should consist of broad-spectrum coverage of both gram-positive cocci and gram-negative bacilli. As culture data become available, antibiotic coverage should be narrowed accordingly. Duration of therapy is controversial but should probably include 2 to 3 weeks of antimicrobial therapy in the setting of full debridement, and 4 to 6 weeks if residual infection is suspected at the time of debridement.

The mortality associated with deep sternal wound infection can be as high as 50%,[109,124,125] and independent risk factors for death are detailed in **Box 7**.[125]

Mediastinitis represents a significant increase in length of stay and a 2- to 3-fold increase in the total cost of hospitalization.[109]

Leg Wound Complications

The incidence of leg wound complications after saphenous vein graft harvesting varies widely, with reported percentages anywhere from 1% to 24%.[126–132] The most common of these complications include infection (cellulitis), dermatitis, neuropathy of the saphenous nerve, and lymphocele. Of these complications, those requiring surgery are rare, and one study found that of 3525 CABG procedures, only 0.65% needed surgical intervention.[128]

Bacteremia

Bloodstream infection or bacteremia occurs in approximately 3% of patients after undergoing CABG, is associated with a greater than 4-fold increase in mortality, and is most pronounced when the bacteremia is due to gram-negative bacteria or *S aureus*.[133] Bacteremia in postoperative cardiac surgery patients is thus an important consideration when considering possible infectious etiology.

Box 7
Independent predictors of death in mediastinitis

Delay in sternal closure after debridement (>3 days)

Age older than 65 years

Stay in intensive care unit immediately before sternal debridement

Serum creatinine greater than 2 mg/dL before debridement

Infectious pathogen identified as methicillin-resistant *Staphylococcus aureus*

HEMATOLOGY
Anemia/Transfusion

Postoperative anemia in cardiac surgery patients is a common occurrence, and is often treated with perioperative transfusion. Since the advent of blood conservation and transfusion guidelines, one study has found that the reported rate of patients receiving transfusion who have undergone CABG has decreased from 68% (in the 1990s) to approximately 30% in 2001.[134] However, there is wide variability reported to the Society of Thoracic Surgery Adult Cardiac Surgery Database, with values ranging from 8% to 90% of patients receiving transfusion following CABG.[135] The risk factors for transfusion are listed in **Box 8**.[136]

The risks and benefits of transfusion should be weighed carefully, as there is clear evidence showing worsened outcomes in patients receiving transfusion.[137] In an examination of the literature including the TRACS trial, the TRIC trial, and recommendations of the American College of Chest Physicians, the Society of Thoracic Surgeons, and the Society of Cardiovascular Anesthesiologists, the hemoglobin level to be used as a transfusion trigger is not clearly stated. The data appear to point toward a more restrictive transfusion strategy, with 6 to 8 g/dL being a more favorable trigger than 10 g/dL.[136–138] In a summary of the data, the Society of Thoracic Surgeons and the Society of Cardiovascular Anesthesiologists have recommended the transfusion triggers for cardiac surgery patients (**Box 9**).

Surgical Hemostasis

Postoperative bleeding is often characterized and divided into medical or surgical bleeding. The distinction between the two is a reflection of the definitive treatment of the bleeding.

Rates of surgical bleeding requiring surgical reexploration vary in the literature, but most fall in the range of 2% to 6%, with more recent studies showing a decreasing rate of reexploration of around 2% for CABG.[139,140] Reexploration causes a significant increase in mortality of approximately 10% and increased use of hospital resources, length of stay, and blood-product usage.[141] The decreasing rate in the need for surgical reexploration has been credited to improvements in surgical technique, the increased use of antifibrinolytics, and improved postoperative care.[139–141]

Box 8
Risk factors for perioperative transfusion in patients undergoing cardiac surgery

Lower preoperative hemoglobin

Lower weight

Older age

Female gender

Perioperative use of antiplatelet or antithrombotic drugs

Reoperation

Acquired or congenital clotting/coagulation abnormalities

Complex procedures

Emergency operations

> **Box 9**
> **Transfusion triggers in patients undergoing cardiac surgery**
>
> Hemoglobin less than 6 g/dL: transfusion reasonable and possibly life-saving
>
> Hemoglobin less than 7 g/dL: transfusion reasonable, but supporting high-level evidence not available
>
> Hemoglobin 7 to 10 g/dL: transfusion not unreasonable in selected patients

Hypocoagulability

Platelet dysfunction following cardiopulmonary bypass in cardiac surgery is a well-known, if only partially understood, phenomenon. Exposure to the foreign substrate of the CPB circuit, hypothermia, and acidosis are all thought to play a role in the functional disturbance of platelets during cardiac surgery.[142] In addition to the effects of CPB, perioperative medications can play an important role. Preoperatively used aspirin, adenosine diphosphate receptor inhibitors (clopidogrel, prasugrel, ticagrelor), and glycoprotein IIB/IIIA inhibitors (abciximab, eptifibatide) are commonly encountered in the cardiac surgery patient, and can significantly contribute to postoperative platelet dysfunction. The timing of discontinuation before cardiac surgery is controversial, and some of these agents may play an important role in postoperative bleeding.[143,144]

Although heparin dosing based on weight, activated clotting time (ACT), and optimal protamine reversal dosing are well established, a residual heparin effect should always be a consideration in the postoperative cardiac surgery patient with bleeding. Continued ACT monitoring, thromboelastography, and activated partial thromboplastin time can be useful tools to help evaluate this effect.[145]

Thrombocytopenia

Cardiac surgery patients are especially prone to the development of thrombocytopenia in the postoperative period. There can be many causes for this. Cardiopulmonary bypass itself can reduce platelet count by 30% to 50% owing to the release of platelet factor 4 (PF4), along with hemodilution and mechanical destruction of platelets in the bypass circuit. Other factors that may play a role in this setting include the use of an intra-aortic balloon pump along with a host of medications including antibiotics, antiarrhythmics, heparin, thienopyridines, and glycoprotein IIb/IIIa inhibitors.[146] Whereas most of these factors are transient and self-limited, heparin-induced thrombocytopenia (HIT) is potentially fatal and requires active therapeutic intervention.

The diagnosis of HIT is particularly difficult in the postoperative cardiac surgical patient because of the myriad of potential causes already outlined. Because the usual decrease in platelets that accompanies use of the CPB circuit does not usually persist beyond 72 hours, HIT should be suspected for thrombocytopenia that persists or worsens beyond this time frame. Of course, any unusual thrombosis or multiple thrombotic events should also make the diagnosis suspect. There are several laboratory tests available, with varying degrees of sensitivity and specificity. Testing for PF4 antibodies using an enzyme-linked immunosorbent assay has an approximately 90% negative predictive value and is a good screening test. Because the specificity of this test is low, a serotonin-releasing assay (SRA) will be more diagnostic. In one study of surgical ICU patients, 81% had a false-positive PF4 with a negative SRA.[147]

Treatment consists of stopping all sources of heparin, including any low molecular weight heparin, heparin flushes for arterial lines, and heparin-coated catheters. Because of the high risk for thrombotic events, an alternative anticoagulant should

---

Box 10
Factors associated with an increased risk of sustaining a neurologic problem

Advanced age

Valvular procedure

Combined coronary artery bypass grafting/valve procedure

Prior neurologic event

Duration of aortic cross-clamping

Diabetes mellitus

Data from Boeken U, Litmathe J, Feindt J, et al. Neurological complications after cardiac surgery: risk factors and correlation to the surgical procedure. Thorac Cardiovasc Surg 2005;53(1):33–6.

---

be started. The 2 most common agents are bivalirudin and argatroban, both direct thrombin inhibitors.[148,149] Platelets should not be transfused unless active bleeding is occurring, owing to the fear that they may contribute to the precipitation of further thrombotic events. Transition to warfarin can occur when the patient has been successfully anticoagulated with a direct thrombin inhibitor and the platelet count has reached at least 150,000/μL.[150,151]

NEUROLOGIC COMPLICATIONS

Neurologic problems can occur following cardiac surgical procedures of all types, and are a significant source of increased morbidity and mortality. These complications can lead to lifelong functional disability, often requiring increased consumption of health care resources and placement in a long-term care facility.

The overall incidence of postoperative neurologic complications ranges from 1% to 2% in low-risk patients up to 6% to 8% for those at high risk (**Box 10**).

Strokes are clearly the most devastating neurologic complication. Strokes may arise from either systemic hypoperfusion occurring in the perioperative period, or as a result of particulate emboli. The latter may arise from a variety of sources, including atheromatous plaque, trapped air, clots, or fat particles. Far more common than strokes, however, are a spectrum of disorders of consciousness, which may include varying degrees of cognitive dysfunction without evidence of motor involvement.

Prolonged emergence, delirium, stupor, or prolonged cognitive dysfunction may be present in up to 10% of postoperative cardiac surgery patients. The etiology of this set of conditions is often difficult to isolate, and is probably multifactorial. Hypoperfusion, microemboli, hypoxia, cerebral edema, and effects of pharmacologic agents have all been thought to play a role in the development of the encephalopathic process. Although CPB and the associated risk of microemboli has been thought to increase the risk of adverse cognitive outcomes, Jensen and colleagues[151] have shown that this has not been necessarily the case. Short-term cognitive defects usually resolve within 1 to 3 months, and long-term risks are not clearly defined.

SUMMARY

Caring for the postoperative cardiac surgical patient is challenging because of the number and severity of potential complications. By definition, the patient presents preoperatively with some degree of cardiac dysfunction, and the procedure itself may cause (at least transiently) further deterioration. The sequelae of the resultant malperfusion state can lead to increased morbidity and mortality. Patients presenting for cardiac surgical procedures are older and with more comorbidities, and the procedures themselves are more complex with the increased use of technology. The physician caring for the postoperative cardiac surgical patient must be cognizant of the myriad of problems with which these patients may present, and be able to marshal the resources necessary to provide effective treatment.

REFERENCES

1. Eltzschig HK, Rosenberger P, Loffler M, et al. Impact of intraoperative transesophageal echocardiography on surgical decisions in 12,566 patients undergoing cardiac surgery. Ann Thorac Surg 2008;85:845–53.
2. Practice guidelines for perioperative transesophageal echocardiography. Anesthesiology 2010;112(5).
3. Shernan S. Perioperative myocardial ischemia reperfusion injury. Anesthesiol Clin North America 2003;21:466.
4. Suleiman MS, Zacharowski K, Gangelini GD. Inflammatory response and cardioprotection during open-heart surgery: the importance of anesthetics. Br J Pharmacol 2008;153:21–33.
5. Yau JM, Alexander JH, Hafley G, et al, PREVENT IV Investigators. Impact of perioperative myocardial infarction on angiographic and clinical outcomes following coronary artery bypass grafting [from project of ex-vivo vein graft engineering via transfection (PREVENT) IV]. Am J Cardiol 2008;102:546–51.
6. Hirsch WS, Ledley GS, Kotler MN. Acute ischemic syndromes following coronary artery bypass graft surgery. Clin Cardiol 1998;21:625–32.
7. Russo AM, O'Connor WH, Waxman HL. Atypical presentations and echocardiographic findings in patients with cardiac tamponade occurring early and late after cardiac surgery. Chest 1993;104:71–8.
8. Rozental T, Shore-Lesserson L. Postoperative bleeding, coagulopathy, and blood transfusion in the cardiac surgical patient. In: Sladen RN, Fanshawe M, editors. Postoperative cardiac care. Baltimore (MD): Lippincott Williams & Wilkins; 2011. p. 231–52.
9. Ibrahim M, Rao C, Ashrafian H, et al. Modern management of systolic anterior motion of the mitral valve. Eur J Cardiothorac Surg 2012;6:1260–70.
10. Shoaib RF, Anwar F, Nyawo B, et al. Bilateral tension pneumothoraces following coronary artery bypass grafting. J Coll Physicians Surg Pak 2009;19(7):444–6.
11. Stevenson LW. Clinical use of inotropic therapy for heart failure: looking backward or forward? Part I: inotropic infusions during hospitalization. Circulation 2003;108:367–72.
12. Christakis GT, Fremes SE, Koch JP, et al. Determinants of low systemic vascular resistance during cardiopulmonary bypass. Ann Thorac Surg 1994;58:1040.
13. Sladen RN. Pharmacotherapy of the failing heart. In: International Anesthesiology Research Society (IARS) review lectures. 2006. p. 117–22.
14. Bristow MR, Ginsburg R, Minobe W. Decreased catecholamine sensitivity and β-adrenergic-receptor density in failing human hearts. N Engl J Med 1982;307:205–11.
15. Brodde OE, Schuler S, Kretsch R, et al. Regional distribution of β-adrenoceptors in the human heart: coexistence of function of β1- and β2-adrenoceptors in both atria and ventricles in severe congestive cardiomyopathy. J Cardiovasc Pharmacol 1986;8:1235–42.

16. Milano CA, Kesler K, Archibald N, et al. Mediastinitis after coronary artery bypass graft surgery. Risk factors and long-term survival. Circulation 1995;92: 2245.
17. Sanders D, Dudley M, Groban L. Diastolic dysfunction, cardiovascular aging, and the anesthesiologist. Anesthesiol Clin 2009;27(3):497–517.
18. Flynn BC. Postoperative pulmonary hypertension: etiologies, sequelae, and management. In: Sladen RN, Fanshawe M, editors. Postoperative cardiac care. Baltimore (MD): Lippincott Williams & Wilkins; 2011. p. 75–91.
19. Patti G, Chello M, Candura D, et al. Randomized trial of atorvastatin for reduction of postoperative atrial fibrillation in patients undergoing cardiac surgery. Circulation 2006;114:1455–61.
20. Rho R. The management of atrial fibrillation after cardiac surgery. Heart 2009;95: 422–9.
21. Daoud EG, Strickberger SA, Man KC, et al. Preoperative amiodarone as prophylaxis against atrial fibrillation after heart surgery. N Engl J Med 1997;337(25): 1785–91.
22. Koniarik I, Apostolakis E, Rogkakou C, et al. Pharmacologic prophylaxis for atrial fibrillation following cardiac surgery: a systematic review. J Cardiothorac Surg 2010;5:121.
23. El-Chami MF, Sawaya FJ, Kilgo P, et al. Ventricular arrhythmia after cardiac surgery. J Am Coll Cardiol 2012;60(25):2664–71.
24. Merin O, Ilan M, Oren A, et al. Permanent pacemaker implantation following cardiac surgery: indications and long-term follow-up. Pacing Clin Electrophysiol 2009;32:7–12.
25. Miller RH, Horneffer PJ, Gardner TJ, et al. The epidemiology of the postpericardiotomy syndrome: a common complication of cardiac surgery. Am Heart J 1988;116:1323–9.
26. Khan AH. The postcardiac injury syndromes. Clin Cardiol 1992;15:67–72.
27. Gaudino M, Anselmi A, Pavone N, et al. Constrictive pericarditis after cardiac surgery. Ann Thorac Surg 2013;95(20):731–6.
28. Yetkin U, Kestelli M, Yilik L, et al. Recent surgical experience in chronic constrictive pericarditis. Tex Heart Inst J 2003;30(1):27–30.
29. Gomes WJ, Carvalho AC, Palma JH, et al. Vasoplegic syndrome: a new dilemma. J Thorac Cardiovasc Surg 1994;107(3):942–3.
30. Carrel T, Englberger L, Mohacsi P, et al. Low systemic vascular resistance after cardiopulmonary bypass: incidence, etiology, and clinical importance. J Card Surg 2000;15(5):347–53.
31. Sun X, Zhang L, Hill PC, et al. Is incidence of postoperative vasoplegic syndrome different between off-pump and on-pump coronary artery bypass grafting surgery? Eur J Cardiothorac Surg 2008;34(4):820–5.
32. Fischer GW, Levin MA. Vasoplegia during cardiac surgery: current concepts and management. Semin Thorac Cardiovasc Surg 2010;22(2):140–4.
33. Landry DW, Levin HR, Gallant EM, et al. Vasopressin deficiency contributes to the vasodilation of septic shock. Circulation 1997;95:1122–5.
34. Weiner MM, Lin HM, Danforth D, et al. Methylene blue is associated with poor outcomes in vasoplegic shock. J Cardiothorac Vasc Anesth 2013;27:1233–8. http://dx.doi.org/10.1053/j.jvca.2013.02.026 pii:S1053-0770(13)00129-8.
35. Papadopoulos G, Sintou E, Siminelakis S, et al. Perioperative infusion of low-dose of vasopressin for prevention and management of vasodilatory vasoplegic syndrome in patients undergoing coronary artery bypass grafting. J Cardiothorac Surg 2010;28(5):17. http://dx.doi.org/10.1186/1749-8090-5-17.

36. Ozal E, Kuralay E, Yildirim V, et al. Preoperative methylene blue administration in patients at high risk for vasoplegic syndrome during cardiac surgery. Ann Thorac Surg 2005;79(5):1615–9.

37. Adabag AS, Wassif HS, Rice K, et al. Preoperative pulmonary function and mortality after cardiac surgery. Am Heart J 2010;159(4):691–7.

38. Weissman C. Pulmonary complications after cardiac surgery. Semin Cardiothorac Vasc Anesth 2004;8(3):185–211.

39. Labidi M, Baillot R, Dionne B, et al. Pleural effusions following cardiac surgery. Chest 2009;136:1604–11.

40. Aguirre VJ, Sinha P, Zimmet A, et al. Phrenic nerve injury during cardiac surgery: mechanism, management and prevention. Heart Lung Circ 2013;22:895–902.

41. Messent M, Sullivan K, Keogh BF, et al. Adult respiratory distress syndrome following cardiopulmonary bypass: incidence and prediction. Anaesthesia 1992;47:267–8.

42. Rady MY, Ryan T, Starr NJ. Early onset of acute pulmonary dysfunction after cardiovascular surgery: risk factors and clinical outcome. Crit Care Med 1997;25:1831–9.

43. Tonz M, Mihaljevic T, von Segesser LK, et al. Acute lung injury during cardiopulmonary bypass: are the neutrophils responsible? Chest 1995;108:1551–6.

44. Royston D, Fleming JS, Desai JB, et al. Increased production of peroxidation products associated with cardiac operations. Evidence for free radical generation. J Thorac Cardiovasc Surg 1986;91:759–66.

45. Kirklin JK, Westaby S, Blackstone EH, et al. Complement and the damaging effects of cardiopulmonary bypass. J Thorac Cardiovasc Surg 1983;86:845–57.

46. Koch C, Li L, Figueroa P, et al. Transfusion and pulmonary morbidity after cardiac surgery. Ann Thorac Surg 2009;88:1410–8.

47. Popovsky M. Transfusion-related acute lung injury: incidence, pathogenesis and the role of multicomponent apheresis in its prevention. Transfus Med Hemother 2008;35:76–9.

48. Toy P, Lowell C. TRALI—definition, mechanisms, incidence and clinical relevance. Best Pract Res Clin Anaesthesiol 2007;21:183–93.

49. Bojar RN. Respiratory management. In: Manual of perioperative care in adult cardiac surgery. 5th edition. Oxford (United Kingdom): Wiley-Blackwell; 2011. p. 385–436.

50. Siddiqui MA, Paras I, Jalal A. Risk factors of prolonged mechanical ventilation following open heart surgery: what has changed over the last decade? Cardiovasc Diagn Ther 2012;2(3):192–9.

51. Hashemzadeh K, Hashemzadeh S. Predictors and outcome of gastrointestinal complications after cardiac surgery. Minerva Chir 2012;67(4):327–35.

52. Mangi AA, Christison-Lagay ER, Torchiana DF, et al. Gastrointestinal complications in patients undergoing heart operation: an analysis of 8709 consecutive cardiac surgical patients. Ann Surg 2005;241(6):895–901 [discussion: 901–4].

53. Yilmaz AT, Arslan M, Demirkilç U, et al. Gastrointestinal complications after cardiac surgery. Eur J Cardiothorac Surg 1996;10(9):763–7.

54. Nilsson J, Hansson E, Andersson B. Intestinal ischemia after cardiac surgery: analysis of a large registry. J Cardiothorac Surg 2013;8:156.

55. Ohri SK, Velissaris T. Gastrointestinal dysfunction following cardiac surgery. Perfusion 2006;21:215–23.

56. Rodriguez R, Robich MP, Plate JF, et al. Gastrointestinal complications following cardiac surgery: a comprehensive review. J Card Surg 2010;25(2):188–97.

57. Sanisoglu I, Guden M, Bayramoglu Z, et al. Does off-pump CABG reduce gastrointestinal complications? Ann Thorac Surg 2004;77(2):619–25.

58. Poirier B, Baillot R, Bauset R, et al. Abdominal complications associated with cardiac surgery. Review of a contemporary surgical experience and of a series done without extracorporeal circulation. Can J Surg 2003;46(3):176–82.

59. Musleh GS, Patel NC, Grayson AD, et al. Off-pump coronary artery bypass surgery does not reduce gastrointestinal complications. Eur J Cardiothorac Surg 2003;23(2):170–4.

60. Clavien PA, Muller C, Harder F. Treatment of mesenteric infarction. Br J Surg 1987;74:500–3.

61. Abboud B, Daher R, Boujaoude J. Acute mesenteric ischemia after cardiopulmonary bypass surgery. World J Gastroenterol 2008;14(35):5361–70.

62. van der Voort PH, Zandstra DF. Pathogenesis, risk factors, and incidence of upper gastrointestinal bleeding after cardiac surgery: is specific prophylaxis in routine bypass procedures needed? J Cardiothorac Vasc Anesth 2000;14:293–9.

63. Bateman BT, Bykov K, Choudhry NK, et al. Type of stress ulcer prophylaxis and risk of nosocomial pneumonia in cardiac surgical patients: cohort study. BMJ 2013;347:f5416.

64. Alhazzani W, Alenezi F, Jaeschke RZ, et al. Proton pump inhibitors versus histamine 2 receptor antagonists for stress ulcer prophylaxis in critically ill patients: a systematic review and meta-analysis. Crit Care Med 2013;41(3):693–705.

65. Cook D, Guyatt G, Marshall J, et al. A comparison of sucralfate and ranitidine for the prevention of upper gastrointestinal bleeding in patients requiring mechanical ventilation. N Engl J Med 1998;338:791–7.

66. Shaw A. Update on acute kidney injury after cardiac surgery. J Thorac Cardiovasc Surg 2012;143:676–81.

67. Alsabbagh MM, Asmar A, Ejaz N, et al. Update on clinical trials for the prevention of acute kidney injury in patients undergoing cardiac surgery. Am J Surg 2013;206:86–95.

68. Kuitunen A, Vento A, Suojaranta-Ylinen R, et al. Acute renal failure after cardiac surgery: evaluation of the RIFLE classification. Ann Thorac Surg 2006;81:542–6.

69. Rosner MD, Okusa MD. Acute kidney injury associated with cardiac surgery. Clin J Am Soc Nephrol 2006;1:19–32.

70. Hudson C, et al. Emerging concepts in acute kidney injury following cardiac surgery. Semin Cardiothorac Vasc Anesth 2008;12:320–30.

71. Coleman MD, Shaefi S, Sladen RN. Preventing acute kidney injury after cardiac surgery. Curr Opin Anesthesiol 2011;24:70–6.

72. Bellomo R, Ronco C, Kellum JA, et al. Acute renal failure: definition, outcome measures, animal models, fluid therapy and information technology needs: the Second International Consensus Conference on the Acute Dialysis Quality Initiative (ADQI) Group. Crit Care 2004;8:R204–12.

73. Mehta RL, Kellum JA, Shah SV, et al. Acute Kidney Injury Network: report of an initiative to improve outcomes in acute kidney injury. Crit Care 2007;11:R31.

74. Morgan DJ, Ho KM. A comparison of nonoliguric and oliguric severe acute kidney injury according to the risk injury failure loss end-stage (RIFLE) criteria. Nephron Clin Pract 2010;115:c59–65.

75. Yan X, Jia S, Meng X, et al. Acute kidney injury in adult postcardiotomy patients with extracorporeal membrane oxygenation: evaluation of the RIFLE classification and the Acute Kidney Injury Network criteria. Eur J Cardiothorac Surg 2010;37:334–8.

76. Chertow GM, Lazarus JM, Christiansen CL, et al. Preoperative renal risk stratification. Circulation 1997;95:878–84.

77. Lassnigg A, Schmid ER, Hiesmayr M, et al. Impact of minimal increases in serum creatinine on outcome in patients after cardiothoracic surgery: do we have to revise current definitions of acute renal failure? Crit Care Med 2008;36:1129–37.
78. Mahesh B, Yim B, Robson D, et al. Does furosemide prevent renal dysfunction in high-risk cardiac surgical patients? Results of a double-blinded prospective randomized trial. Eur J Cardiothorac Surg 2008;33:370–6.
79. Del Duca D, Iqbal S, Rahme E, et al. Renal failure after cardiac surgery: timing of cardiac catheterization and other perioperative risk factors. Ann Thorac Surg 2007;84:1264–71.
80. Mueller C, Beurkle G, Buettner HJ, et al. Prevention of contrast media-associated nephropathy: randomized comparison of 2 hydration regimens in 1620 patients undergoing coronary angioplasty. Arch Intern Med 2002;162: 329–36.
81. Kambhampati G, Ross EA, Alsabbagh MM, et al. Perioperative fluid balance and acute kidney injury. Clin Exp Nephrol 2012;16:730–8.
82. Stewart RM, Park PK, Hunt JP, et al. Less in more: improved outcomes in surgical patients with conservative fluid administration and central venous catheter monitoring. J Am Coll Surg 2009;208:725–35.
83. Valentine RJ, Duke ML, Imman MH, et al. Effectiveness of pulmonary artery catheters in aortic surgery: a randomized trial. J Vasc Surg 1998;27:203–11.
84. Perner A, Haase N, Guttormsen AB, et al. Hydroxyethyl starch 130/0.4 versus Ringer's acetate in severe sepsis. N Engl J Med 2012;367:124–34.
85. Van den Berghe G, Wouters P, Weekers F, et al. Intensive insulin therapy in the critically ill patients. N Engl J Med 2001;345:1359–67.
86. NICE-SUGAR Study Investigators, Finfer S, Chittock DR, et al. Intensive versus conventional glucose control in critically ill patients. N Engl J Med 2009;360: 1283–97.
87. Lassnigg A, Donner E, Grubhofer G, et al. Lack of renoprotective effects of dopamine and furosemide during cardiac surgery. J Am Soc Nephrol 2000; 11:97–104.
88. McGuinness SP, Parke RL, Bellomo R, et al. Sodium bicarbonate infusion to reduce cardiac surgery-associated acute kidney injury: a phase II multicenter double-blind randomized controlled trial. Crit Care Med 2013;41:1599–607.
89. Haase M, Haase-Fielitz A, Plass M, et al. Prophylactic perioperative sodium bicarbonate to prevent injury following open heart surgery: a multicenter double-blinded randomized controlled trial. PLoS Med 2013;10(4):e1001426.
90. Stafford-Smith M, Newman MF. What effects do hemodilution and blood transfusion during cardiopulmonary bypass have on renal outcomes? Nat Clin Pract Nephrol 2006;2:188–9.
91. Adbag AS, Ishani A, Bloomfield HE, et al. Efficacy of N-acetylcysteine in preventing renal injury after heart surgery: a systemic review of randomized trials. Eur Heart J 2009;30:1910–7.
92. Landoni G, Biondi-Zoccai GG, Marino G, et al. Fenoldopam reduces the need for renal replacement therapy and in-hospital death in cardiovascular surgery: a meta-analysis. J Cardiothorac Vasc Anesth 2008;22:27–33.
93. Zangrillo A, Biondi-Zoccai GG, Frati E, et al. Fenoldopam and acute renal failure in cardiac surgery: a meta-analysis of randomized placebo-controlled trials. J Cardiothorac Vasc Anesth 2012;26:407–13.
94. Ranucci M, Soro G, Barzaghi N, et al. Fenoldopam prophylaxis of postoperative acute renal failure in high-risk cardiac surgery patients. Ann Thorac Surg 2004; 78:1332–7.

95. Lamy A, Devereaux PJ, Prabhakaran D, et al. Off-pump or on-pump coronary-artery bypass grafting at 30 days. N Engl J Med 2012;366:1489–97.
96. Durmaz I, Yagdi T, Calkavur T, et al. Prophylactic dialysis in patients with renal dysfunction undergoing on-pump coronary artery bypass surgery. Ann Thorac Surg 2003;75(3):859–64.
97. Bent P, Tan HK, Bellomo R, et al. Early and intensive continuous hemofiltration for severe renal failure after cardiac surgery. Ann Thorac Surg 2001;71(3): 832–7.
98. Schiffl H, Lang SM, Fischer R. Daily hemodialysis and the outcome of acute renal failure. N Engl J Med 2002;346(5):305–10.
99. Rabindranath K, Adams J, Macleod AM, et al. Intermittent versus continuous renal replacement therapy for acute renal failure in adults. Cochrane Database Syst Rev 2007;(3):CD003773.
100. Rosas MM, Goicoecha-Turcott EW, Ortiz PA, et al. Glycemic control in cardiac surgery. In: Perioperative considerations in cardiac surgery. Rijeka, Croatia: Intech; 2012.
101. Devos P, Preiser JC, Melot C. Impact of tight glycemic control by intensive insulin therapy on ICU mortality and the rate of hypoglycemia: final results of the Glucontrol study. Intensive Care Med 2007;33(Suppl 2):S189.
102. Gandhi GY, Nuttall GA, Abel MD, et al. Intensive intraoperative insulin therapy versus conventional glucose management during cardiac surgery: a randomized trial. Ann Intern Med 2007;146:233–43.
103. Lazar HL, McDonnell M, Chipkin SR, et al. The Society of Thoracic Surgeons practice guidelines series: blood glucose management during adult cardiac surgery. Ann Thorac Surg 2009;87:663–9.
104. Specifications Manual for National Hospital Inpatient Quality Measures. The Joint Commission. SCIP-Inf-4-1 – SCIP-Inf-4-9, September 2013.
105. Oliveira DC, Oliveira Filho JB, Silva RF, et al. Sepsis in the postoperative period of cardiac surgery: problem description. Arq Bras Cardiol 2010;94(3):332–6.
106. Segers P, Speekenbrink RG, Ubbink DT, et al. Prevention of nosocomial infection in cardiac surgery. JAMA 2006;296(20):2460–6.
107. Michalopoulos A, Stavridis G, Geroulanos S. Severe sepsis in cardiac surgical patients. Eur J Surg 1998;164(3):217–22.
108. Lola I, Levidiotou S, Petrou A, et al. Are there independent predisposing factors for postoperative infections following open heart surgery? J Cardiothorac Surg 2011;6:151.
109. Loop FD, Lytle BW, Cosgrove DM, et al. J. Maxwell Chamberlain memorial paper. Sternal wound complications after isolated coronary artery bypass grafting: early and late mortality, morbidity, and cost of care. Ann Thorac Surg 1990; 49:179.
110. Baldwin RT, Radovancevic B, Sweeney MS, et al. Bacterial mediastinitis after heart transplantation. J Heart Lung Transplant 1992;11:545.
111. Griffith BP, Kormos RL, Hardesty RL, et al. The artificial heart: infection-related morbidity and its effect on transplantation. Ann Thorac Surg 1988;45:409.
112. Borger MA, Rao V, Weisel RD, et al. Deep sternal wound infection: risk factors and outcomes. Ann Thorac Surg 1998;65:1050.
113. Braxton JH, Marrin CA, McGrath PD, et al. Mediastinitis and long-term survival after coronary artery bypass graft surgery. Ann Thorac Surg 2000;70: 2004–7.
114. Bitkover CY, Gårdlund B. Mediastinitis after cardiovascular operations: a case-control study of risk factors. Ann Thorac Surg 1998;65:36.

115. Trick WE, Scheckler WE, Tokars JI, et al. Modifiable risk factors associated with deep sternal site infection after coronary artery bypass grafting. J Thorac Cardiovasc Surg 2000;119:108.
116. Furnary AP, Zerr KJ, Grunkemeier GL, et al. Continuous intravenous insulin infusion reduces the incidence of deep sternal wound infection in diabetic patients after cardiac surgical procedures. Ann Thorac Surg 1999;67:352.
117. Wouters R, Wellens F, Vanermen H, et al. Sternitis and mediastinitis after coronary artery bypass grafting. Analysis of risk factors. Tex Heart Inst J 1994; 21:183.
118. Blasco-Colmenares E, Perl TM, Guallar E, et al. Aspirin plus clopidogrel and risk of infection after coronary artery bypass surgery. Arch Intern Med 2009;169:788.
119. Fariñas MC, Gald Peralta F, Bernal JM, et al. Suppurative mediastinitis after open-heart surgery: a case-control study covering a seven-year period in Santander, Spain. Clin Infect Dis 1995;20:272.
120. Bor DH, Rose RM, Modlin JF, et al. Mediastinitis after cardiovascular surgery. Rev Infect Dis 1983;5:885.
121. Jolles H, Henry DA, Roberson JP, et al. Mediastinitis following median sternotomy: CT findings. Radiology 1996;201:463.
122. Fowler VG Jr, Kaye KS, Simel DL, et al. *Staphylococcus aureus* bacteremia after median sternotomy: clinical utility of blood culture results in the identification of postoperative mediastinitis. Circulation 2003;108:73.
123. El Oakley RM, Wright JE. Postoperative mediastinitis: classification and management. Ann Thorac Surg 1996;61:1030.
124. Risnes I, Abdelnoor M, Almdahl SM, et al. Mediastinitis after coronary artery bypass grafting risk factors and long-term survival. Ann Thorac Surg 2010; 89:1502.
125. Karra R, McDermott L, Connelly S, et al. Risk factors for 1-year mortality after postoperative mediastinitis. J Thorac Cardiovasc Surg 2006;132:537.
126. L'Ecuyer PB, Murphy D, Little JR, et al. The epidemiology of chest and leg wound infections following cardiothoracic surgery. Clin Infect Dis 1996;22:424.
127. Slaughter MS, Olson MM, Lee JT Jr, et al. A fifteen-year wound surveillance study after coronary artery bypass. Ann Thorac Surg 1993;56:1063.
128. Paletta CE, Huang DB, Fiore AC, et al. Major leg wound complications after saphenous vein harvest for coronary revascularization. Ann Thorac Surg 2000;70:492.
129. Kiaii B, Moon BC, Massel D, et al. A prospective randomized trial of endoscopic versus conventional harvesting of the saphenous vein in coronary artery bypass surgery. J Thorac Cardiovasc Surg 2002;123:204.
130. Schurr UP, Lachat ML, Reuthebuch O, et al. Endoscopic saphenous vein harvesting for CABG—a randomized, prospective trial. Thorac Cardiovasc Surg 2002;50:160.
131. Dacey LJ, Braxton JH Jr, Kramer RS, et al. Long-term outcomes of endoscopic vein harvesting after coronary artery bypass grafting. Circulation 2011;123: 147.
132. Swenne CL, Lindholm C, Borowiec J, et al. Surgical-site infections within 60 days of coronary artery by-pass graft surgery. J Hosp Infect 2004;57:14.
133. Olsen MA, Krauss M, Agniel D, et al. Mortality associated with bloodstream infection after coronary artery bypass surgery. Clin Infect Dis 2008;46:1537.
134. Karkouti K, Cohen MM, McCluskey SA, et al. A multivariable model for predicting the need for blood transfusion in patients undergoing first-time elective coronary bypass graft surgery. Transfusion 2001;41:1193.

135. Bennett-Guerrero E, Zhao Y, O'Brien SM, et al. Variation in use of blood transfusion in coronary artery bypass graft surgery. JAMA 2010;304:1568.
136. Society of Thoracic Surgeons Blood Conservation Guideline Task Force, Ferraris VA, et al. Perioperative blood transfusion and blood conservation in cardiac surgery: the Society of Thoracic Surgeons and the Society of Cardiovascular Anesthesiologists clinical practice guideline. Ann Thorac Surg 2007;83:S27.
137. Hajjar LA, Vincent JL, Galas FR, et al. Transfusion requirements after cardiac surgery: the TRACS randomized controlled trial. JAMA 2010;304:1559.
138. Hébert PC, Wells G, Blajchman MA, et al. A multicenter, randomized, controlled clinical trial of transfusion requirements in critical care. N Engl J Med 1999; 340(6):409–17.
139. Sellman M, Intonti MA, Ivert T. Reoperations for bleeding after coronary artery bypass procedures during 25 years. Eur J Cardiothorac Surg 1997;11:521.
140. Munoz JJ, Birkmeyer NJ, Dacey LJ, et al. Trends in rates of reexploration for hemorrhage after coronary artery bypass surgery. Northern New England Cardiovascular Disease Study Group. Ann Thorac Surg 1999;68:1321.
141. Dacey LJ, Munoz JJ, Baribeau YR, et al. Reexploration for hemorrhage following coronary artery bypass grafting: incidence and risk factors. Arch Surg 1998; 133:442–7.
142. Harker LA, Malpass TW, Branson HE, et al. Mechanism of abnormal bleeding in patients undergoing cardiopulmonary bypass: acquired transient platelet dysfunction associated with selective alpha-granule release. Blood 1980;56(5):824–34.
143. Eagle KA, Guyton RA, Davidoff R, et al. ACC/AHA 2004 guideline update for coronary artery bypass graft surgery: summary article. A report of the American College of Cardiology/American Heart Association task force on practice guidelines (Committee to update the 1999 guidelines for coronary artery bypass graft surgery). J Am Coll Cardiol 2004;44:e213.
144. Becker RC, Meade TW, Berger PB, et al. The primary and secondary prevention of coronary artery disease: American College of Chest Physicians evidence-based clinical practice guidelines (8th edition). Chest 2008;133:776S.
145. Lincoff AM, LeNarz LA, Despotis GJ, et al. Abciximab and bleeding during coronary surgery: results from the EPILOG and EPISTENT trials. Improve long-term outcome with abciximab GP IIb/IIIa blockade. Evaluation of platelet IIb/IIIa inhibition in STENTing. Ann Thorac Surg 2000;70:516.
146. Matthai WH. Thrombocytopenia in cardiovascular patients. Chest 2005;127: 46S–52S.
147. Berry C, Tcherniantchouk O, Ley EJ, et al. Overdiagnosis of heparin-induced thrombocytopenia in surgical ICU patients. J Am Coll Surg 2011;213(1):10–7.
148. Warkentin TE, Greinacher A, Koster A, et al. Treatment and prevention of heparin-induced thrombocytopenia: American College of Chest Physicians evidence-based clinical practice guidelines (8th edition). Chest 2008; 133(Suppl 6):340S.
149. Lewis BE, Wallis DE, Leya F, et al. Argatroban anticoagulation in patients with heparin-induced thrombocytopenia. Arch Intern Med 2003;163(15):1849.
150. Linkins LA, Dans AL, Moores LK, et al. Treatment and prevention of heparin-induced thrombocytopenia: antithrombotic therapy and prevention of thrombosis, 9th ed: American College of Chest Physicians evidence-based clinical practice guidelines. Chest 2012;141(Suppl 2):e495S.
151. Jensen BO, Rasmussen LS, Steinbruchel DA. Cognitive outcomes in elderly high-risk patients 1 year after off-pump versus on-pump coronary artery bypass grafting. A randomized trial. Eur J Cardiothorac Surg 2008;34(5):1016–21.

Neurologic Aspects of Cardiac Emergencies

Lauren Ng, MD, MPH[a,b], Jing Wang, PhD[c], Laith Altaweel, MD[d],
M. Kamran Athar, MD[b,e],*

KEYWORDS

- Cardiac emergencies • Neurologic complications • Stroke • Acute brain injury

KEY POINTS

- Therapeutic hypothermia has improved neurologic outcomes after cardiac arrest, with newer prognostication models emerging.
- Hemorrhagic and ischemic stroke and transient ischemic attack are the most common neurologic complications associated with aortic dissection, ventricular assist devices and coronary artery bypass grafting.
- Neurologic complications occur in 20–40% of cases of infective endocarditis and include stroke, intracerebral hemorrhage, meningitis, brain abscess and intracranial mycotic aneurysms.
- There is a lack of data on the management of aortic dissection, ventricular assist devices, coronary artery bypass grafting and infective endocarditis in the setting of neurologic complications.
- Neurogenic stunned myocardium is an important disease entity that can mimic an acute myocardial infarction, but is a stress cardiomyopathy related to neurologic illness.

INTRODUCTION

Cardiac emergencies can be associated with a wide variety of neurologic complications and sequelae. These sequelae can be the most important factor in determining patient outcomes, including long-term functional outcomes. In this review, the important topic of cardiac arrest are discussed, with a focus on neuroprognostication and

[a] Division of Critical Care and Neurotrauma and Cerebrovascular Diseases, Department of Neurology, Thomas Jefferson University, 901 Walnut Street, 4th Floor, Philadelphia, PA 19107, USA; [b] Division of Critical Care and Neurotrauma, Department of Neurological Surgery, Thomas Jefferson University, 901 Walnut Street, 3rd Floor, Philadelphia, PA 19107, USA; [c] Department of Medicine, Inova Fairfax Hospital, 3300 Gallows Road, Falls Church, VA 22042, USA; [d] Neuroscience Intensive Care, Department of Medicine, Inova Fairfax Hospital, 3300 Gallows Road, Falls Church, VA 22042, USA; [e] Department of Medicine, Jefferson College of Medicine, Thomas Jefferson University, 1025 Walnut Street, Philadelphia, PA 19107, USA
* Corresponding author. Division of Critical Care and Neurotrauma, Departments of Neurological Surgery and Medicine, Jefferson College of Medicine, Thomas Jefferson University, 901 Walnut Street, 3rd Floor, Philadelphia, PA 19107.
E-mail address: Muhammad.athar@jefferson.edu

Crit Care Clin 30 (2014) 557–584
http://dx.doi.org/10.1016/j.ccc.2014.03.002
0749-0704/14/$ – see front matter © 2014 Elsevier Inc. All rights reserved.
criticalcare.theclinics.com

the emerging data, with regard to identifying more accurate predictors of neurologic outcomes in the era of therapeutic hypothermia (TH). Some of the recent controversies with regard to targeted temperature management in comatose survivors of cardiac arrest are also discussed. The next section focuses on neurologic complications associated with surgical disease and procedures, namely aortic dissection, infective endocarditis (IE), left ventricular (LV) assist devices (LVADs), and coronary artery bypass grafting (CABG). We believed that these topics should be discussed given the complexities in their management. In the final section of the review, the cause, pathogenesis, and management of neurogenic stunned myocardium (NSM), an important clinical entity, are discussed.

ANOXIC-ISCHEMIC ENCEPHALOPATHY
Epidemiology

About 450,000 Americans have cardiac arrest (CA) annually.[1] Eighty percent of CAs occur at home, and mortality for such arrests is more than 90%.[1,2] More than half the survivors have permanent brain damage of varying degrees.[3,4] The outcomes for in-hospital arrests are better, with restoration of spontaneous circulation in 44% of patients and survival to discharge in 17% of patients. Survivors of CA who remain comatose are presumed to have anoxic-ischemic encephalopathy. A wide range of neurologic outcomes is possible in such patients, ranging from brain death to good recovery.

Neuroprognostication and Predictors of Poor Outcome

The American Academy of Neurology has identified several predictors of poor neurologic outcome to assist with prognostication.[5] These predictors include absent pupillary or corneal reflexes at day 3 after CA, absent or extensor motor responses at day 3,[6–8] bilateral absent N20 responses of somatosensory evoked potentials on days 1 to 3,[9–12] serum neuron-specific enolase (NSE) greater than 33 ng/mL at days 1 to 3,[7,13] and the presence of myoclonus status epilepticus within 24 hours.[7,14]

In prospective studies involving 491 patients,[6,15–19] all 108 patients who had absent pupillary light reflex (PLR) at day 3 after CA had poor outcomes. Absent corneal reflex at 72 hours was shown to be associated with poor outcomes in 2 prospective studies.[6,7] In another prospective study of 407 patients, myoclonic status epilepticus at 24 hours after CA was associated with no false-positive results for poor outcomes (95% confidence interval [CI], 0–14).[7] Several prospective studies have shown that a motor response to noxious stimuli that was no better than extensor posturing at 72 hours was associated with poor outcome.[6,7,16] However, these indicators of poor prognosis are derived from patients not treated with TH.

Several recent studies have looked into the accuracy of these predictors in the era of TH after CA. Fugate and colleagues[20] found that absent PLR, absent corneal reflexes, and motor response no better than extensor at day 3 remained predictive of a poor outcome in patients who received TH. Similarly, absent N20 responses were still predictive of poor outcome. However, an increased NSE level measured 1 to 3 days after CA was a less reliable predictor of poor outcome in such patients. However, pharmacologic sedation related to TH may influence prognostication of neurologic outcomes after CA. Recovery of motor responses, especially, may be delayed. A small study of 37 patients[21] showed that 2 of 14 patients who had a motor response no better than extensor posturing on day 3 showed some recovery of consciousness on day 6. **Table 1** compares the predictors of poor outcome both before and after the era of TH.

More recently, Oddo and Rossetti[22] adopted a multimodal approach for outcome prediction after CA and TH. These investigators found that clinical examination, which

Table 1 Predictors of poor outcome after CA	
Before TH	**After TH**
Absent PLR	Absent PLR
Absent corneal reflexes	Absent corneal reflexes
Motor response no better than extensor	Motor response no better than extensor[a]
Absent N20 response	Absent N20 responses[a]
Myoclonic status epilepticus	Serum NSE >33 ng/mL[a]
Serum NSE >33 ng/mL	

[a] Data on these responses remain controversial.

included incomplete recovery of brainstem reflexes and myoclonus, nonreactive hypothermic electroencephalography and serum NSE levels greater than 33 μg/L were independent predictors of poor outcome in comatose patients after CA and the combination of the 3 had the highest specificity (100%) and positive predictive value for poor outcome.

Hypothermia After CA

TH affects multiple pathways involved in ischemia-reperfusion injury after CA, and neurologic outcomes after CA have improved with the introduction of TH. Two major studies changed clinical practice in the management of out-of-hospital CA. The first study led by Bernard,[23] was performed in Australia between 1996 and 1999 on patients presenting with ventricular fibrillation (VF) and return of spontaneous circulation (ROSC) with persistent coma. Randomization occurred in the field, and a total of 84 patients were enrolled. Patients in the hypothermia arm were cooled to 33°C beginning in the field with ice bags. In the multivariate analysis, the odds ratio (OR) for a good outcome (defined as survival to hospital discharge to either home or a rehabilitation facility) in the hypothermia group compared with the normothermia group was 5.75 (CI 1.47–18.76; $P = .011$). The difference in mortality in the 2 groups was not significant.

The second study was completed by the Hypothermia After Cardiac Arrest Study Group.[24] This study enrolled patients in the emergency department who had witnessed CA caused by VF or pulseless ventricular tachycardia (VT) with ROSC within 60 minutes and no response to verbal commands. Two hundred and seventy-five patients were enrolled, and in the hypothermia arm, patients were cooled to 32°C to 34°C using an external cooling device as well as ice packs. The primary outcome was a favorable neurologic outcome at 6 months using the Pittsburgh cerebral performance category (**Table 2**) of 1 or 2 of 5. Patients were not randomized well in this study, but

Table 2 Pittsburgh Cerebral Performance Category Scale	
CPC 1	None to mild disability, able to work, may have mild neurologic or psychological deficit
CPC 2	Moderate disability, able to complete independent activities of daily life and work in a sheltered environment
CPC 3	Severe disability, dependent on daily support. Ranges from ambulatory to severe dementia to paralysis
CPC 4	Coma or vegetative state
CPC 5	Brain death

the rate of favorable neurologic outcome and mortality at 6 months were improved. There was no statistical difference in rate of complications in either group, although there was a trend toward increased rates of infection in the hypothermia arm.

TH is routinely performed in patients who present with CA and ROSC, given its neuroprotective effects. A prospective study looked at the cognitive outcomes of patients undergoing hypothermia after CA[25] and reported that 79% of patients who were working at the time of CA returned to work. This study supports the view that those who survive are likely to have a good outcome.

Although these studies support the use of TH, a recent study conducted by the Targeted Temperature Management Trial Investigators[26] that compared targeted temperature management of 33°C with 36°C after CA showed no difference in outcome. In this study, 75% of patients had VT or VF arrest, and 25% presented with pulseless electrical activity. This finding is in contrast to previous studies in which all patients had VT/VF arrest. The study suggests that controlled normothermia and fever control are what confer outcome benefit and that maintaining temperatures of 36°C after CA is all that is needed. Additional studies need to be performed before there is a change in practice.

Despite advances in emergency services and advanced cardiac life support, survival from CA remains low. For comatose survivors of CA, chances of long-term survival without significant neurologic deficits also remain low. Predicting neurologic outcomes after CA is challenging. Several variables of poor neurologic outcome have been identified. There is emerging evidence that in the era of TH, a multimodal approach incorporating clinical examination, electrophysiologic variables, and serologic data may be more beneficial in accurately predicting neurologic outcomes in comatose survivors of CA treated with TH. In addition, there is no doubt that temperature control in the period immediately after CA and prevention of hyperthermia is important to improve outcomes. Whether normothermia confers the same benefit as induced hypothermia is open to debate.

SURGICAL DISEASE
Neurologic Complications After Aortic Dissection

Introduction
Stroke is the most common neurologic complication of aortic dissection, and is the initial presenting symptom in 5% to 29% of cases, mainly resulting from supraaortic arch involvement.[27–31] Often, the diagnosis of aortic dissection is missed in patients who present with stroke, because only two-thirds of patients presenting with neurologic symptoms had any chest or back pain, whereas 94.4% of patients without neurologic symptoms experienced pain.[27,28] In 1 study, the average mean National Institutes of Health Stroke Scale (NIHSS) (**Table 3**) on admission was 12.9.[29] Right hemispheric strokes are more common, with an incidence of 69.2% to 81%, compared with 13% for left hemispheric strokes and 6% for bilateral strokes.[27,29] Other neurologic symptoms reported with aortic dissection are listed in **Box 1**.[27,30,32] These symptoms are believed to result from either extension of the dissection flap and occlusion of the true lumen or hypoperfusion syndromes as a result of hypotension and shock.[27,30] In patients who underwent surgery, 47.5% had postoperative neurologic complications, with stroke being the most common diagnosis.

Aortic dissection repair and neurologic outcomes
Optimal treatment of aortic arch dissection in patients with neurologic deficits is not clear. Patients with ascending aortic dissection who present with stroke and coma are less likely to go to surgery and have higher hospital mortality.[28] Multiple studies

Table 3 NIHSS		
Item	**Points**	**Description**
1a. LOC	0	Alert
	1	Drowsy
	2	Obtunded
	3	Coma
1b. LOC questions	0	Answers both questions correctly
	1	Answers 1 question correctly
	2	Answers neither question correctly
1c. LOC commands	0	Performs both tasks correctly
	1	Performs 1 task correctly
	2	Performs neither task correctly
2. Best gaze	0	Normal horizontal movements
	1	Partial gaze palsy
	2	Compete gaze palsy
3. Visual field	0	No visual field defect
	1	Partial hemianopia
	2	Complete hemianopia
	3	Bilateral hemianopia
4. Facial movement	0	Normal
	1	Minor facial weakness
	2	Partial facial weakness
	3	Complete unilateral palsy
5. Arm motor function	0	No drift
a. Left	1	Drifts before 5 s
b. Right	2	Falls before 10 s
	3	No effort against gravity
	4	No movement
6. Leg motor function	0	No drift
a. Left	1	Drifts before 5 s
b. Right	2	Falls down before 5 s
	3	No effort against gravity
	4	No movement
7. Limb ataxia	0	Absent
	1	Present in 1 limb
	2	Present in 2 limbs
8. Sensory	0	No sensory loss
	1	Mild to moderate sensory loss
	2	Severe to total sensory loss
9. Best language	0	Normal
	1	Mild aphasia
	2	Severe aphasia
	3	Mute or global aphasia
10. Articulation	0	Normal
	1	Mild to moderate dysarthria
	2	Severe dysarthria
11. Extinction and inattention	0	No abnormality
	1	Mild loss of 1 sensory modality
	2	Severe loss of 2 modalities

Abbreviation: LOC, level of consciousness.

Box 1
Neurologic symptoms in aortic dissection

- Stroke
- Spinal ischemia
- Ischemic neuropathy
- Hypoxic encephalopathy
- Syncope
- Tonic-clonic seizures
- Somnolence
- Coma
- Transient global amnesia

---

have looked into the safety of surgery and risk factors for transient neurologic dysfunction (TND) and permanent neurologic dysfunction (PND). In a retrospective study of 1873 patients,[28] 100% of patients with coma and 76.2% with stroke died with medical management alone. In the surgical arm, mortality decreased to 44% in those with preoperative coma and 27% in patients with stroke. There was postoperative improvement in symptoms in 74.2% of patients with coma and 80.4% with stroke. This study concluded that surgery was protective against mortality in patients with preoperative brain injury and a reversal of the injury can occur with surgery. These findings are supported by the German Registry for Acute Aortic Dissection Type A, which found that 62.1% of those with preoperative neurologic dysfunction had resolution of symptoms after surgery, with hemiparesis resolving in 70.5%, paraparesis in 78.8%, aphasias in 80.6%, and coma in 70.9%.[33]

In addition, spinal cord injury (SCI) is an important complication of thoracic aortic aneurysm repair, complicating 20% of open repair and 3.88% of thoracic endovascular aortic repair (TEVAR).[34] Three randomized control trials[35–37] have suggested that prophylactic cerebrospinal fluid (CSF) drainage reduces the risk of perioperative SCI in open repair of thoracic aortic aneurysms. However, in the setting of TEVAR, there have been conflicting data on the use of prophylactic CSF drainage. In a recent systematic review,[34] SCI after routine prophylactic drainage was 3.2% compared with 3.47% in patients without routine prophylactic drainage and 5.60% in patients with selective prophylactic drainage; however, there was evidence of bias in the selective drainage group. Thus, although prophylactic CSF drainage can be recommended in patients undergoing open repair, more research needs to be undertaken on the use of prophylactic drainage in TEVAR.

Predictors of neurologic outcome after aortic surgery
Baseline NIHSS and time to surgery seem to be the most important predictors of neurologic improvement postoperatively. In a retrospective study of 41 patients,[38] recovery was seen in 88% of patients with NIHSS less than 11% and 85% if the time to surgery was less than 9.1 hours. In a subgroup analysis[38] combining the 2 risk factors for poor outcome (NIHSS >11 and time to surgery >9.1 hours), recovery was 100% in patients with no risk factors, 75% in patients with 1 risk factor, and 0% in those with both risk factors. This finding is consistent with the results by Estrera and colleagues,[29] in which 80% of patients who underwent surgery in less than 10 hours had neurologic improvement, in contrast to no improvement in symptoms for those operated on after 10 hours.

Other factors that have been identified to imply poor neurologic recovery are preoperative cerebral malperfusion syndrome, use of deep hypothermic circulatory arrest, and duration of cardiopulmonary bypass (CPB) and circulatory arrest.[33,39,40] No single surgical cerebral protection strategy has proved to be superior to another. An increase in mortality has been noted if bypass was performed for greater than 30 minutes without the use of anterior cerebral perfusion and greater than 60 minutes if cerebral perfusion was used.[41]

In patients without previous neurologic deficits, factors associated with TND and PND include poor preoperative mental status, male gender, diabetes and peripheral artery disease, EuroSCORE, aortic cross-clamp time, and femoral cannulation.[42] Data regarding the effect of age on neurologic dysfunction are variable; some studies show age as a risk factor, whereas others do not.[40,43]

Overall, stroke is a common presenting symptom of aortic dissection and must be recognized immediately. Current literature seems to support early surgery in patients with neurologic dysfunction, but this warrants further study. Risk factors for the development of neurologic dysfunction after aortic dissection repair include preoperative cerebral malperfusion syndrome, duration of CPB, circulatory arrest, time to surgery, and baseline NIHSS score (**Box 2**).

Neurologic Complications of Ventricular Assist Devices

Stroke and transient ischemic attack

Stroke and transient ischemic attacks (TIAs) are the most common neurologic complications after placement of a ventricular assist device, with incidence ranging from 2.7% to 48% of patients.[44–47] Other neurologic events that have been described include air embolism, seizures, brain abscess, metabolic encephalopathy, bilateral tremors, dementia, and anoxic brain injury secondary to CA.[48–50] In many cases, there were multiple events per patient. The time course of neurologic complications after LVAD placement is variable, with events occurring from 3 to 368 days after implantation. In most studies, the highest incidence is within 30 days of placement.[49,51,52] Patients with early complications occurring less than 14 days after implantation had 67% mortality, and 1 study reported stroke as cause of death in 8% of patients.[53,54]

Pathogenesis and risk factors

Thromboembolism is the leading cause of neurologic events.[44,49,53] Emboli are believed to emanate from the pump itself, with deposits found on the inflow valves in explanted devices, although LV thrombus and heart valves can contribute.[44,55] It is postulated that the ventricular assist devices alter the coagulation and fibrinolytic

---

Box 2
Risk factors for neurologic dysfunction after aortic dissection repair

- Baseline NIHSS greater than 11
- Time to surgery greater than 10 hours
- Preoperative malperfusion syndrome
- Use of deep hypothermic circulatory arrest
- Duration of CPB and CA
- History of diabetes
- Male gender
- Peripheral artery disease

systems, leading to increased platelet, coagulant, and fibrinolytic activities (**Fig. 1**).[44,56,57] This finding is secondary to foreign and irregular surfaces on the device, which lead to turbulent blood flow and shear stress, resulting in hypercoagulability, stasis, and device-related infection.[49] Infection has been associated with increased risk of neurologic complications and is believed to cause changes in the microvascular structure and reactivity, leading to coagulation abnormalities.[58] Other risk factors for postoperative stroke are listed in **Box 3**.[45,53,58]

The rates of neurologic complications differ based on the device implanted, with the HeartMate (Thoratec Corp, Pleasanton, CA, USA) device having a lower incidence of stroke compared with ThoratecBiVAD (Thoratec Corp, Pleasanton, CA, USA), Thoratec LVAD (Thoratec Corp, Pleasanton, CA, USA), and Novacor (WorldHeart, Oakland, CA, USA), with 75%, 64%, 63%, and 33% freedom from stroke at 6 months, respectively.[51] This situation is possibly caused by the biointimal surface on the HeartMate, which reduces the risk of thromboembolism.[44] However, the HeartMatell (Thoratec Corp, Pleasanton, CA, USA) has seen a sharp increase in the rate of thrombosis since 2011 occurring about 1 month after implantation, and it is unknown what the inciting factor is.[55]

Intracerebral hemorrhage

Intracerebral hemorrhage (ICH) is also a complication with LVAD, given the concomitant use of both anticoagulants and antiplatelet therapy.[59,60] However, there is little in the literature on how to manage these patients. The largest study included 330 patients with an LVAD, of whom 36 (11%) had ICH (defined as subarachnoid, subdural, or intraparenchymal hemorrhage).[60] All patients were on warfarin and aspirin at the time of presentation, with a mean international normalized ratio of 1.6, although

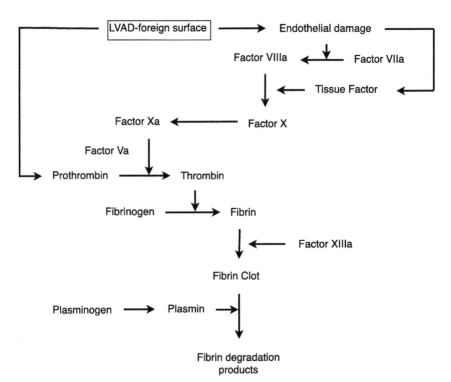

Fig. 1. Mechanism of thrombus formation in LVAD.

Box 3
Risk factors for stroke after LVAD implantation

- Infection
- Subtherapeutic international normalized ratio
- Atrial fibrillation
- Heparin-induced thrombocytopenia
- Baseline cardiomyopathy
- Higher mean right atrial pressure preoperatively
- Lower total protein after surgery
- Larger right ventricular end-diastolic dimension preoperatively
- History of stroke
- INTERMACS profile of 1 or 2

---

patients presenting with subarachnoid or subdural hemorrhage also had a history of fall or trauma.[60] In general, those with intraparenchymal hemorrhage as well as low Glasgow Coma Scale score had higher mortality and morbidity than those presenting with subarachnoid hemorrhage (SAH) or subdural hematoma.[60] Aspirin and warfarin were both stopped for a median time of 6 days and 10.5 days, respectively, in these patients, with no pump failure or ischemic events observed and no delayed rehemorrhage when resumed.[60] This study suggests that withholding aspirin for about a week and warfarin for about 10 days was adequate to prevent rehemorrhage as well as prevent pump failure and ischemic events.[60] Given the limited data, more studies are needed in this area.

Stroke and TIA are the most common neurologic complications after ventricular assist device placement and are mainly thromboembolic in nature. Major risk factors for neurologic complications include the type of device implanted, infection, and subtherapeutic anticoagulation.

Neurologic Complications of IE

Incidence

IE remains a major clinical problem, with mortality of 20% to 40%.[61,62] Neurologic complications occur in about 20% to 40% of cases of IE during the active course of the disease.[61,63] In ICE-PCS (International Collaboration on Endocarditis-Prospective Cohort Study),[62] the incidence of stroke was 17%. Sonneville and colleagues[64] found a 55% incidence of neurologic events among 198 patients with IE admitted to the intensive care unit (ICU).

Risk Factors

Several risk factors have been found to influence the occurrence of neurologic complications in IE (**Box 4**). Risk of cerebral embolism (CE) is higher with mitral valve disease and is maximal when vegetations involve the anterior mitral valve leaflet.[65] Vegetations greater than 10 to 15 mm and mobile vegetations are also associated with an increased risk of CE.[65–67] In a prospective study of 384 patients who underwent transesophageal echocardiography, size of the vegetation (10 mm) and its mobility were independent predictors of CE. Frequency of neurologic complications is 2 to 3 times more with *Staphylococcus aureus* infection than with other pathogens.[63,68] In some studies, it has been identified as the most important risk factor

---

Box 4
Risk factors for neurologic complications in IE

- Mitral valve vegetation, particularly anterior mitral valve leaflet
- Vegetations greater than 10 to 15 mm
- Mobile vegetations
- *Staphylococcus aureus* infection

---

for neurologic complications.[68] However, despite adequate antibiotic therapy, new embolic events are still observed in about 7% of cases.[69] If anticoagulant treatment is necessary, it is particularly associated with ICH.[68]

Complications

Ischemic events
Stroke or TIAs account for 40% to 60% of neurologic complications of IE[68] and result from dislodgement or fragmentation of endocardial vegetations. In addition, clinically silent CE is increasingly being reported and may be detected in up to 30% of patients with left-sided endocarditis using repeated brain magnetic resonance imaging.[70] However, the clinical importance of silent CE is unclear.

ICH
ICH complicates about 5% of cases of IE.[64,71–74] Mechanisms include hemorrhagic transformation of septic embolic infarcts, rupture of intracranial mycotic aneurysms (ICMAs), and erosion of arterial wall with subsequent hemorrhage. Erosion of arterial wall with subsequent hemorrhage is seen mostly in patients with *S aureus* IE. Risk factors for ICH include anticoagulant treatment, *S aureus* infection, and severe thrombocytopenia.[75]

Meningitis
Meningitis occurs in 2% to 20% of patients with IE. It results from dissemination of emboli into meningeal vessels. In most case series, it is diagnosed by presence of CSF pleocytosis with or without isolation of causative microorganism on culture.

Brain abscess
Brain abscess is a rare complication of IE, occurring in less than 5% of patients with IE. Garcia-Cabrera and colleagues[68] found 2 cases of brain abscess in a cohort of 1345 patients with IE. In the critically ill, it was observed in 14 (13%) of 108 patients with IE.[64] IE should be suspected in the absence of an obvious source of brain abscess and when multiple abscesses are present. *S aureus* is the most common pathogen for brain abscess in the setting of IE.

ICMAs
ICMAs account for 2% to 4% of neurologic complications of IE. The incidence is likely underestimated, because cerebral angiography is not performed regularly.[76] The pathologic mechanism of ICMA is from septic embolization to the vasa vasorum with destruction of the adventitia and the intima. ICMAs are multiple in 20% to 25% cases and are mostly located on the distal bifurcations of middle cerebral artery. Four-vessel cerebral angiography is the gold standard for diagnosis of ICMAs. However, magnetic resonance angiography has high sensitivity (90%–95%) and is especially useful for follow-up.[76]

Serial imaging can be used to follow small or unruptured ICMAs, because most resolve with antibiotic therapy. Treatment options for ruptured ICMAs or aneurysms that are enlarging or persistent despite appropriate antimicrobial therapy include endovascular coiling or surgical clipping.

Most neurologic complications occur before or during the first week of treatment. Once appropriate antimicrobial therapy is started, the incidence gradually decreases during the following weeks. In ICE-PCS,[77] the crude incidence of stroke decreased from 4.82/1000 patient days in the first week of therapy to 1.71/1000 patient days in the second week of treatment. This rate continued to decline with additional therapy.

The decrease in the rate of neurologic complications after a week of treatment was less pronounced when vegetations were greater than 1 cm in diameter.[59] In cases of vegetations greater than 3 cm, risk of embolic events remained high (20%). This is an important consideration when deciding on timing of cardiac surgery.

Impact of Neurologic Complications on Outcomes

Overall mortality for IE ranges from 20% to 40%.[62,78–81] Functional outcomes have also been evaluated in small observational studies. Sonneville and colleagues[64] found that only 31 of 106 patients in the ICU with IE and neurologic complications had a modified Rankin Scale lower than 3 at follow-up (3.9 months [3–8.5]) (**Table 4**). In another cohort of 68 patients,[82] full neurologic recovery was observed in 78% of patients with NIHSS at admission of 4 to 9 but in only 33% when the score was greater than 15.

Timing of Cardiac Surgery

The indications for surgery are listed in **Box 5**. The timing of valvular surgery in case of IE complicated by stroke is controversial, because of concern regarding the safety of CPB in patients with stroke. Anticoagulation during cardiac surgery may increase the risk of hemorrhage after cerebral infarction. Hypercoagulability or hypotension during CPB may exacerbate preexisting ischemic brain lesions. Earlier studies[82–84] have reported high rates of postoperative morbidity and mortality. However, more recent studies[85,86] have suggested better outcomes of patients with IE with stroke who underwent cardiac surgery, particularly in the presence of ischemic rather than hemorrhagic stroke.

Piper and colleagues[85] found the risk of neurologic deterioration to be low when surgery was performed within 72 hours. Barsic and colleagues[86] showed that in patients with IE and ischemic stroke, there was a nonsignificant trend toward increased

Table 4 Modified Rankin Scale	
Grade	Description
0	No symptoms at all
1	No significant disability despite symptoms; able to carry out all usual duties and activities
2	Slight disability; unable to carry out all previous activities, but able to look after own affairs without assistance
3	Moderate disability; requiring some help, but able to walk without assistance
4	Moderately severe disability; unable to walk without assistance and unable to attend to own bodily needs without assistance
5	Severe disability; bedridden, incontinent, and requiring constant nursing care and attention
6	Dead

Adapted from Van Swieten JC, Koudstaal PJ, Visser MC, et al. Interobserver agreement for the assessment of handicap in stroke patients. Stroke 1988;19:604–7.

Box 5
Indications for surgery in IE

- Hemodynamic failure related to valve destruction
- Persistent fever despite appropriate antibiotic therapy
- Development of abscesses or fistulas caused by perivalvular spread of infection
- Highly resistant organisms (*Coxiella burnetii*, *Brucella*, aggressive staphylococcal strains, fungi)
- Prosthetic valve endocarditis, particularly in the early postoperative phase
- Large vegetations with high risk of embolism (10 mm and mobile)
- Vegetations with size increasing despite appropriate antibiotic therapy

---

in-hospital mortality in the early surgery (surgery within 1–7 days of an ischemic stroke) group. However, 1-year mortality was similar in both groups. This study excluded patients with hemorrhagic stroke.

Current recommendations, which are not based on prospective data, are to delay surgery for 2 to 4 weeks in the case of large cerebral infarction and for 4 weeks in the event of ICH, unless a delay in surgery puts the patient at immediate risk of death.[87–89]

Neurologic complications are common in patients with IE. Mitral valve disease, vegetations greater than 10 to 15 mm, and mobile vegetations are associated with the greatest risk of CE. The risk of embolism decreases gradually once antimicrobial therapy is initiated. Timing of cardiac surgery is controversial, although there is recent literature showing that early surgery may be performed safely in selected patients with ischemic stroke. In patients with hemorrhagic stroke, surgery is usually delayed for at least 4 weeks.

Neurologic Complications of CABG

Incidence

Neurologic events complicating CABG are varied, with stroke being an important cause of morbidity and mortality. These neurologic complications are listed in **Table 5**, using the classification from Roach and colleagues.[90] The incidence of stroke ranges from 0.9% to 16% of cases, with 30% to 60% of patients developing neuropsychological changes.[91–94] Studies have observed a 10-fold increase in in-hospital mortality in patients developing type I outcomes and a 5-fold increase in type II outcomes, as well as mortality ranging from 0% to 38% from stroke in patients with CABG with an increased length of ICU stay, hospital stay, and cost.[90,93–95]

Risk Factors

Several studies have focused on identifying risk factors for stroke after cardiac surgery, which are listed in **Box 6**.[90–93,95,96] Bucerius and colleagues[97] prospectively

---

Table 5
Neurologic complications of CABG

Type I	Type II
Death caused by stroke or hypoxic encephalopathy	New deterioration in intellectual function
	Confusion
Nonfatal stroke	Agitation
TIA	Disorientation
Stupor or coma at discharge	Memory deficit
	Seizure without focal injury

> **Box 6**
> **Risk factors for neurologic events in CABG**
>
> - Age older than 60 years
> - History of stroke or TIA
> - Carotid bruits or carotid occlusion
> - Peripheral vascular disease
> - History of hypertension
> - Pulmonary disease
> - Ascending aortic disease
> - Perioperative myocardial infarction
> - Low LV ejection fraction
> - Perioperative hypotension

evaluated the incidence and predictors of perioperative stroke among 16,184 consecutive adult patients undergoing cardiac surgery. The overall incidence of stroke was 4.6%, but varied according to procedure, with valvular surgery having the highest rate and beating heart CABG with the lowest incidence of stroke. In multivariate analysis,[97] independent risk factors for stroke included history of cerebrovascular disease, peripheral vascular disease, diabetes, hypertension, previous cardiac surgery, preoperative infection, urgent operation, CPB time more than 2 hours, need for intraoperative hemofiltration, and high transfusion requirement. In this analysis, a history of cerebrovascular disease was the strongest preoperative predictor of stroke. Redmond and colleagues[92] looked at patients with a history of stroke and observed a higher incidence of stroke, TND, depressed level of consciousness, confusion, longer time to awaken from anesthesia, longer to wean from mechanical ventilation, higher incidence of aspiration and reintubation, longer ICU stay, and higher mortality. This situation is believed to be caused by increased vulnerability and susceptibility to the effects of CPB in previously injured brain tissue.

Intraoperative Factors

Additional intraoperative factors that are associated with increased stroke risk are listed in **Box 7**.[94,96,98] Several studies have looked at off-pump CABG with CPB (OPCAB) versus conventional CABG with CPB (CCAB) to decrease the risk of stroke and neurocognitive outcomes. Although there is some evidence to suggest that OPCAB decreases the risk of stroke, mortality, and delirium in patients undergoing CABG, the data have been controversial.[99–102] In 2 studies, OPCAB was associated with fewer embolic phenomena as observed on intraoperative transcranial Doppler, but they had differing results with regard to neurocognitive testing.[103,104] One failed to show any difference in neurocognitive testing in the CCAB group, whereas the other showed better neurocognitive function at discharge, but this effect dissipated at 6 weeks and 6 months.[103,104]

Several randomized control trials Veterans Affairs Randomized On/Off Bypass, CABG Off or On Pump Revascularization Study, German Off-Pump Coronary Artery Bypass Grafting in Elderly Patients (ROOBY, CORONARY, and GOPCABE) have failed to show any difference in morbidity or mortality, including stroke and neurocognitive function, at 30 days and 1 year.[105–108] However, these trials have inherent selection bias, either excluding many of the sicker or older patients or placing them in the

---

Box 7
Intraoperative risk factors for stroke in CABG

- Cold cardioplegia
- Intraoperative or postoperative IABP
- Duration on CPB
- Return to CPB after initial separation
- Extensive aortic manipulation
- Prolonged inotrope use
- Atrial fibrillation
- Low cardiac output syndrome
- Ventricular or atrial thrombus

CCAB group. Thus, the results of decreased mortality and complications may be a result of different patient populations as opposed to surgical modality. The ROOBY trial noted that enrolled patients had a significantly lower predicted risk of death than those who were excluded, and the GOPCABE Study Group also noted that excluded patients were more likely to have an ejection fraction (EF) less than 30% and to be in critical condition before surgery.[105,108] Thus, there is not enough strong evidence to suggest that OPCAB versus CCAB leads to decreased mortality, stroke, and delirium.

NSM
Synopsis

NSM resembling acute coronary syndrome or acute myocardial infarction (AMI) can occur in the setting of acute brain injury, predominantly in patients with poor grade aneurysmal SAH, namely Hunt Hess scale greater than 3 (**Table 6**).[109] Patients with SAH who developed NSM have substantially higher mortality and morbidity. Prompt recognition and early intervention of NSM in patients with SAH are key to improving clinical outcomes. The main aspects of managing NSM include treatment of underlying neurologic conditions, hemodynamic support with vasopressors, and supportive care.

Introduction

NSM is an acquired reversible LV cardiomyopathy in the absence of atherosclerotic coronary artery disease.[110,111] NSM is also known by several other names (**Box 8**),

---

Table 6
Hunt Hess Scale

Grade	Clinical Description
1	Asymptomatic or minimal headache and slight nuchal rigidity
2	Moderate to severe headache, nuchal rigidity, no neurologic deficit other than cranial nerve palsy
3	Drowsiness, confusion, or mild focal deficit
4	Stupor, moderate to severe hemiparesis, possibly early decerebrate rigidity, and vegetative disturbances
5	Deep coma, decerebrate rigidity, moribund

Adapted from Hunt WE, Hess RM. Surgical risk as related to time of intervention in the repair of intracranial aneurysms. J Neurosurg 1968;28(1):14–20.

Box 8
Interchangeable nomenclature in the literature

- NSM
- Takotsubo cardiomyopathy
- Stress-induced cardiomyopathy
- Reversible LV dysfunction
- Transient apical ballooning
- Broken heart syndrome
- Ampulla cardiomyopathy

---

and is associated with numerous acute physical or psychological conditions (**Box 9**). The pathophysiology of NSM relates to excessive catecholamine release at the time of a stressor, which results in a clinical syndrome similar to an AMI. The syndrome presents with chest pain, electrocardiographic (EKG) abnormalities, increased troponin (TnI) levels, and abnormal echocardiogram. There are important distinguishing features, such as reversible regional wall motion abnormalities, which do not adhere to 1 coronary vascular territory. Yet, although NSM is reversible, it is associated with worse outcomes in brain-injured patients.

This discussion focuses on aneurysmal SAH. SAH is a condition that afflicts more than 30,000 Americans per year and is associated with significant morbidity and mortality. Clinically, the rupture of an aneurysm and extravasation of blood into the subarachnoid space results in sudden headache, syncope, and even death caused by the sudden increase of intracranial pressure (ICP). This acute stressor likely contributes to the pathogenesis of NSM. Early recognition and treatment by securing the aneurysm, either by coiling or clipping, CSF diversion, and management of increased ICP are critical to improving patient outcomes. Approximately 3 to 14 days after onset of SAH, up to one-third of patients develop delayed cerebral ischemia (DCI), or transient neurologic deficits or stroke, which further adversely affects morbidity and mortality. The treatment of DCI includes medical therapy such as intravenous fluid administration and blood

---

Box 9
Common neurologic conditions triggering NSM

- Aneurysmal SAH[2–5]
- ICH[6]
- Ischemic stroke
- Traumatic brain injury[5,7]
- Status epilepticus[7]
- Encephalitis[8,9]
- Acute myelitis[8,9]
- Guillain-Barré syndrome[10]
- Acute hydrocephalus and ventriculoperitoneal shunt malfunction[11–13]
- Reversible posterior leukoencephalopathy syndrome[14]
- Acute spinal cord infarction[14]
- Metastatic brain tumors[15]

pressure augmentation with vasopressors and, in certain cases, endovascular rescue therapy. The relationship among NSM, SAH, and DCI is discussed in this context.

PATHOGENESIS

The pathogenesis of NSM is still not fully understood but is believed to be related to excessive catecholamine release at the time of acute physical or psychological stress. **Fig. 2** outlines a general pathway of cardiac injury. As shown in **Fig. 2**, acute stress results in stimulation or injury to autonomic centers of the brain, such as the right insular cortex, amygdale, and hypothalamus, resulting in excessive sympathetic outflow.[112–114] This situation leads to catecholamine release at the sympathetic nerve terminals that act on α and β receptors and Ca^{2+} channels on myocytes to induce excessive Ca^{2+} influx and production of oxidative free radicals,[115] culminating in reduced ventricular function. Other mechanisms contributing to cardiac injury include[116,117]: (1) coronary artery spasm; (2) coronary microvascular dysfunction; and (3) neuroinflammation. The combination of these mechanisms contributes to reduced cardiac function noted in NSM.

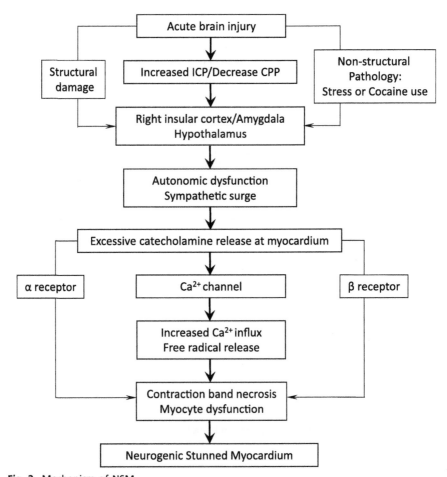

Fig. 2. Mechanism of NSM.

Incidence

The incidence of NSM is unclear, because most studies are retrospective. One prospective study found that 28% of patients with SAH have some degree of regional wall motion abnormality (RWMA) consistent with NSM.[118–121] NSM seemed to occur most commonly within the first 2 days after SAH, and there was a trend toward greater mortality when compared with SAH without RWMA (25 vs 15%, $P = .13$).[118] Other studies have found a similar trend of increased mortality associated with NSM after SAH.[122]

Risk Factors

Risk factors for females with NSM include, poor Hunt Hess grade aneurysmal SAH,[118] young age, posterior circulation aneurysms, poor Fisher grade SAH, and the presence of hydrocephalus.[123] Certain β_1, β_2, and α_2 genetic polymorphisms are also associated with NSM in the setting of SAH.[124] Severe RWMA was associated with increased risk for DCI in at least 1 study.[125] Risk of NSM is even higher in those who develop vasospasm and DCI (39% compared with 13% in the non-NSM group).[124]

Diagnosis and Management

Diagnosis of NSM

Diagnosis of NSM requires a high level of clinical suspicion and exclusion of AMI based on clinical, laboratory, EKG, and echocardiography results (**Table 7**). The diagnosis of NSM requires an inciting psychological or physical stress, which commonly results in dynamic EKG changes, increases in biomarkers of cardiac injury, and reversible dysfunction in LV wall motion, involving multiple coronary vascular territories. In some cases, cardiac catheterization may be necessary to exclude significant coronary artery occlusion. **Fig. 3** outlines the clinical decision tree in differentiating NSM from myocardial infarction (MI).

Table 7 Key clinical and diagnostic features of NSM	
Triggering event	Psychological or physical stress
Clinical characteristics	Female predominance AMI or acute coronary syndrome–like presentation, such as chest pain or dyspnea Hemodynamic instability if cardiogenic shock occurs Sudden death
Diagnostic features	No previous history of CAD/CHF Mild increase of cardiac TnI (typically <2.8 ng/mL): increases as early as day 1, peaks ≤3 d; normalizes in 3–8 d Increased BNP (up to >1000 pg/mL, normally <100 pg/mL), as early as day 1 EKG abnormalities: arrhythmias, QT interval prolongation, ST segment elevation/depression, and T-wave inversions in anterior precordial leads New-onset echocardiogram-proven global wall motion abnormality or RWMA not specific to a coronary distribution or systolic or diastolic LV/RV dysfunction Chest radiography: pulmonary edema Negative coronary angiography Complete or partial resolution of cardiac abnormalities on follow-up EKG and echocardiography

Abbreviations: CAD, coronary artery disease; CHF, congestive heart failure; RV, right ventricle.

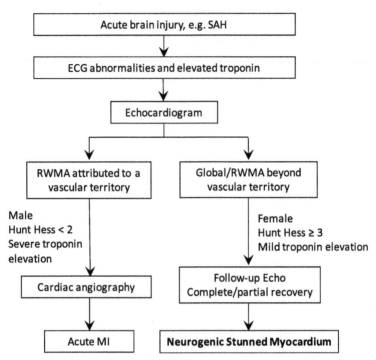

Fig. 3. Steps involved in the diagnosis of NSM.

EKG AND SERUM MARKERS

The association of aneurysmal SAH with EKG and echocardiographic abnormalities has been well noted. EKG changes have been found in 50% to 90% of patients with aneurysmal SAH.[118,126–129] Common EKG abnormalities include arrhythmia and QT interval prolongation, ST segment elevation or depression, and T-wave inversions, which can also be seen with MI.

Levels of TnI, a serum marker of myocardial injury, are increased in 20% to 68% patients after SAH,[109,130,131] with levels peaking by day 2.[130] Peak levels tend to be mild, with 18% to 25% levels of TnI greater than 10.[123,130] Increased TnI levels are commonly seen in the setting of poor Hunt Hess grade, female gender, hypotension, and increased vasopressor requirement and are associated with LV dysfunction, DCI, and death.[123,130,132] Similarly, an increase in B-type natriuretic peptide (BNP) has been associated with RWMA, cardiac dysfunction, pulmonary edema, need for neuro-interventional treatment of DCI, and in-hospital mortality.[132,133]

ECHOCARDIOGRAPHY

Recognizing echocardiography changes is critical to identifying NSM. In NSM, dilated apical or midapical LV segments with hypokinesis or akinesis extend beyond a single coronary artery distribution in the absence of coronary artery obstruction. In a prospective study of 300 patients with SAH, RWMA were found in 26%, with 8% having a significant reduction in EF of less than 50%.[134] Reduced EF was associated with reduced blood pressure and greater vasopressor requirement, although whether the vasopressor reduced EF by increasing afterload or was required because of reduced

EF-associated hypotension is unclear.[132] Unlike AMI, echocardiographic changes in NSM are partially or completely reversible in weeks.

COMPLICATIONS CAUSED BY NSM

Although associated with a greater disease severity at SAH presentation, NSM is an independent predictor of death with an OR of 2.71 (95% CI 1.012–7.288).[120] A possible explanation for this finding may be that NSM-related RWMA can result in moderate or severe reduction in LV function, potentially reducing cerebral blood flow, and putting patients at risk for DCI and death.[123] Other less commonly described complications are listed in **Box 10**.[135,136]

MANAGEMENT OF NSM

Management of NSM in the setting of SAH is mainly supportive and relates to the phase of neurologic injury (**Fig. 4**). Initial therapy should be aimed at reducing the inciting neurologic injury whenever possible. Increased ICP should be treated aggressively with hyperosmolar therapy, CSF diversion, and surgical evacuation of hematoma, as necessary. Approximately 3 to 14 days after SAH, the risk for developing DCI is highest. Once DCI develops, treatment consists of intravenous fluid administration and vasopressor administration. This therapy in the setting of reduced LV function may be counterproductive by increasing afterload with vasopressors and preload with fluids, resulting in congestive heart failure, pulmonary edema, and potentially exacerbating cerebral hypoperfusion. By contrast, managing congestive heart failure with diuresis increases the risk for DCI. Administration of inotropes, such as milrinone or dobutamine, with the aid of cardiac output monitoring with a Swan-Ganz catheter can be considered.[137] In more severe cases of LV dysfunction, an intra-aortic balloon pump can be considered.[138,139] Endovascular treatment of DCI, typically reserved for failure of vasopressors and fluids to resolve DCI, may need to be considered sooner in cases of reduced LV function.

NSM is a well-recognized complication of acute brain injury related in part to excessive stress-induced catecholamine release. Patients with NSM present with symptoms, ECG findings, and TnI levels similar to AMI. However, on echocardiogram, regional wall motion abnormalities involve multiple vascular territories and can be moderate to severe in 10% of patients with SAH. Abnormal cardiac function can contribute to DCI and complicate therapy.

Box 10
In-hospital complications of NSM

- Death
- RWMA, heart failure
- Cardiogenic shock
- Atrial fibrillation
- Ventricular arrhythmia
- LV thrombosis
- Severe mitral regurgitation
- LV outflow tract obstruction
- DCI

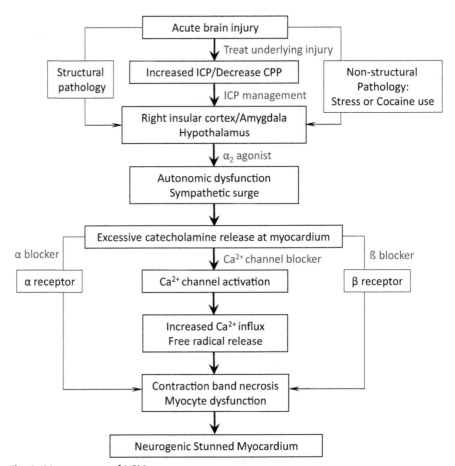

Fig. 4. Management of NSM.

SUMMARY

Cardiac emergencies and cardiovascular procedures can have significant neurologic implications. Both in-hospital and out-of-hospital CA and its neurologic sequelae remain major clinical problems. Recent advances in postresuscitative care, including TH, have improved outcomes after adult CA over the past decade. Data continue to emerge regarding identifying more reliable predictors of neurologic outcomes as well as the optimum strategy for targeted temperature management in the post-CA setting. The management strategy remains controversial for patients with type A aortic dissection who have cerebrovascular involvement, with observational data showing that early surgery may improve survival and reverse some of the neurologic deficits. Stroke and TIAs remain the most common neurologic complications associated with LVAD placement and CABG. Newer LVADs with biointimal surface may reduce the risk of embolic complications. However, management of ICH associated with LVADs remains challenging, with limited data suggesting that withholding aspirin for a week and anticoagulation for 10 days may be safe. There are good data showing that OPCAB is associated with a lower risk of embolic complications, with conflicting data regarding its beneficial effect on long-term cognitive outcomes. IE continues to be associated with significant neurologic sequelae. Early initiation of antimicrobial treatment significantly decreases the risk of recurrent embolic events. Timing of cardiac surgery remains controversial, with recent data showing that early surgery may be performed safely in selected patients with ischemic strokes. Our understanding of the pathophysiology of NSM and its effects on patient outcomes continues to improve.

REFERENCES

1. Callans DJ. Out-of-hospital cardiac arrest–the solution is shocking. N Engl J Med 2004;351(7):632–4.
2. Albert CM, Chae CU, Grodstein F, et al. Prospective study of sudden cardiac death among women in the United States. Circulation 2003;107(16):2096–101.
3. Pusswald G, Fertl E, Faltl M, et al. Neurological rehabilitation of severely disabled cardiac arrest survivors. Part II. Life situation of patients and families after treatment. Resuscitation 2000;47(3):241–8.
4. Herlitz J, Andersson E, Bang A, et al. Experiences from treatment of out-of-hospital cardiac arrest during 17 years in Goteborg. Eur Heart J 2000;21(15):1251–8.
5. Wijdicks EF, Hijdra A, Young GB, et al. Practice parameter: prediction of outcome in comatose survivors after cardiopulmonary resuscitation (an evidence-based review): report of the Quality Standards Subcommittee of the American Academy of Neurology. Neurology 2006;67(2):203–10.
6. Levy DE, Caronna JJ, Singer BH, et al. Predicting outcome from hypoxic-ischemic coma. JAMA 1985;253(10):1420–6.
7. Zandbergen EG, Hijdra A, Koelman JH, et al. Prediction of poor outcome within the first 3 days of postanoxic coma. Neurology 2006;66(1):62–8.
8. Edgren E, Hedstrand U, Kelsey S, et al. Assessment of neurological prognosis in comatose survivors of cardiac arrest. BRCT I Study Group. Lancet 1994;343(8905):1055–9.
9. Chen R, Bolton CF, Young B. Prediction of outcome in patients with anoxic coma: a clinical and electrophysiologic study. Crit Care Med 1996;24(4):672–8.
10. Bassetti C, Bomio F, Mathis J, et al. Early prognosis in coma after cardiac arrest: a prospective clinical, electrophysiological, and biochemical study of 60 patients. J Neurol Neurosurg Psychiatry 1996;61(6):610–5.
11. Logi F, Fischer C, Murri L, et al. The prognostic value of evoked responses from primary somatosensory and auditory cortex in comatose patients. Clin Neurophysiol 2003;114(9):1615–27.
12. Gendo A, Kramer L, Hafner M, et al. Time-dependency of sensory evoked potentials in comatose cardiac arrest survivors. Intensive Care Med 2001;27(8):1305–11.
13. Fogel W, Krieger D, Veith M, et al. Serum neuron-specific enolase as early predictor of outcome after cardiac arrest. Crit Care Med 1997;25(7):1133–8.
14. Wijdicks EF, Parisi JE, Sharbrough FW. Prognostic value of myoclonus status in comatose survivors of cardiac arrest. Ann Neurol 1994;35(2):239–43.
15. Berek K, Lechleitner P, Luef G, et al. Early determination of neurological outcome after prehospital cardiopulmonary resuscitation. Stroke 1995;26(4):543–9.
16. Edgren E, Hedstrand U, Nordin M, et al. Prediction of outcome after cardiac arrest. Crit Care Med 1987;15(9):820–5.
17. Krumholz A, Stern BJ, Weiss HD. Outcome from coma after cardiopulmonary resuscitation: relation to seizures and myoclonus. Neurology 1988;38(3):401–5.

18. Kano T, Shimoda O, Morioka T, et al. Evaluation of the central nervous function in resuscitated comatose patients by multilevel evoked potentials. Resuscitation 1992;23(3):235–48.

19. Earnest MP, Breckinridge JC, Yarnell PR, et al. Quality of survival after out-of-hospital cardiac arrest: predictive value of early neurologic evaluation. Neurology 1979;29(1):56–60.

20. Fugate JE, Wijdicks EF, Mandrekar J, et al. Predictors of neurologic outcome in hypothermia after cardiac arrest. Ann Neurol 2010;68(6):907–14.

21. Al Thenayan E, Savard M, Sharpe M, et al. Predictors of poor neurologic outcome after induced mild hypothermia following cardiac arrest. Neurology 2008;71(19):1535–7.

22. Oddo M, Rossetti AO. Early multimodal outcome prediction after cardiac arrest in patients treated with hypothermia. Crit Care Med 2014. [Epub ahead of print].

23. Bernard SA, Gray TW, Buist MD, et al. Treatment of comatose survivors of out-of-hospital cardiac arrest with induced hypothermia. N Engl J Med 2002;346(8): 557–63.

24. Hypothermia after Cardiac Arrest Study Group. Mild therapeutic hypothermia to improve the neurologic outcome after cardiac arrest. N Engl J Med 2002;346(8): 549–56.

25. Fugate JE, Moore SA, Knopman DS, et al. Cognitive outcomes of patients undergoing therapeutic hypothermia after cardiac arrest. Neurology 2013;81(1):40–5.

26. Nielsen N, Wetterslev J, Cronberg T, et al. Targeted temperature management at 33 degrees C versus 36 degrees C after cardiac arrest. N Engl J Med 2013; 369(23):2197–206.

27. Gaul C, Dietrich W, Friedrich I, et al. Neurological symptoms in type A aortic dissections. Stroke 2007;38(2):292–7.

28. Di Eusanio M, Patel HJ, Nienaber CA, et al. Patients with type A acute aortic dissection presenting with major brain injury: should we operate on them? J Thorac Cardiovasc Surg 2013;145(Suppl 3):213–21.e1.

29. Estrera AL, Garami Z, Miller CC, et al. Acute type A aortic dissection complicated by stroke: can immediate repair be performed safely? J Thorac Cardiovasc Surg 2006;132(6):1404–8.

30. Blanco M, Diez-Tejedor E, Larrea JL, et al. Neurologic complications of type I aortic dissection. Acta Neurol Scand 1999;99(4):232–5.

31. Hagan PG, Nienaber CA, Isselbacher EM, et al. The International Registry of Acute Aortic Dissection (IRAD): new insights into an old disease. JAMA 2000; 283(7):897–903.

32. Lynch DR, Dawson TM, Raps EC, et al. Risk factors for the neurologic complications associated with aortic aneurysms. Arch Neurol 1992;49(3):284–8.

33. Conzelmann LO, Hoffmann I, Blettner M, et al. Analysis of risk factors for neurological dysfunction in patients with acute aortic dissection type A: data from the German Registry for Acute Aortic Dissection type A (GERAADA). Eur J Cardiothorac Surg 2012;42(3):557–65.

34. Wong CS, Healy D, Canning C, et al. A systematic review of spinal cord injury and cerebrospinal fluid drainage after thoracic aortic endografting. J Vasc Surg 2012;56(5):1438–47.

35. Svensson LG, Hess KR, D'Agostino RS, et al. Reduction of neurologic injury after high-risk thoracoabdominal aortic operation. Ann Thorac Surg 1998;66(1):132–8.

36. Coselli JS, LeMaire SA, Köksoy C, et al. Cerebrospinal fluid drainage reduces paraplegia after thoracoabdominal aortic aneurysm repair: results of a randomized clinical trial. J Vasc Surg 2002;35(4):631–9.

37. Reitz BA, Crawford ES, Svensson LG, et al. A prospective randomized study of cerebrospinal fluid drainage to prevent paraplegia after high-risk surgery on the thoracoabdominal aorta. J Vasc Surg 1991;13(1):36–46.
38. Morimoto N, Okada K, Okita Y. Lack of neurologic improvement after aortic repair for acute type A aortic dissection complicated by cerebral malperfusion: predictors and association with survival. J Thorac Cardiovasc Surg 2011;142(6): 1540–4.
39. Czerny M, Fleck T, Zimpfer D, et al. Risk factors of mortality and permanent neurologic injury in patients undergoing ascending aortic and arch repair. J Thorac Cardiovasc Surg 2003;126(5):1296–301.
40. Krähenbühl ES, Immer FF, Stalder M, et al. Temporary neurological dysfunction after surgery of the thoracic aorta: a predictor of poor outcome and impaired quality of life. Eur J Cardiothorac Surg 2008;33(6):1025–9.
41. Kruger T, Weigang E, Hoffmann I, et al. Cerebral protection during surgery for acute aortic dissection type A: results of the German Registry for Acute Aortic Dissection Type A (GERAADA). Circulation 2011;124(4):434–43.
42. Haldenwang PL, Wahlers T, Himmels A, et al. Evaluation of risk factors for transient neurological dysfunction and adverse outcome after repair of acute type A aortic dissection in 122 consecutive patients. Eur J Cardiothorac Surg 2012; 42(5):e115–20.
43. Rylski B, Hoffmann I, Beyersdorf F, et al. Acute aortic dissection type A: age-related management and outcomes reported in the German Registry for Acute Aortic Dissection type A (GERAADA) of over 2000 patients. Ann Surg 2014; 259(3):598–604.
44. Piccione W Jr. Left ventricular assist device implantation: short and long-term surgical complications. J Heart Lung Transplant 2000;19(Suppl 8):S89–94.
45. Nakajima I, Kato TS, Komamura K, et al. Pre- and post-operative risk factors associated with cerebrovascular accidents in patients supported by left ventricular assist device. Circ J 2011;75(5):1138–46.
46. Schmid C, Weyand M, Nabavi DG, et al. Cerebral and systemic embolization during left ventricular support with the Novacor N100 device. Ann Thorac Surg 1998;65(6):1703–10.
47. Popov AF, Hosseini MT, Zych B, et al. Clinical experience with HeartWare left ventricular assist device in patients with end-stage heart failure. Ann Thorac Surg 2012;93(3):810–5.
48. Lazar RM, Shapiro PA, Jaski BE, et al. Neurological events during long-term mechanical circulatory support for heart failure: the Randomized Evaluation of Mechanical Assistance for the Treatment of Congestive Heart Failure (REMATCH) experience. Circulation 2004;109(20):2423–7.
49. Pae WE, Connell JM, Boehmer JP, et al. Neurologic events with a totally implantable left ventricular assist device: European LionHeart Clinical Utility Baseline Study (CUBS). J Heart Lung Transplant 2007;26(1):1–8.
50. Copeland JG, Copeland H, Gustafson M, et al. Experience with more than 100 total artificial heart implants. J Thorac Cardiovasc Surg 2012;143(3):727–34.
51. Tsukui H, Abla A, Teuteberg JJ, et al. Cerebrovascular accidents in patients with a ventricular assist device. J Thorac Cardiovasc Surg 2007;134(1):114–23.
52. Yuan N, Arnaoutakis GJ, George TJ, et al. The spectrum of complications following left ventricular assist device placement. J Card Surg 2012;27(5): 630–8.
53. Thomas CE, Jichici D, Petrucci R, et al. Neurologic complications of the Novacor left ventricular assist device. Ann Thorac Surg 2001;72(4):1311–5.

54. Dell'Aquila AM, Schneider SR, Schlarb D, et al. Initial clinical experience with the HeartWare left ventricular assist system: a single-center report. Ann Thorac Surg 2013;95(1):170–7.
55. Starling RC, Moazami N, Silvestry SC, et al. Unexpected abrupt increase in left ventricular assist device thrombosis. N Engl J Med 2014;370(1):33–40.
56. John R, Panch S, Hrabe J, et al. Activation of endothelial and coagulation systems in left ventricular assist device recipients. Ann Thorac Surg 2009;88(4):1171–9.
57. Spanier T, Oz M, Levin H, et al. Activation of coagulation and fibrinolytic pathways in patients with left ventricular assist devices. J Thorac Cardiovasc Surg 1996; 112(4):1090–7.
58. Kato TS, Schulze PC, Yang J, et al. Pre-operative and post-operative risk factors associated with neurologic complications in patients with advanced heart failure supported by a left ventricular assist device. J Heart Lung Transplant 2012; 31(1):1–8.
59. Vermes E, Kirsch M, Farrokhi T, et al. Management of intracranial hemorrhage in patients with mechanical circulatory support: a role for low-molecular-weight heparins? ASAIO J 2005;51(4):485–6.
60. Wilson TJ, Stetler WR Jr, Al-Holou WN, et al. Management of intracranial hemorrhage in patients with left ventricular assist devices. J Neurosurg 2013;118(5): 1063–8.
61. Galvez-Acebal J, Rodriguez-Bano J, Martinez-Marcos FJ, et al. Prognostic factors in left-sided endocarditis: results from the Andalusian multicenter cohort. BMC Infect Dis 2010;10:17.
62. Murdoch DR, Corey GR, Hoen B, et al. Clinical presentation, etiology, and outcome of infective endocarditis in the 21st century: the International Collaboration on Endocarditis-Prospective Cohort Study. Arch Intern Med 2009;169(5): 463–73.
63. Heiro M, Nikoskelainen J, Engblom E, et al. Neurologic manifestations of infective endocarditis: a 17-year experience in a teaching hospital in Finland. Arch Intern Med 2000;160(18):2781–7.
64. Sonneville R, Mirabel M, Hajage D, et al. Neurologic complications and outcomes of infective endocarditis in critically ill patients: the ENDOcardite en REAnimation prospective multicenter study. Crit Care Med 2011;39(6):1474–81.
65. Pruitt AA, Rubin RH, Karchmer AW, et al. Neurologic complications of bacterial endocarditis. Medicine (Baltimore) 1978;57(4):329–43.
66. Anderson DJ, Goldstein LB, Wilkinson WE, et al. Stroke location, characterization, severity, and outcome in mitral vs aortic valve endocarditis. Neurology 2003;61(10):1341–6.
67. Vilacosta I, Graupner C, San Roman JA, et al. Risk of embolization after institution of antibiotic therapy for infective endocarditis. J Am Coll Cardiol 2002;39(9): 1489–95.
68. Garcia-Cabrera E, Fernandez-Hidalgo N, Almirante B, et al. Neurological complications of infective endocarditis: risk factors, outcome, and impact of cardiac surgery: a multicenter observational study. Circulation 2013;127(23):2272–84.
69. Thuny F, Di Salvo G, Belliard O, et al. Risk of embolism and death in infective endocarditis: prognostic value of echocardiography: a prospective multicenter study. Circulation 2005;112(1):69–75.
70. Snygg-Martin U, Gustafsson L, Rosengren L, et al. Cerebrovascular complications in patients with left-sided infective endocarditis are common: a prospective study using magnetic resonance imaging and neurochemical brain damage markers. Clin Infect Dis 2008;47(1):23–30.

71. Salgado AV, Furlan AJ, Keys TF, et al. Neurologic complications of endocarditis: a 12-year experience. Neurology 1989;39(2 Pt 1):173–8.
72. Hart RG, Foster JW, Luther MF, et al. Stroke in infective endocarditis. Stroke 1990;21(5):695–700.
73. Horstkotte D, Follath F, Gutschik E, et al. Guidelines on prevention, diagnosis and treatment of infective endocarditis executive summary; the task force on infective endocarditis of the European Society of Cardiology. Eur Heart J 2004;25(3):267–76.
74. Thuny F, Avierinos JF, Tribouilloy C, et al. Impact of cerebrovascular complications on mortality and neurologic outcome during infective endocarditis: a prospective multicentre study. Eur Heart J 2007;28(9):1155–61.
75. Mourvillier B, Trouillet JL, Timsit JF, et al. Infective endocarditis in the intensive care unit: clinical spectrum and prognostic factors in 228 consecutive patients. Intensive Care Med 2004;30(11):2046–52.
76. Peters PJ, Harrison T, Lennox JL. A dangerous dilemma: management of infectious intracranial aneurysms complicating endocarditis. Lancet Infect Dis 2006; 6(11):742–8.
77. Dickerman SA, Abrutyn E, Barsic B, et al. The relationship between the initiation of antimicrobial therapy and the incidence of stroke in infective endocarditis: an analysis from the ICE Prospective Cohort Study (ICE-PCS). Am Heart J 2007; 154(6):1086–94.
78. Netzer RO, Zollinger E, Seiler C, et al. Infective endocarditis: clinical spectrum, presentation and outcome. An analysis of 212 cases 1980-1995. Heart 2000; 84(1):25–30.
79. Mylonakis E, Calderwood SB. Infective endocarditis in adults. N Engl J Med 2001;345(18):1318–30.
80. Hoen B, Alla F, Selton-Suty C, et al. Changing profile of infective endocarditis: results of a 1-year survey in France. JAMA 2002;288(1):75–81.
81. Beynon RP, Bahl VK, Prendergast BD. Infective endocarditis. BMJ 2006; 333(7563):334–9.
82. Gillinov AM, Shah RV, Curtis WE, et al. Valve replacement in patients with endocarditis and acute neurologic deficit. Ann Thorac Surg 1996;61(4):1125–9 [discussion: 1130].
83. Maruyama M, Kuriyama Y, Sawada T, et al. Brain damage after open heart surgery in patients with acute cardioembolic stroke. Stroke 1989;20(10): 1305–10.
84. Eishi K, Kawazoe K, Kuriyama Y, et al. Surgical management of infective endocarditis associated with cerebral complications. Multi-center retrospective study in Japan. J Thorac Cardiovasc Surg 1995;110(6):1745–55.
85. Piper C, Wiemer M, Schulte HD, et al. Stroke is not a contraindication for urgent valve replacement in acute infective endocarditis. J Heart Valve Dis 2001;10(6): 703–11.
86. Barsic B, Dickerman S, Krajinovic V, et al. Influence of the timing of cardiac surgery on the outcome of patients with infective endocarditis and stroke. Clin Infect Dis 2013;56(2):209–17.
87. Habib G, Hoen B, Tornos P, et al. Guidelines on the prevention, diagnosis, and treatment of infective endocarditis (new version 2009): the Task Force on the Prevention, Diagnosis, and Treatment of Infective Endocarditis of the European Society of Cardiology (ESC). Endorsed by the European Society of Clinical Microbiology and Infectious Diseases (ESCMID) and the International Society of Chemotherapy (ISC) for Infection and Cancer. Eur Heart J 2009;30(19):2369–413.

88. Baddour LM, Wilson WR, Bayer AS, et al. Infective endocarditis: diagnosis, antimicrobial therapy, and management of complications: a statement for healthcare professionals from the Committee on Rheumatic Fever, Endocarditis, and Kawasaki Disease, Council on Cardiovascular Disease in the Young, and the Councils on Clinical Cardiology, Stroke, and Cardiovascular Surgery and Anesthesia, American Heart Association: endorsed by the Infectious Diseases Society of America. Circulation 2005;111(23):e394–434.

89. Angstwurm K, Borges AC, Halle E, et al. Timing the valve replacement in infective endocarditis involving the brain. J Neurol 2004;251(10):1220–6.

90. Roach GW, Kanchuger M, Mangano CM, et al. Adverse cerebral outcomes after coronary bypass surgery. Multicenter Study of Perioperative Ischemia Research Group and the Ischemia Research and Education Foundation Investigators. N Engl J Med 1996;335(25):1857–63.

91. Mickleborough LL, Walker PM, Takagi Y, et al. Risk factors for stroke in patients undergoing coronary artery bypass grafting. J Thorac Cardiovasc Surg 1996; 112(5):1250–8 [discussion: 1258–9].

92. Redmond JM, Greene PS, Goldsborough MA, et al. Neurologic injury in cardiac surgical patients with a history of stroke. Ann Thorac Surg 1996;61(1):42–7.

93. Puskas JD, Winston AD, Wright CE, et al. Stroke after coronary artery operation: incidence, correlates, outcome, and cost. Ann Thorac Surg 2000;69(4):1053–6.

94. Wolman RL, Nussmeier NA, Aggarwal A, et al. Cerebral injury after cardiac surgery: identification of a group at extraordinary risk. Stroke 1999;30(3): 514–22.

95. McKhann GM, Goldsborough MA, Borowicz LM Jr, et al. Predictors of stroke risk in coronary artery bypass patients. Ann Thorac Surg 1997;63(2):516–21.

96. Kapetanakis EI, Stamou SC, Dullum MK, et al. The impact of aortic manipulation on neurologic outcomes after coronary artery bypass surgery: a risk-adjusted study. Ann Thorac Surg 2004;78(5):1564–71.

97. Bucerius J, Gummert JF, Borger MA, et al. Stroke after cardiac surgery: a risk factor analysis of 16,184 consecutive adult patients. Ann Thorac Surg 2003; 75(2):472–8.

98. Likosky DS, Leavitt BJ, Marrin CAS, et al. Intra- and postoperative predictors of stroke after coronary artery bypass grafting. Ann Thorac Surg 2003;76(2): 428–34.

99. Bucerius J, Gummert JF, Borger MA, et al. Predictors of delirium after cardiac surgery delirium: effect of beating-heart (off-pump) surgery. J Thorac Cardiovasc Surg 2004;127(1):57–64.

100. Cleveland JC Jr, Shroyer AL, Chen AY, et al. Off-pump coronary artery bypass grafting decreases risk-adjusted mortality and morbidity. Ann Thorac Surg 2001;72(4):1282–8 [discussion: 1288–9].

101. Stamou SC, Jablonski KA, Pfister AJ, et al. Stroke after conventional versus minimally invasive coronary artery bypass. Ann Thorac Surg 2002;74(2):394–9.

102. Patel NC, Grayson AD, Jackson M, et al. The effect off-pump coronary artery bypass surgery on in-hospital mortality and morbidity. Eur J Cardiothorac Surg 2002;22(2):255–60.

103. Motallebzadeh R, Bland JM, Markus HS, et al. Neurocognitive function and cerebral emboli: randomized study of on-pump versus off-pump coronary artery bypass surgery. Ann Thorac Surg 2007;83(2):475–82.

104. Stroobant N, Van Nooten G, Van Belleghem Y, et al. Relation between neurocognitive impairment, embolic load, and cerebrovascular reactivity following on- and off-pump coronary artery bypass grafting. Chest 2005;127(6):1967–76.

105. Diegeler A, Borgermann J, Kappert U, et al. Off-pump versus on-pump coronary-artery bypass grafting in elderly patients. N Engl J Med 2013;368(13): 1189–98.
106. Lamy A, Devereaux PJ, Prabhakaran D, et al. Off-pump or on-pump coronary-artery bypass grafting at 30 days. N Engl J Med 2012;366(16):1489–97.
107. Lamy A, Devereaux PJ, Prabhakaran D, et al. Effects of off-pump and on-pump coronary-artery bypass grafting at 1 year. N Engl J Med 2013;368(13):1179–88.
108. Shroyer AL, Grover FL, Hattler B, et al. On-pump versus off-pump coronary-artery bypass surgery. N Engl J Med 2009;361(19):1827–37.
109. Tung P, Kopelnik A, Banki N, et al. Predictors of neurocardiogenic injury after subarachnoid hemorrhage. Stroke 2004;35(2):548–51.
110. Porto I, Della Bona R, Leo A, et al. Stress cardiomyopathy (tako-tsubo) triggered by nervous system diseases: a systematic review of the reported cases. Int J Cardiol 2013;167(6):2441–8.
111. Maron BJ, Towbin JA, Thiene G, et al. Contemporary definitions and classification of the cardiomyopathies: an American Heart Association Scientific Statement from the Council on Clinical Cardiology, Heart Failure and Transplantation Committee; Quality of Care and Outcomes Research and Functional Genomics and Translational Biology Interdisciplinary Working Groups; and Council on Epidemiology and Prevention. Circulation 2006;113(14):1807–16.
112. Nguyen H, Zaroff JG. Neurogenic stunned myocardium. Curr Neurol Neurosci Rep 2009;9(6):486–91.
113. Cheung RT, Hachinski V. The insula and cerebrogenic sudden death. Arch Neurol 2000;57(12):1685–8.
114. Masuda T, Sato K, Yamamoto S, et al. Sympathetic nervous activity and myocardial damage immediately after subarachnoid hemorrhage in a unique animal model. Stroke 2002;33(6):1671–6.
115. Bolli R, Marban E. Molecular and cellular mechanisms of myocardial stunning. Physiol Rev 1999;79(2):609–34.
116. Lee VH, JK O, SL M, et al. Mechanisms in neurogenic stress cardiomyopathy after aneurysmal subarachnoid hemorrhage. Neurocrit Care 2006;5(3): 243–9.
117. Previtali M, Repetto A, Panigada S, et al. Left ventricular apical ballooning syndrome: prevalence, clinical characteristics and pathogenetic mechanisms in a European population. Int J Cardiol 2009;134(1):91–6.
118. Banki N, Kopelnik A, Tung P, et al. Prospective analysis of prevalence, distribution, and rate of recovery of left ventricular systolic function in patients with aneurysmal subarachnoid hemorrhage. J Neurosurg 2006;105(1):15–20.
119. Bybee KA, Prasad A. Stress-related cardiomyopathy syndromes. Circulation 2008;118(4):397–409.
120. Lee VH, Connolly HM, Fulgham JR, et al. Tako-tsubo cardiomyopathy in aneurysmal subarachnoid hemorrhage: an underappreciated ventricular dysfunction. J Neurosurg 2006;105(2):264–70.
121. Donaldson JW, Pritz MB. Myocardial stunning secondary to aneurysmal subarachnoid hemorrhage. Surg Neurol 2001;55(1):12–6 [discussion: 16].
122. Kilbourn KJ, Levy S, Staff I, et al. Clinical characteristics and outcomes of neurogenic stress cardiomyopathy in aneurysmal subarachnoid hemorrhage. Clin Neurol Neurosurg 2013;115(7):909–14.
123. Temes RE, Tessitore E, Schmidt JM, et al. Left ventricular dysfunction and cerebral infarction from vasospasm after subarachnoid hemorrhage. Neurocrit Care 2010;13(3):359–65.

124. Zaroff JG, Pawlikowska L, Miss JC, et al. Adrenoceptor polymorphisms and the risk of cardiac injury and dysfunction after subarachnoid hemorrhage. Stroke 2006;37(7):1680–5.
125. Mayer SA, Lin J, Homma S, et al. Myocardial injury and left ventricular performance after subarachnoid hemorrhage. Stroke 1999;30(4):780–6.
126. Sakr YL, Lim N, Amaral AC, et al. Relation of ECG changes to neurological outcome in patients with aneurysmal subarachnoid hemorrhage. Int J Cardiol 2004;96(3):369–73.
127. Lanzino G, Kongable GL, Kassell NF. Electrocardiographic abnormalities after nontraumatic subarachnoid hemorrhage. J Neurosurg Anesthesiol 1994;6(3): 156–62.
128. Davies KR, Gelb AW, Manninen PH, et al. Cardiac function in aneurysmal subarachnoid haemorrhage: a study of electrocardiographic and echocardiographic abnormalities. Br J Anaesth 1991;67(1):58–63.
129. Brouwers PJ, Wijdicks EF, Hasan D, et al. Serial electrocardiographic recording in aneurysmal subarachnoid hemorrhage. Stroke 1989;20(9):1162–7.
130. Naidech AM, Kreiter KT, Janjua N, et al. Cardiac troponin elevation, cardiovascular morbidity, and outcome after subarachnoid hemorrhage. Circulation 2005; 112(18):2851–6.
131. Horowitz MB, Willet D, Keffer J. The use of cardiac troponin-I (cTnI) to determine the incidence of myocardial ischemia and injury in patients with aneurysmal and presumed aneurysmal subarachnoid hemorrhage. Acta Neurochir (Wien) 1998; 140(1):87–93.
132. Yarlagadda S, Rajendran P, Miss JC, et al. Cardiovascular predictors of inpatient mortality after subarachnoid hemorrhage. Neurocrit Care 2006;5(2): 102–7.
133. Tung PP, Olmsted E, Kopelnik A, et al. Plasma B-type natriuretic peptide levels are associated with early cardiac dysfunction after subarachnoid hemorrhage. Stroke 2005;36(7):1567–9.
134. Kothavale A, Banki NM, Kopelnik A, et al. Predictors of left ventricular regional wall motion abnormalities after subarachnoid hemorrhage. Neurocrit Care 2006;4(3):199–205.
135. Madhavan M, Prasad A. Proposed Mayo Clinic criteria for the diagnosis of takotsubo cardiomyopathy and long-term prognosis. Herz 2010;35(4):240–3.
136. Brenner R, Weilenmann D, Maeder MT, et al. Clinical characteristics, sex hormones, and long-term follow-up in Swiss postmenopausal women presenting with takotsubo cardiomyopathy. Clin Cardiol 2012;35(6):340–7.
137. Naidech A, Du Y, Kreiter KT, et al. Dobutamine versus milrinone after subarachnoid hemorrhage. Neurosurgery 2005;56(1):21–61 [discussion: 26–7].
138. Lazaridis C, Pradilla G, Nyquist PA, et al. Intra-aortic balloon pump counterpulsation in the setting of subarachnoid hemorrhage, cerebral vasospasm, and neurogenic stress cardiomyopathy. Case report and review of the literature. Neurocrit Care 2010;13(1):101–8.
139. Apostolides PJ, Greene KA, Zabramski JM, et al. Intra-aortic balloon pump counterpulsation in the management of concomitant cerebral vasospasm and cardiac failure after subarachnoid hemorrhage: technical case report. Neurosurgery 1996;38(5):1056–9 [discussion: 1059–60].

Mechanical Circulatory Devices in Acute Heart Failure

Jeffrey J. Teuteberg, MD[a],*, Josephine C. Chou, MD, MS[b]

KEYWORDS

- Cardiogenic shock • Acute heart failure • Mechanical circulatory support
- Ventricular assist device

KEY POINTS

- Cardiogenic shock can complicate acute myocardial infarction, occur after cardiac surgery, and develop in the setting of chronic heart failure.
- Temporary ventricular assist devices (VAD) provide rapid hemodynamic stabilization and can improve survival in certain causes of cardiogenic shock.
- Indications for temporary mechanical support are bridge to decision in patients whose candidacy for advanced heart failure therapies is uncertain; bridge to transplant or durable VAD; or bridge to recovery of native cardiac function.
- Common complications of temporary ventricular device therapy are bleeding, infection, thromboembolism, and limb ischemia.

INTRODUCTION

Cardiogenic shock is defined as myocardial dysfunction causing decreased cardiac output and tissue hypoxia despite adequate intravascular volume.[1] It is determined by various clinical and hemodynamic parameters. Hemodynamic criteria include sustained hypotension (systolic blood pressure [SBP] less than 90 mm Hg for greater than 30 minutes or the need for supportive measures to maintain SBP >90 mm Hg) or reduced cardiac index (<2.2 L/min/m^2) with an elevated pulmonary capillary wedge pressure (>15 mm Hg).[2] Clinical criteria include evidence of end-organ

---

Conflicts of interest: Dr J.J. Teuteberg: HeartWare, advisory board, speaking; Sunshine Heart, consultant; XDx, advisory board; Abiomed, advisory board; Dr J.C. Chou: none.
Funding: none.
[a] Heart and Vascular Institute, University of Pittsburgh Medical Center, Scaife Hall, Suite 556, 200 Lothrop Street, Pittsburgh, PA 15213, USA; [b] Heart and Vascular Institute, University of Pittsburgh Medical Center, 200 Lothrop Street, B-571.3 Scaife Hall, Pittsburgh, PA 15213, USA
* Corresponding author.
E-mail address: teutebergjj@upmc.edu

Crit Care Clin 30 (2014) 585–606
http://dx.doi.org/10.1016/j.ccc.2014.04.002
0749-0704/14/$ – see front matter © 2014 Elsevier Inc. All rights reserved.

hypoperfusion, such as cool extremities, low urine output (less than 30 mL/h), altered mental status, pulmonary congestion, elevated lactate, and mixed venous saturation less than 65%.[3]

Causes of Cardiogenic Shock

The most common cause of cardiogenic shock is acute myocardial infarction (MI). It can also be caused by mechanical complications of MI, such as acute mitral regurgitation or rupture of the interventricular septum or the free wall. Nonischemic causes of shock include acute decompensation of a chronic cardiomyopathy, myocarditis, postcardiotomy syndrome, and cardiac allograft dysfunction. The various causes of cardiogenic shock are summarized in **Table 1**. Although left ventricular (LV) dysfunction is the most common cause of cardiogenic shock, right ventricular failure (RVF) (whether isolated or contributing to biventricular failure) can also produce shock and is discussed in subsequent sections.

Continuum of Cardiogenic Shock

The severity of cardiogenic shock covers a wide spectrum (**Fig. 1**). Patients in mild shock can be adequately treated with low-dose inotropes and vasopressors, such as dobutamine, dopamine, and norepinephrine. Patients in more profound shock refractory to additional inotropes and vasopressors require mechanical circulatory support (MCS) to maintain adequate systemic perfusion.[4] With worsening cardiac failure, cardiac output decreases, LV filling pressures increase and if the shock becomes profound then a vasodilatory state ensues. The most common initial device used in shock is the intra-aortic balloon pump (IABP), however the IABP only modestly augments cardiac output and reduces LV filling pressures. It functions as a volume-displacement device, with IABP deflation lowering aortic pressure and, thus, afterload resulting in improved forward flow. Extracorporeal membrane oxygenation (ECMO) can provide total cardiopulmonary support; it has significant drawbacks, including significant bleeding risk, activation of inflammatory cascades, potentially inadequate ventricular unloading when placed peripherally, and vascular injury or insufficiency from the large-bore peripheral catheters required during implantation.[5] A temporary ventricular assist device (VAD) provides the ventricular unloading and hemodynamic support needed in patients with severe refractory cardiogenic shock.

BENEFITS OF MCS

The main goal of MCS is to decompress the failing ventricle and augment systemic perfusion.[6] Mechanical unloading of the LV decreases pulmonary congestion, reduces pulmonary arterial pressure, and improves RV function. These hemodynamic benefits are also associated with favorable cellular changes. Normalization of LV pressure reduces neurohormonal activation, which decreases catecholaminergic excess that is myotoxic.[7] LV decompression reduces myocardial oxygen consumption and promotes myocardial recovery.[8] Cardiac myocytes from VAD-supported patients have less fibrosis and collagen content in the cardiac extracellular matrix when compared with nonsupported patients, indicating a reduction in reverse remodeling.[9] They also have improved myocyte contractile properties, such as increased magnitude of contraction with shortened time to peak contraction, and reversed downregulation of beta-receptors with increased response to beta-adrenergic stimulation.[10,11] These findings suggest that mechanical support may help reverse some cardiac dysfunction in heart failure.

Table 1
Causes of cardiogenic shock

Cause of Cardiogenic Shock	Underlying Causes or Diseases
Acute MI	• Ruptured unstable plaque • Coronary vasospasm • Myocardial bridging
Mechanical complications of acute MI	• Myocardial stunning • Tamponade • Papillary muscle rupture with severe mitral regurgitation • Postinfarction ventricular septal defect • Ventricular free wall rupture
Acute decompensation of chronic heart failure	• Dilated cardiomyopathy (ischemic or nonischemic) • Hypertrophic cardiomyopathy with LV outflow tract obstruction • Congenital heart disease
Postcardiotomy syndrome	• Postcardiopulmonary bypass
Cardiac graft failure	• Donor-recipient mismatch • Rejection-related failure (early or late) • Insufficient allograft preservation
Acute heart failure	• Myocarditis (ie, viral, giant cell) • Postpartum cardiomyopathy • Takotsubo syndrome • Myocardial contusion • Pulmonary embolism (causing acute right heart failure)
Acute arrhythmias	• Ventricular fibrillation • Ventricular tachycardia • Intractable atrial fibrillation with rapid ventricular response
Valvular disease	• Severe aortic stenosis • Prosthetic valve failure • Endocarditis • Rheumatic heart disease
Impaired ventricular filling	• Constrictive pericarditis • Cardiac tamponade • Restrictive cardiomyopathy (ie, amyloidosis)
Systemic metabolic dysfunction	• Hypothermia • Hypoxemia • Electrolyte imbalance • Intoxication (beta-blockers, cocaine, carbon monoxide) • Pheochromocytoma • Septicemia • Thyrotoxicosis • Anemia

Adapted from Koerner MM, Jahanyar J. Assist devices for circulatory support in therapy-refractory acute heart failure. Curr Opin Cardiol 2008;23:399–406; with permission.

MECHANICS OF TEMPORARY VAD SYSTEMS
Introduction to Continuous Flow Devices

Continuous flow pumps have a continuously spinning rotor or impeller that produces forward flow by pulling blood from the ventricle and ejecting it into arterial system, typically the proximal aorta. The pump operates at a speed set by the clinician, with higher speeds delivering more flow. The devices are valveless, so retrograde flow is possible

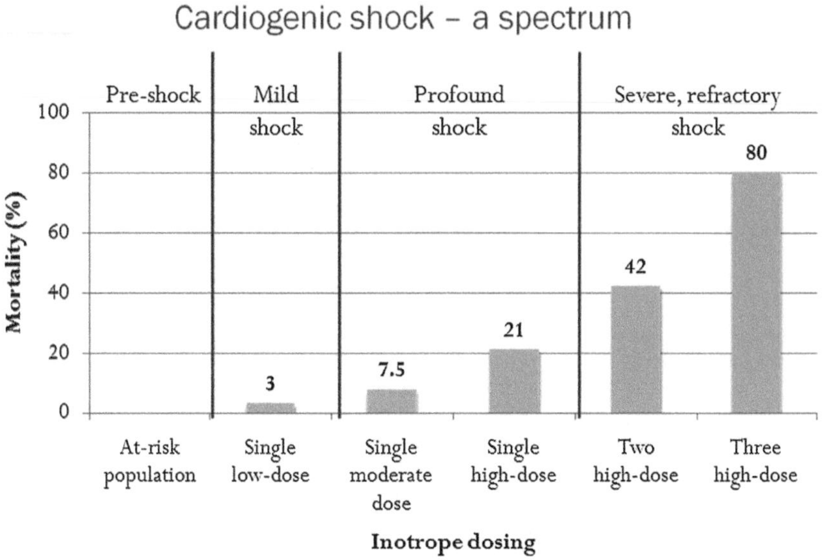

Cardiogenic shock – a spectrum

Fig. 1. Continuum of cardiogenic shock. ECMO, extracorporeal membrane oxygenation; IABP, intra-aortic balloon pump. (*Data from* Samuels LE, Kaufman MS, Thomas MP, et al. Pharmacologic criteria for ventricular assist device insertion following postcardiotomy shock: experience with the Abiomed BVS system. J Card Surg 1999;14:288–93.)

if the pump speed is inadequate or in pump failure.[12] The two types of continuous flow devices are axial and centrifugal flow. Axial flow pumps have an impeller in the same axis as the blood flow, which accelerates blood and provides flow. Centrifugal pumps have a rotor that is suspended by a fluid layer or magnetically levitated within an outer casing in which in the inflow of blood is perpendicular to the impeller.

Impella

The Impella systems (Abiomed, Inc, Danvers, MA) are a set of percutaneously placed microaxial VADs used to provide rapid, short-term support during high-risk percutaneous interventions, acute heart failure, acute MI, or during/after cardiac surgery.[13] They are inserted retrograde across the aortic valve with the caged inlet within the LV cavity and the outflow in the ascending aorta.[14] Blood is aspirated by an electrically driven motor from the LV and pumped into the aorta.[15] Impella pumps are continuously purged with a heparinized dextrose solution to prevent blood from entering the motor and forming thrombus; system anticoagulation is not usually necessary, though some centers maintain patients on systemic heparin.[13–15] Pressure transducers within the cannula verify cannula placement by measuring pressures on both sides of the aortic valve. Transthoracic echocardiography may also be used to assist in repositioning the device, although repositioning can be performed without visualization by pulling the cannula back until the diastolic pressure increases back to baseline.[14]

The Impella is available in 3 configurations 2.5, CP, and 5.0. The 2.5 (**Fig. 2**A, B) is the smallest in the series; it is inserted through a 12F femoral artery sheath and can generate up to 2.5 L/min of flow.[14] The Impella 5.0 is available for percutaneous delivery or via a vascular graft (LD) and provides up to 5.0 L/min of flow. The LP 5.0 is a larger version of the LP 2.5 that is inserted through a 21F sheath and requires

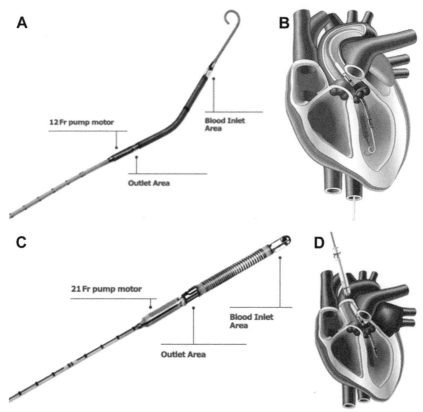

Fig. 2. (*A*) Impella LP 2.5 pump. (*B*) Impella LP 2.5 inserted from femoral artery across aortic valve. (*C*) Impella LD pump. (*D*) Impella LD inserted through ascending aorta. (*Courtesy of Abiomed, Inc, Danvers, MA; with permission.*)

surgical cutdown of the femoral artery for placement. The LD (see **Fig. 2**C, D) is inserted directly into the ascending aorta through a 10-mm vascular graft.[15] The CP is the most recent Food and Drug Administration–approved Impella Recover pump. It provides approximately 3.5 L/min of flow and is inserted via a femoral artery 14F sheath (**Table 2**). The pump catheters are controlled and powered by a bedside console. The console displays a pressure waveform to monitor pump placement, a motor current tracing, the pump power level, and a calculated cardiac output.

The Impella cannot be used in patients with heavily calcified aortic valves or prosthetic aortic valves. Although severe aortic regurgitation is not an absolute contraindication, it may reduce the efficacy of the pump.[16] Severe peripheral vascular disease may preclude femoral insertion.[5,13,15] Patients with femoral insertion are immobilized during support to prevent pump displacement. Additionally, the head of the bed cannot be raised more than 30°, and a knee immobilizer can be used to avoid bending the catheter at the insertion site.[14] However, if the device is placed through a graft sutured to the subclavian artery, the patient can be mobilized while on support.

TandemHeart

The TandemHeart (CardiacAssist, Inc, Pittsburgh, PA) is a percutaneous centrifugal pump (**Fig. 3**). The pump houses a 6-blade rotor that can generate up to 5.0 L/min

Table 2
Comparison of IABP with available percutaneous ventricular assist devices

Pump Characteristics	IABP	Impella LP 2.5[a]	Impella LP 5.0[a]	Impella LD[a]	TandemHeart[b]	CentriMag[c]
Pump mechanism	Pneumatic	Axial	Axial	Axial	Centrifugal	Centrifugal
Arterial or outflow insertion	7–9F Femoral artery	12F Femoral artery	21F Femoral artery	10-mm Graft ascending aorta	15–17F Femoral artery	22F LVAD: ascending aorta RVAD: main pulmonary artery
Venous or inflow insertion	N/A	N/A	N/A	N/A	21F Femoral vein to left atrium via transseptal puncture	32F LVAD: left ventricle apex or left atrium RVAD: right atrium
Amount of support	0.5 L/min	2.5 L/min	5.0 L/min	5.0 L/min	5.0 L/min	10 L/min
Maximal duration of support	10 d	5 d	5 d	7 d	14 d	30 d
Contraindications	• Moderate to severe aortic regurgitation • Aortic dissection • Unable to tolerate anticoagulation	• Severe aortic stenosis • Prosthetic aortic valve replacement • Hypertrophic cardiomyopathy • Left ventricular thrombus • Ventricular septal defect • Peripheral arterial disease • Right ventricular failure			• Severe aortic regurgitation • Aortic dissection • Peripheral arterial disease • Right ventricular failure • Ventricular septal defect	• Unable to tolerate anticoagulation
Major complications	• Thromboembolism • Air embolism (caused by IABP rupture) • Aortic injury, dissection, or rupture • Branch artery obstruction (caused by device malposition) • Limb ischemia • Infection • Bleeding	• Hemolysis • Bleeding • Limb ischemia (peripheral insertion) • Device malpositioning • Endocardial or valvular injury caused by suction events • Thromboembolism • Infection			• Bleeding • Thromboembolism • Infection • Aortic root puncture • Right atrial perforation • Coronary sinus perforation	• Bleeding • Thromboembolism • Infection

Abbreviations: IABP, intra-aortic balloon pump; LVAD, left ventricular assist device; N/A, not applicable; RVAD, right ventricular assist device.
[a] Abiomed, Inc, Danvers, MA.
[b] CardiacAssist, Inc, Pittsburgh, PA.
[c] Thoratec Corp, Pleasanton, CA.
Adapted from Basra SS, Loyalka P, Kar B. Current status of percutaneous ventricular assist devices for cardiogenic shock. Curr Opin Cardiol 2011;26:548–54; with permission.

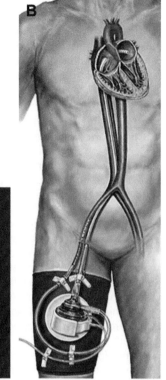

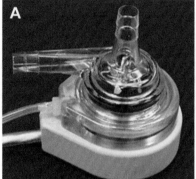

Fig. 3. (*A*) TandemHeart pump. (*B*) TandemHeart system. (*Courtesy of* CardiacAssist, Inc, Pittsburg, PA; with permission.)

at 7500 rpm. The inflow cannula is a 21F polyurethane tube with an end hole and multiple side holes that are inserted through the femoral vein into the left atrium via a transseptal puncture approach. Blood is returned to patients by the outflow cannula (either one 17F cannula or two 15F cannulas connected to a Y catheter) in the contralateral femoral artery. Insertion via the axillary artery and vein has also been reported.[17] An ultrasonic flow probe in the outflow cannula measures device output, which registers on the control console. Once the pump is in place, systemic anticoagulation with heparin is required to prevent pump thrombosis.[14]

Complications associated with the transseptal puncture are perforation of the aortic root, coronary sinus, or posterior right atrial free wall.[18] Long-term disposition of the transseptal puncture is unknown, but echocardiographic studies have not shown any significant left-to-right shunting after removal of the transseptal catheter.[19] The control console continuously displays the pump flow rate, pump speed, and purge fluid pressures. Unlike the Impella system, the TandemHeart system does not use pressure tracings to monitor the cannula position.[14] Cannula dislodgement is diagnosed by arterial gas measurement, chest radiograph, or echocardiogram. Repositioning of the cannulae must be performed in the catheterization laboratory.[14] Widespread use of the Tandem-Heart has been limited by the need for transseptal placement of the inflow catheter, which, if not done during cardiovascular surgery, requires the expertise of a certified interventional cardiologist.[16]

The TandemHeart is contraindicated in patients with ventricular septal defect (risk of hypoxemia caused by right-to-left shunting with LV unloading) and aortic insufficiency. Severe peripheral vascular disease may prevent TandemHeart insertion.[20] While on support, patients are immobilized to avoid damage to the cannulae entry sites or dislodgement of the left atrial inflow cannula.[14] Insertion via the axillary vessels allows patients to sit up and partially mobilize.[17]

CentriMag

The CentriMag (Thoratec Corp, Pleasanton, CA) is a surgically implanted centrifugal pump with a bearingless, magnetically levitated rotor (**Fig. 4**A). It was specifically designed for extracorporeal circulatory support applications, such as cardiopulmonary bypass (CPB) or ventricular assistance.[21] The pump has no contact between the impeller and the rest of the pump components, thus, creating a frictionless motor that does not generate heat or wear of the components, which leads to lower rates of hemolysis and pump thrombosis.[14] The pump can provide up to 10 L/min of flow and is intended for up to 14 days of support.[5] A console displays the pump's rotational speed and flow rate. The CentriMag system is versatile and can support a variety of patients. It can be used for univentricular or biventricular support. In LV support, the inflow cannula is placed in the left atrium or LV and the outflow cannula into the ascending aorta; in RV support, the inflow is placed in the right atrium and the outflow cannula in the main pulmonary artery (see **Fig. 4**B). Although insertion is usually via a sternotomy, peripheral cannulation via the femoral artery and vein has also been reported.[22] If full cardiopulmonary support is needed, an oxygenator can be added to the circuit to adapt it for ECMO.[23]

Even though the blood pump itself is minimally thrombogenic, the combined surface area of the pump, cannulas, and tubing are still susceptible to thrombus formation. Low pump flow states, such as hypovolemia or during pump weaning, also increase the risk of thrombosis.[14] Because of this reason, patients are maintained on systemic anticoagulation while on CentriMag support. Some centers delay initiation of anticoagulation for up to 24 hours postoperatively to reduce the risk of bleeding.[24,25] If bleeding occurs while on support, anticoagulation has been held for up to 72 hours while maintaining higher pump flows, without signs of pump malfunction caused by thrombosis.[26]

Compared with the Impella and TandemHeart, the CentriMag system can provide longer-term support. Although the system is typically used for less than 1 week, the

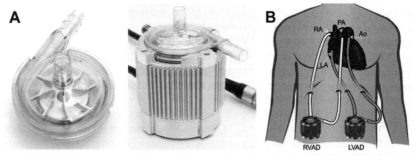

Fig. 4. (*A*) CentriMag pump and pump with motor. (*B*) Common CentriMag cannulation configurations for univentricular or biventricular support. Ao, aorta; LA, left atrium; LVAD, left VAD; PA, pulmonary artery; RA, right atrium; RVAD, right VAD. (*Courtesy of* Thoratec Corporation, Pleasanton, CA; with permission.)

CentriMag has been reported to provide more than 100 days of support, with pumps exchanged every 4 to 6 weeks to prevent fibrin formation.[27] The pumps can be exchanged at the bedside or in the operating room.[15] Additionally, with central cannulation through the chest wall, patients can be mobilized and may even be able to participate in limited physical therapy, with proper perfusionist supervision.[27]

Bio-Medicus

The Bio-Medicus pump (Medtronic, Inc, Minneapolis, MN) is a versatile pump that can be used for ventricular assistance, cardiopulmonary bypass, and ECMO. It can be inserted centrally (left atrium to pulmonary vein for left VAD [LVAD] support and right atrium to pulmonary artery for right VAD [RVAD] support) or peripherally (femoral artery to femoral vein). However, it is meant for short-term use, limited by bleeding complications and a hemolysis rate that is double that of the CentriMag.[21]

HEMODYNAMIC CHANGES IN PATIENTS WITH VAD
Decreased Arterial Pulse Pressure

Because a VAD provides continuous blood flow through all phases of the cardiac cycle, it creates flow during both systole and diastole, thus, decreasing the pulse pressure.[28] With the continuous unloading of the ventricle, the LV contracts against very low volumes, which does not generate sufficient pressure to allow it to eject during systole, which further contributes to a decreased or absent pulse pressure.

Systemic pressure is measured as a mean arterial pressure (MAP); there is no ideal pressure value, though in general a MAP of 70 to 90 mm Hg is typically targeted.[29] On invasive arterial pressure monitoring, the arterial waveform may be virtually flat and patients often do not have a palpable peripheral pulse. Changes in arterial pressures or morphology waveforms may indicate acute blood loss, volume overload, impaired pump flow, or changes in cardiac function (**Fig. 5**).[12]

Afterload Sensitive, Preload Insensitive System

Flow through a continuous flow pump depends on the pressure differential across the pump. For an LVAD, this is the difference between the left heart (ventricle or atria depending location of inflow) and aortic pressures; for an RVAD, it is the difference between the right heart (ventricle or atria, depending on the location of inflow) and pulmonary arterial pressures. All pumps require adequate preload into the chamber from which the inflow cannula/inlet withdraws blood for proper functioning. Low volumes cause negative pressure and collapse of the chamber, resulting in a suction event, which causes total occlusion of the inlet cannula and compromises forward flow from the VAD. Increased afterload pressures decreases flow through the VAD and, therefore, the amount of support provided by the device. Hence, effective afterload reduction is required during support for optimal pump function.[12,14]

COMPLICATIONS OF TEMPORARY VAD THERAPY
Bleeding

Bleeding is the most common complication in temporary VAD therapy.[30] Patients may require continuous anticoagulation to prevent device and cannula thrombus formation. Those who have recently undergone CPB have a higher risk for postoperative bleeding.[14] Lastly, comorbidities such as malnutrition, the use of chronic

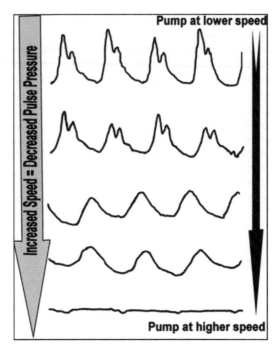

Fig. 5. Effect of pump speed on arterial pulse pressure waveforms. (*From* Christensen DM. Physiology of continuous-flow pumps. AACN Adv Crit Care 2012;23(1):46–54; with permission.)

anticoagulation, or organ malperfusion from shock may result in liver dysfunction, which further increases their risk of bleeding.[31]

Most of the bleeding in temporary VAD support is not device related.[32,33] Nonetheless, any bleeding increases patient morbidity and mortality. Blood transfusions predispose patients to infection and transfusion reactions. In LVAD recipients, the large volumes of blood products may increase their risk of developing RV failure and systemic volume overload, especially in the immediate postoperative period. This complication may cause hepatic congestion and dysfunction, leading to coagulopathy and further increased bleeding risk. In patients deemed transplant candidates, transfusions increase the risk of allosensitization that can delay or prevent successful transplantation.[30]

There are several strategies to reduce the risk of bleeding after VAD implant. If time allows, preoperative administration of vitamin K, especially if liver dysfunction is present, may reduce postoperative bleeding.[34] If renal dysfunction exists, desmopressin (DDAVP) can also be considered to optimize platelet function.[30] Postoperatively, peripheral cannulation sites are common sites of bleeding and should be checked regularly, especially if covered by bulkier dressings. If transfusions are needed, leuko-reduced packed red blood cells and single donor platelets should be preferentially used in transplant candidates to reduce the risk of allosensitization.

Infection

Infections are another common complication in temporary VAD patients. The highest risk of infection is in the early postoperative period when patients may be intubated and have multiple central venous catheters.[35] The incidence of infection increases with the duration of support; patients on LVAD therapy support for more than 60 days have twice the infection rate of patients supported for less than 30 days.[36] Multiorgan dysfunction, malnutrition, surgery and reoperations, multiple intravascular lines, endotracheal tubes, urinary catheters, and chest tubes all predispose these patients to localized and systemic infections. Postoperative bleeding contributes to the infection risk by increasing exposure via reoperation and blood transfusions.[35]

Most infections are bacterial, with typical pathogens consisting of *coagulase-negative staphylococcus*, *Staphylococcus aureus*, and *Pseudomonas aeruginosa*.[37] Fungal colonization is common in VAD patients, but fungal infections only occur when there is fungal overgrowth and/or impaired host immunity. Once established, fungi adhere to foreign material more readily than bacteria and are, therefore, much more difficult to eradicate.[38]

Strategies to reduce infectious complications include minimizing indwelling lines and catheters. Preoperative antibiotics are standard in surgically implanted VADs and may be considered before implantation of percutaneously inserted devices if time allows. The use of prophylactic antibiotic and antifungal use after temporary VAD insertion is not routine because of concern of development of resistant organisms. Several studies report routine antibiotic or antifungal therapy as long as invasive devices are required.[35,39–41] Although overt sepsis is a contraindication to transplantation, a successful transplant may be performed after infection is resolved. Surprisingly, patients with infections while on VAD support have similar rates of posttransplant infectious complications and no difference in long-term survival.[35,42]

Hemolysis

Hemolysis is a relatively uncommon complication of temporary VAD therapy. It occurs in 4% to 7% of Impella and TandemHeart patients.[33,43–46] The CentriMag device, with its bearingless magnetically levitated rotor, has been shown to cause less blood trauma compared with other centrifugal devices.[21,47,48] Many CentriMag studies do not report hemolysis rates; of those with hemolysis data, the reported incidence is low at 0% to 5%.[32,49] Causes of hemolysis include high impeller speeds, device malposition, or suction events caused by inadequate LV preload.[14,50,51] Prolonged support has not been associated with a greater incidence or severity of hemolysis.[45] Hemolysis is detected by hematologic indicators of blood trauma, such as decreased hemoglobin/hematocrit, increased lactate dehydrogenase levels, and increased plasma-free hemoglobin.[52] In most cases the degree of hemolysis is minimal and no intervention is required, though persistent severe hemolysis may require device removal.[51]

Thromboembolism

Overall rates of clinically observed thromboembolisms (ie, cerebrovascular event, pulmonary embolism) while on temporary VAD support are low, occurring in 1% to 11% of patients.[25,49,53] Autopsy studies show that the subclinical thromboembolic event rates are much higher, up to 54%.[25] The surface areas of the devices, cannulas, and tubing are all susceptible to thrombus formation. Prevention of thromboembolism is largely dependent on maintaining adequate anticoagulation and pump flow.

Peripheral Vascular Complications

Limb ischemia is a concern in peripherally inserted temporary VADs, especially in patients with small arteries or peripheral arterial disease. It is more common in the TandemHeart and Impella LP 5.0, which have larger-bore insertion cannulas.[54–56]

Treatment options are cannula removal or implantation of an accessory antegrade cannula in the ischemic limb.[55] Visualizing the femoral arteries by dye injection under fluoroscopy before cannula insertion may help prevent this complication.[55] Another complication of peripheral insertion is femoral artery dissection, which usually necessitates surgical repair.[57]

CLINICAL SCENARIOS FOR MECHANICAL SUPPORT IN LV FAILURE
Acute MI

Cardiogenic shock complicates 7% to 10% of ST elevation MI (STEMI).[58] Mortality rates are high at 60% to 80%, even with prompt revascularization.[59] IABP support has traditionally been recommended as the first-line MCS of cardiogenic shock in STEMI.[60] Recently, it has been shown that IABP use did not reduce 30-day mortality in patients with shock and early revascularization. It also failed to improve other secondary end points, such as hemodynamic stabilization and renal function.[61] In patients in whom IABP provides inadequate hemodynamic support, a temporary VAD should be considered.[60]

Temporary VAD systems have been successfully used in STEMI without cardiogenic shock and high-risk percutaneous intervention.[62–64] In cardiogenic shock, they can be quickly inserted to provide rapid hemodynamic stabilization.[44] However, despite improved hemodynamics, patients placed on temporary mechanical support continue to have high mortality rates. Randomized controlled trials comparing IABP with Impella or TandemHeart have consistently shown that temporary VADs improve hemodynamics but fail to improve 30-day mortality.[45,46,56] However, these trials are small and possibly underpowered to detect a mortality benefit. A meta-analysis of these trials still did not demonstrate lower mortality with temporary VAD support.[65] Longer duration of support with the CentriMag system also does not significantly improve survival.[26]

Although survival rates with the percutaneous devices studied in shock are similar to historical rates, the patients in these studies were often in profound shock on multiple pressors, had failed IABP and often had undergone CPR. The outcomes with these devices in less advanced degrees of shock, particularly in the absence of systemic vasodilation, is still being studied.[5] Additionally, there are several systemic perturbations that occur after acute MI that affect survival. Large systemic insults, such as a large acute MI, produce a systemic inflammatory response. Patients with large MIs have leukocytosis, fever, and elevated levels of various inflammatory markers, such as interleukins, C-reactive protein, and complement. These cytokines stimulate cellular production of toxic levels of nitric oxide (NO) and the cytotoxic NO-derived peroxynitrite, which have several deleterious effects on the cardiovascular system, including direct inhibition of myocardial contractility and inappropriate systemic vasodilation.[66] Improving systemic perfusion with a VAD may further promote systemic inflammation by increasing cytokine circulation and subsequent progression to multiorgan failure.[56] There are some data to suggest that the continuous flow provided by an LVAD may be detrimental to myocardial recovery. A smaller difference between systolic and diastolic flow may stagnate flows in stenotic regions, which can cause platelet adhesion and thrombus formation and, therefore, stent or graft occlusion.[67,68] This conclusion is highly controversial because the reduced coronary blood flow may be caused by the decreased myocardial oxygen consumption from LV unloading.[69,70] Current data do not demonstrate a survival benefit with the use of temporary LVADs in cardiogenic shock after acute MI despite improved hemodynamics, but it is unclear whether this is because of confounding factors, the advanced degree of shock seen in the studies, or a true lack of benefit.

Postcardiotomy Shock

Postcardiotomy cardiogenic shock (PCCS) is a leading cause of death after cardiac surgery, with an incidence of 0.2% to 6% and mortality rates around 75%.[71–74] It is defined as the inability to successfully wean from CPB despite maximal inotropic and IABP support either in the operating room or in the early postoperative period.[29] The first devices used for mechanical support in PCCS were the centrifugal pumps used in CPB (eg, Bio-Pump [Medtronic, Minneapolis, MN], Sarns [Terumo Corp, Somerset, NJ]) but with low survival rates of 16% to 40%. The use of paracorporeal pumps (eg, Abiomed AB5000 [Abiomed Inc, Danvers, MA], Thoratec PVAD [Thoratec Corp, Pleasanton, CA]) have improved survival to 29% to 50%. Their use has been limited by device bulk, need for high-dose anticoagulation, and extensive reoperation for device removal.[71]

The new temporary VADs are smaller and easier to implant with lower operative times and surgical trauma. The CentriMag was one of the first temporary devices to be used in PCS. Early studies showed improvement in mortality (43%–50% 30-day survival).[25,53] Subsequent studies evaluating the efficacy of the TandemHeart and Impella LP 5.0/LD systems have yielded similar survival rates.[31,33,75] Native cardiac function was recovered in most patients with explant rates of 60% to 93%, although some patients eventually required transplant.[31,53,75]

Immediate postoperative hemodynamics while on temporary VAD support is predictive of success of device explant and patient survival in PCCS.[76] Earlier initiation of circulatory support provides hemodynamic stabilization postoperatively, thus, preserving end-organ function and improving overall survival.[33] Another contributing factor is that patients who are unable to respond to mechanical support may have little recoverable myocardium, which is associated with significantly poorer survival.[75] Thus, patients at high risk for developing PCCS, such as those with systolic dysfunction or renal impairment, should be considered for early or even prophylactic temporary VAD implant directly from CPB.[77,78]

Acute on Chronic Systolic Heart Failure

Heart transplantation is currently the standard treatment of end-stage cardiomyopathy, though surgically implanted durable LVADs are quickly becoming an equal alternative as destination therapy. The options are limited for patients with end-stage heart failure who present with cardiogenic shock. Their candidacy for transplant or durable LVAD implant is often unclear because of coexisting medical issues (eg, neurologic status, sepsis). Additionally, these patients have poor survival after transplant and after durable LVAD implant, with mortality rates of 64% to 80%.[79,80]

In such patients, temporary LVADs have been successfully used as a bridge to decision by providing hemodynamic stabilization while the patients' candidacy for advanced heart failure therapies is evaluated. Both short-term support with TandemHeart and longer support with CentriMag (up to 87.6 days) have been reported.[32,57,81,82] In patients deemed appropriate candidates, temporary LVADs maintain end-organ function and prevent the development of more profound shock, thus, improving surgical mortality.[57] Survival rates of these patients after transplant and after permanent LVAD implant were 73.3% to 85.7% at 30 days and 64.9% to 66.7% at 6 months. Despite severe hemodynamic compromise and end-organ dysfunction in these patients, these survival rates are comparable with stable patients with advanced heart failure undergoing permanent LVAD implant.[83]

Cardiac Allograft Rejection

The incidence of cardiac allograft rejection has decreased with improvements in immunosuppression; however, its occurrence is complicated by high mortality and morbidity. It is often resistant to medical therapy, requiring mechanical support until recovery or retransplant can occur. There are several case reports of successful use of the Impella LP 5.0 and TandemHeart for cellular or humoral rejection causing acute heart failure occurring months to years after the initial transplant.[84–87] Patients were treated with aggressive antirejection medications while on mechanical support, and devices were explanted after echocardiography demonstrated improvement in cardiac function.

Acute Fulminant Myocarditis

Lymphocytic myocarditis can cause LV dysfunction, which is fully recoverable in about half of patients. Patients with fulminant myocarditis have excellent long-term prognosis if they survive the acute illness.[41] Temporary mechanical support with the TandemHeart and CentriMag systems has been successfully used to provide aggressive hemodynamic support as a bridge to recovery.[32,88] Many of these patients have biventricular dysfunction as a result of the diffuse inflammatory condition and may require ECMO or biventricular support rather than LVAD support alone. The Impella LP 2.5 has been used in conjunction with ECMO to provide LV decompression and facilitated earlier ECMO weaning.[89] These devices can also be used as a bridge to transplant or durable LVAD implant if recovery does not occur.[32,90]

Biventricular Failure

The most common cause of RVF is LV dysfunction. If RV dysfunction persists after reversal of LV failure, then biventricular support needs to be considered. The Centri-Mag system has been used as a bridge to recovery, transplant, or durable LVAD implant in cardiogenic shock caused by acute MI and decompensated chronic heart failure.[26,27] It has also been used in acute allograft failure for a bridge to recovery or retransplant.[25] There are case reports of successful use of the TandemHeart used for RV support in conjunction with other forms of LV support: Impella LP 2.5 for cardiac allograft rejection and IABP for cardiogenic shock caused by acute MI.[91,92] Typically, in the setting of severe biventricular failure, ECMO or as a biventricular assist device (BiVAD) CentriMag is required.

MECHANICAL SUPPORT IN RVF

Acute RVF can occur in a variety of settings. Cardiogenic shock caused by acute RVF is diagnosed hemodynamically (high central venous pressure, low cardiac output, low RV stroke work index) and by echocardiography (reduced tricuspid annular excursion and low RV tissue Doppler S′). The common causes of primary RV failure are RV infarct and increases in afterload (eg, pulmonary hypertension, pulmonary embolus, after cardiac surgery, and mechanical ventilation).[93] Initial treatment strategies involve volume optimization, enhancing RV inotropy, and reducing RV afterload. In some circumstances, mechanical support has been used to increase RV output when medications and/or other surgical interventions have failed. In cases of increased RV afterload, mechanical support can be used to augment RV function. If the primary problem is afterload resistance, increasing blood flow may actually increase pulmonary arterial pressures and worsen lung injury without increasing cardiac output. In these situations, veno-arterial ECMO is likely a more appropriate means of support.[94]

Mechanical Support Devices

Pulsatile devices are commonly used for long-term RV support. In acute RVF, percutaneous VAD use is increasing because of their rapid insertion and smaller profile.[95] The CentriMag and TandemHeart have been used primarily as bridge-to-recovery devices in RV infarction and after cardiac surgery. The Impella RP is an investigational, dedicated RV axial flow device. It is a 22F pump inserted through the femoral vein via an 11F catheter; it passes through the RV and pumps up to 5 L/min into the pulmonary artery.[96] The RECOVER RIGHT trial is currently underway to assess the efficacy of the Impella RP in RVF after LVAD implant, after cardiotomy shock, and after MI.[97]

Post–Cardiac Surgery RVF

RVF after cardiac surgery can occur after LVAD implant or heart transplant. After LVAD, the incidence of RV failure ranges from 5% to 44% and is associated with up to 70% mortality. Temporary mechanical support (less than 1 week) successfully bridges a substantial percentage of patients with postcardiotomy RVF to recovery. These patients have adequate cardiac output, even despite ongoing RV dysfunction.[74] Bhama and colleagues[24] reported on the use of CentriMag RVAD in patients with RVF caused by PCCS, after transplant, and after LVAD. Thirty-day mortality was 48%, and there was no difference in mortality based on indication for support. Most survivors recovered their RV function and underwent RVAD explant (59%) after a mean of 8 days of support; the other patients required permanent RVAD implant or were bridged to heart transplantation.

RV Infarction

RV infarction complicates up to 50% of inferior wall MI (IWMI) and carries a higher mortality when compared with IWMI without RVF (31% vs 6%).[98] The hemodynamic variations of RV infarcts vary widely. Up to 80% of patients with RV infarction have imaging evidence of RV dilation and wall motion abnormalities, but less than 50% of them present with hemodynamic compromise. Patients with persistent hemodynamic impairment have a higher mortality than those without (24% with vs 7% without).[99]

The TandemHeart was the first percutaneous device used in 2006 for a successful bridge to recovery in RVF after IWMI.[100] It remains an effective option today, with a recent small series reporting an 83% survival to discharge in patients supported by peripherally inserted TandemHeart for RVF in IWMI.[101] The Impella RP has been used as bridge to recovery RVF complicating IWMI in case studies.[96,102] Compared with the TandemHeart, the Impella RP would allow for potentially more rapid insertion without the need for transseptal puncture. Early hemodynamic stabilization with temporary RVAD support in such patients may improve survival.[101] Additionally, unloading the RV with mechanical support, in conjunction with revascularization, may also enhance RV recovery.[101]

GOALS OF THERAPY

The goals of temporary MCS are to restore hemodynamics and organ function to allow for myocardial recovery and device explant. Weaning of VAD support occurs once noncardiac organ systems have recovered. VAD support is decreased gradually (hours to days); if hemodynamics and other organ function remains adequate, the VAD is explanted. If not, patients may need to be considered for heart transplantation or durable VAD implantation. Patients with irrecoverable end-organ and/or neurologic dysfunction are unlikely to benefit from or even survive transplant or VAD implantation; in these patients, candid discussions with family and, if possible, the patients regarding goals of care and possible withdraw of mechanical support should take place.

Currently, there is no risk model or set preoperative variables that predict the success or failure of temporary mechanical support. All patients who receive temporary MCS should be concurrently assessed for candidacy for advanced heart failure therapies, with the work-up beginning ideally as soon as possible after temporary support is initiated. The evaluation of patients' emotional, physical, and social considerations may be just as complex and time consuming, if not more, than their medical and surgical issues. These nonmedical issues include, but are certainly not limited to, the cognitive ability to care for a durable mechanical device or a transplanted heart, the emotional ability to adapt to a new state of health and its complications, and an adequate social network for emergencies and long-term emotional support.

SUMMARY

Since the first clinical LVAD was implanted in 1963 as salvage therapy for postcardiotomy shock,[103] temporary mechanical support today is routinely used to bridge patients with cardiogenic shock facing imminent death to recovery or other long-term advanced heart failure therapies. It is hoped that advances in device design and patient selection will result in further improvements in outcomes with reductions in adverse events.

REFERENCES

1. Hollenberg SM, Kavinsky CJ, Parrillo JE. Cardiogenic shock. Ann Intern Med 1999;131:47–59.
2. Hochman JS, Sleeper LA, Webb JG, et al. Early revascularization in acute myocardial infarction complicated by cardiogenic shock. SHOCK Investigators. Should we emergently revascularize occluded coronaries for cardiogenic shock. N Engl J Med 1999;341:625–34.
3. Cove ME, MacLaren G. Clinical review: mechanical circulatory support for cardiogenic shock complicating acute myocardial infarction. Crit Care 2010; 14:235.
4. Samuels LE, Kaufman MS, Thomas MP, et al. Pharmacological criteria for ventricular assist device insertion following postcardiotomy shock: experience with the Abiomed BVS system. J Card Surg 1999;14:288–93.
5. Garatti A, Russo C, Lanfranconi M, et al. Mechanical circulatory support for cardiogenic shock complicating acute myocardial infarction: an experimental and clinical review. ASAIO J 2007;53:278–87.
6. Dandel M, Weng Y, Siniawski H, et al. Prediction of cardiac stability after weaning from left ventricular assist devices in patients with idiopathic dilated cardiomyopathy. Circulation 2008;118:S94–105.
7. James KB, McCarthy PM, Thomas JD, et al. Effect of the implantable left ventricular assist device on neuroendocrine activation in heart failure. Circulation 1995; 92:II191–5.
8. Allen BS, Okamoto F, Buckberg GD, et al. Reperfusion conditions: critical importance of total ventricular decompression during regional reperfusion. J Thorac Cardiovasc Surg 1986;92:605–12.
9. Li YY, Feng Y, McTiernan CF, et al. Downregulation of matrix metalloproteinases and reduction in collagen damage in the failing human heart after support with left ventricular assist devices. Circulation 2001;104:1147–52.

10. Dipla K, Mattiello JA, Jeevanandam V, et al. Myocyte recovery after mechanical circulatory support in humans with end-stage heart failure. Circulation 1998;97: 2316–22.
11. Ogletree-Hughes ML, Stull LB, Sweet WE, et al. Mechanical unloading restores beta-adrenergic responsiveness and reverses receptor downregulation in the failing human heart. Circulation 2001;104:881–6.
12. Christensen DM. Physiology of continuous-flow pumps. AACN Adv Crit Care 2012;23:46–54.
13. de Souza CF, de Souza Brito F, De Lima VC, et al. Percutaneous mechanical assistance for the failing heart. J Interv Cardiol 2010;23:195–202.
14. Myers TJ. Temporary ventricular assist devices in the intensive care unit as a bridge to decision. AACN Adv Crit Care 2012;23:55–68.
15. Ziemba EA, John R. Mechanical circulatory support for bridge to decision: which device and when to decide. J Card Surg 2010;25:425–33.
16. Koerner MM, Jahanyar J. Assist devices for circulatory support in therapy-refractory acute heart failure. Curr Opin Cardiol 2008;23:399–406.
17. Anyanwu AC, Fischer GW, Kalman J, et al. Preemptive axillo-axillary placement of percutaneous transseptal ventricular assist device to facilitate high-risk reoperative cardiac surgery. Ann Thorac Surg 2010;89:2053–5.
18. Friedman PA, Munger TM, Torres N, et al. Percutaneous endocardial and epicardial ablation of hypotensive ventricular tachycardia with percutaneous left ventricular assist in the electrophysiology laboratory. J Cardiovasc Electrophysiol 2007;18:106–9.
19. Thiele H, Smalling RW, Schuler GC. Percutaneous left ventricular assist devices in acute myocardial infarction complicated by cardiogenic shock. Eur Heart J 2007;28:2057–63.
20. Aragon J, Lee MS, Kar S, et al. Percutaneous left ventricular assist device: "TandemHeart" for high-risk coronary intervention. Catheter Cardiovasc Interv 2005; 65:346–52.
21. Hoshi H, Shinshi T, Takatani S. Third-generation blood pumps with mechanical noncontact magnetic bearings. Artif Organs 2006;30:324–38.
22. Fitzgerald D, Ging A, Burton N, et al. The use of percutaneous ECMO support as a 'bridge to bridge' in heart failure patients: a case report. Perfusion 2010;25: 321–5, 7.
23. Aziz TA, Singh G, Popjes E, et al. Initial experience with CentriMag extracorporal membrane oxygenation for support of critically ill patients with refractory cardiogenic shock. J Heart Lung Transplant 2010;29:66–71.
24. Bhama JK, Kormos RL, Toyoda Y, et al. Clinical experience using the Levitronix CentriMag system for temporary right ventricular mechanical circulatory support. J Heart Lung Transplant 2009;28:971–6.
25. Shuhaiber JH, Jenkins D, Berman M, et al. The Papworth experience with the Levitronix CentriMag ventricular assist device. J Heart Lung Transplant 2008; 27:158–64.
26. John R, Liao K, Lietz K, et al. Experience with the Levitronix CentriMag circulatory support system as a bridge to decision in patients with refractory acute cardiogenic shock and multisystem organ failure. J Thorac Cardiovasc Surg 2007;134:351–8.
27. Haj-Yahia S, Birks EJ, Amrani M, et al. Bridging patients after salvage from bridge to decision directly to transplant by means of prolonged support with the CentriMag short-term centrifugal pump. J Thorac Cardiovasc Surg 2009; 138:227–30.

28. Myers TJ, Bolmers M, Gregoric ID, et al. Assessment of arterial blood pressure during support with an axial flow left ventricular assist device. J Heart Lung Transplant 2009;28:423–7.

29. Paul S, Leacche M, Unic D, et al. Determinants of outcomes for postcardiotomy VAD placement: an 11-year, two-institution study. J Card Surg 2006;21: 234–7.

30. Goldstein DJ, Beauford RB. Left ventricular assist devices and bleeding: adding insult to injury. Ann Thorac Surg 2003;75:S42–7.

31. Pitsis AA, Visouli AN, Burkhoff D, et al. Feasibility study of a temporary percutaneous left ventricular assist device in cardiac surgery. Ann Thorac Surg 2007; 84:1993–9.

32. De Robertis F, Rogers P, Amrani M, et al. Bridge to decision using the Levitronix CentriMag short-term ventricular assist device. J Heart Lung Transplant 2008; 27:474–8.

33. Griffith BP, Anderson MB, Samuels LE, et al. The RECOVER I: a multicenter prospective study of Impella 5.0/LD for postcardiotomy circulatory support. J Thorac Cardiovasc Surg 2013;145:548–54.

34. Kaplon RJ, Gillinov AM, Smedira NG, et al. Vitamin K reduces bleeding in left ventricular assist device recipients. J Heart Lung Transplant 1999;18: 346–50.

35. Myers TJ, Khan T, Frazier OH. Infectious complications associated with ventricular assist systems. ASAIO J 2000;46:S28–36.

36. Piccione W Jr. Left ventricular assist device implantation: short and long-term surgical complications. J Heart Lung Transplant 2000;19:S89–94.

37. Gandelman G, Frishman WH, Wiese C, et al. Intravascular device infections: epidemiology, diagnosis, and management. Cardiol Rev 2007;15:13–23.

38. Goldberg SP, Baddley JW, Aaron MF, et al. Fungal infections in ventricular assist devices. ASAIO J 2000;46:S37–40.

39. Goldstein DJ, el-Amir NG, Ashton RC Jr, et al. Fungal infections in left ventricular assist device recipients. Incidence, prophylaxis, and treatment. ASAIO J 1995; 41:873–5.

40. Holman WL, Skinner JL, Waites KB, et al. Infection during circulatory support with ventricular assist devices. Ann Thorac Surg 1999;68:711–6.

41. McCarthy PM, Schmitt SK, Vargo RL, et al. Implantable LVAD infections: implications for permanent use of the device. Ann Thorac Surg 1996;61:359–65 [discussion: 72–3].

42. Gordon SM, Schmitt SK, Jacobs M, et al. Nosocomial bloodstream infections in patients with implantable left ventricular assist devices. Ann Thorac Surg 2001; 72:725–30.

43. Lauten A, Engstrom AE, Jung C, et al. Percutaneous left-ventricular support with the Impella-2.5-assist device in acute cardiogenic shock: results of the Impella-EUROSHOCK-registry. Circ Heart Fail 2013;6:23–30.

44. Meyns B, Dens J, Sergeant P, et al. Initial experiences with the Impella device in patients with cardiogenic shock - impella support for cardiogenic shock. Thorac Cardiovasc Surg 2003;51:312–7.

45. Seyfarth M, Sibbing D, Bauer I, et al. A randomized clinical trial to evaluate the safety and efficacy of a percutaneous left ventricular assist device versus intra-aortic balloon pumping for treatment of cardiogenic shock caused by myocardial infarction. J Am Coll Cardiol 2008;52:1584–8.

46. Burkhoff D, Cohen H, Brunckhorst C, et al, TandemHeart Investigators Group. A randomized multicenter clinical study to evaluate the safety and efficacy of

the TandemHeart percutaneous ventricular assist device versus conventional therapy with intraaortic balloon pumping for treatment of cardiogenic shock. Am Heart J 2006;152:469.e1–8.

47. Asama J, Shinshi T, Hoshi H, et al. A compact highly efficient and low hemolytic centrifugal blood pump with a magnetically levitated impeller. Artif Organs 2006; 30:160–7.

48. Zhang J, Gellman B, Koert A, et al. Computational and experimental evaluation of the fluid dynamics and hemocompatibility of the CentriMag blood pump. Artif Organs 2006;30:168–77.

49. John R, Long JW, Massey HT, et al. Outcomes of a multicenter trial of the Levitronix CentriMag ventricular assist system for short-term circulatory support. J Thorac Cardiovasc Surg 2011;141:932–9.

50. Jurmann MJ, Siniawski H, Erb M, et al. Initial experience with miniature axial flow ventricular assist devices for postcardiotomy heart failure. Ann Thorac Surg 2004;77:1642–7.

51. Sibbald M, Dzavik V. Severe hemolysis associated with use of the Impella LP 2.5 mechanical assist device. Catheter Cardiovasc Interv 2012;80:840–4.

52. Sobieski MA, Giridharan GA, Ising M, et al. Blood trauma testing of CentriMag and RotaFlow centrifugal flow devices: a pilot study. Artif Organs 2012;36:677–82.

53. De Robertis F, Birks EJ, Rogers P, et al. Clinical performance with the Levitronix Centrimag short-term ventricular assist device. J Heart Lung Transplant 2006; 25:181–6.

54. Engstrom AE, Cocchieri R, Driessen AH, et al. The Impella 2.5 and 5.0 devices for ST-elevation myocardial infarction patients presenting with severe and profound cardiogenic shock: the Academic Medical Center intensive care unit experience. Crit Care Med 2011;39:2072–9.

55. Thiele H, Lauer B, Hambrecht R, et al. Reversal of cardiogenic shock by percutaneous left atrial-to-femoral arterial bypass assistance. Circulation 2001;104: 2917–22.

56. Thiele H, Sick P, Boudriot E, et al. Randomized comparison of intra-aortic balloon support with a percutaneous left ventricular assist device in patients with revascularized acute myocardial infarction complicated by cardiogenic shock. Eur Heart J 2005;26:1276–83.

57. Idelchik GM, Simpson L, Civitello AB, et al. Use of the percutaneous left ventricular assist device in patients with severe refractory cardiogenic shock as a bridge to long-term left ventricular assist device implantation. J Heart Lung Transplant 2008;27:106–11.

58. Goldberg RJ, Gore JM, Alpert JS, et al. Cardiogenic shock after acute myocardial infarction. Incidence and mortality from a community-wide perspective, 1975 to 1988. N Engl J Med 1991;325:1117–22.

59. Holmes DR Jr, Bates ER, Kleiman NS, et al. Contemporary reperfusion therapy for cardiogenic shock: the GUSTO-I trial experience. The GUSTO-I Investigators. Global utilization of streptokinase and tissue plasminogen activator for occluded coronary arteries. J Am Coll Cardiol 1995;26:668–74.

60. American College of Emergency Physicians, Society for Cardiovascular Angiography and Interventions, O'Gara PT, et al. 2013 ACCF/AHA guideline for the management of ST-elevation myocardial infarction: a report of the American College of Cardiology Foundation/American Heart Association Task Force on Practice Guidelines. J Am Coll Cardiol 2013;61:e78–140.

61. Thiele H, Zeymer U, Neumann FJ, et al. Intraaortic balloon support for myocardial infarction with cardiogenic shock. N Engl J Med 2012;367:1287–96.

62. Henriques JP, Remmelink M, Baan J Jr, et al. Safety and feasibility of elective high-risk percutaneous coronary intervention procedures with left ventricular support of the Impella Recover LP 2.5. Am J Cardiol 2006;97:990–2.

63. Sjauw KD, Konorza T, Erbel R, et al. Supported high-risk percutaneous coronary intervention with the Impella 2.5 device the Europella registry. J Am Coll Cardiol 2009;54:2430–4.

64. Sjauw KD, Remmelink M, Baan J Jr, et al. Left ventricular unloading in acute ST-segment elevation myocardial infarction patients is safe and feasible and provides acute and sustained left ventricular recovery. J Am Coll Cardiol 2008; 51:1044–6.

65. Cheng JM, den Uil CA, Hoeks SE, et al. Percutaneous left ventricular assist devices vs. intra-aortic balloon pump counterpulsation for treatment of cardiogenic shock: a meta-analysis of controlled trials. Eur Heart J 2009;30:2102–8.

66. Hochman JS. Cardiogenic shock complicating acute myocardial infarction: expanding the paradigm. Circulation 2003;107:2998–3002.

67. Cao J, Rittgers SE. Particle motion within in vitro models of stenosed internal carotid and left anterior descending coronary arteries. Ann Biomed Eng 1998;26: 190–9.

68. Xydas S, Rosen RS, Pinney S, et al. Reduced myocardial blood flow during left ventricular assist device support: a possible cause of premature bypass graft closure. J Heart Lung Transplant 2005;24:1976–9.

69. Merhige ME, Smalling RW, Cassidy D, et al. Effect of the hemopump left ventricular assist device on regional myocardial perfusion and function. Reduction of ischemia during coronary occlusion. Circulation 1989;80:III158–66.

70. Tuzun E, Eya K, Chee HK, et al. Myocardial hemodynamics, physiology, and perfusion with an axial flow left ventricular assist device in the calf. ASAIO J 2004;50:47–53.

71. Sylvin EA, Stern DR, Goldstein DJ. Mechanical support for postcardiotomy cardiogenic shock: has progress been made? J Card Surg 2010;25:442–54.

72. Goldstein DJ, Oz MC. Mechanical support for postcardiotomy cardiogenic shock. Semin Thorac Cardiovasc Surg 2000;12:220–8.

73. Helman DN, Morales DL, Edwards NM, et al. Left ventricular assist device bridge-to-transplant network improves survival after failed cardiotomy. Ann Thorac Surg 1999;68:1187–94.

74. Moazami N, Pasque MK, Moon MR, et al. Mechanical support for isolated right ventricular failure in patients after cardiotomy. J Heart Lung Transplant 2004;23: 1371–5.

75. Siegenthaler MP, Brehm K, Strecker T, et al. The Impella Recover microaxial left ventricular assist device reduces mortality for postcardiotomy failure: a three-center experience. J Thorac Cardiovasc Surg 2004;127:812–22.

76. Meyns B, Sergeant P, Wouters P, et al. Mechanical support with microaxial blood pumps for postcardiotomy left ventricular failure: can outcome be predicted? J Thorac Cardiovasc Surg 2000;120:393–400.

77. Akay MH, Gregoric ID, Radovancevic R, et al. Timely use of a CentriMag heart assist device improves survival in postcardiotomy cardiogenic shock. J Card Surg 2011;26:548–52.

78. Westaby S, Balacumaraswami L, Evans BJ, et al. Elective transfer from cardiopulmonary bypass to centrifugal blood pump support in very high-risk cardiac surgery. J Thorac Cardiovasc Surg 2007;133:577–8.

79. Farrar DJ. Preoperative predictors of survival in patients with Thoratec ventricular assist devices as a bridge to heart transplantation. Thoratec Ventricular

Assist Device Principal Investigators. J Heart Lung Transplant 1994;13:93–100 [discussion: 100–1].

80. Oz MC, Goldstein DJ, Pepino P, et al. Screening scale predicts patients successfully receiving long-term implantable left ventricular assist devices. Circulation 1995;92:II169–73.

81. Bruckner BA, Jacob LP, Gregoric ID, et al. Clinical experience with the Tandem-Heart percutaneous ventricular assist device as a bridge to cardiac transplantation. Tex Heart Inst J 2008;35:447–50.

82. Gregoric ID, Jacob LP, La Francesca S, et al. The TandemHeart as a bridge to a long-term axial-flow left ventricular assist device (bridge to bridge). Tex Heart Inst J 2008;35:125–9.

83. Rose EA, Gelijns AC, Moskowitz AJ, et al. Long-term use of a left ventricular assist device for end-stage heart failure. N Engl J Med 2001;345:1435–43.

84. Beyer AT, Hui PY, Haeusslein E. The Impella 2.5 L for percutaneous mechanical circulatory support in severe humoral allograft rejection. J Invasive Cardiol 2010; 22:E37–9.

85. Chandola R, Cusimano R, Osten M, et al. Use of Impella 5L for acute allograft rejection postcardiac transplant. Thorac Cardiovasc Surg 2012;60:302–4.

86. Samoukovic G, Al-Atassi T, Rosu C, et al. Successful treatment of heart failure due to acute transplant rejection with the Impella LP 5.0. Ann Thorac Surg 2009;88:271–3.

87. Velez-Martinez M, Rao K, Warner J, et al. Successful use of the TandemHeart percutaneous ventricular assist device as a bridge to recovery for acute cellular rejection in a cardiac transplant patient. Transplant Proc 2011;43:3882–4.

88. Chandra D, Kar B, Idelchik G, et al. Usefulness of percutaneous left ventricular assist device as a bridge to recovery from myocarditis. Am J Cardiol 2007;99: 1755–6.

89. Chaparro SV, Badheka A, Marzouka GR, et al. Combined use of Impella left ventricular assist device and extracorporeal membrane oxygenation as a bridge to recovery in fulminant myocarditis. ASAIO J 2012;58:285–7.

90. Suradi H, Breall JA. Successful use of the Impella device in giant cell myocarditis as a bridge to permanent left ventricular mechanical support. Tex Heart Inst J 2011;38:437–40.

91. Atwater BD, Nee LM, Gimelli G. Long-term survival using intra-aortic balloon pump and percutaneous right ventricular assist device for biventricular mechanical support of cardiogenic shock. J Invasive Cardiol 2008;20:E205–7.

92. Rajagopal V, Steahr G, Wilmer CI, et al. A novel percutaneous mechanical biventricular bridge to recovery in severe cardiac allograft rejection. J Heart Lung Transplant 2010;29:93–5.

93. Lahm T, McCaslin CA, Wozniak TC, et al. Medical and surgical treatment of acute right ventricular failure. J Am Coll Cardiol 2010;56:1435–46.

94. Berman M, Tsui S, Vuylsteke A, et al. Life-threatening right ventricular failure in pulmonary hypertension: RVAD or ECMO? J Heart Lung Transplant 2008;27: 1188–9.

95. Hsu PL, Parker J, Egger C, et al. Mechanical circulatory support for right heart failure: current technology and future outlook. Artif Organs 2012;36:332–47.

96. Margey R, Chamakura S, Siddiqi S, et al. First experience with implantation of a percutaneous right ventricular Impella right side percutaneous support device as a bridge to recovery in acute right ventricular infarction complicated by cardiogenic shock in the United States. Circ Cardiovasc Interv 2013;6:e37–8.

97. Available at: http://clinicaltrials.gov/ct2/show/NCT01777607?term=impella+rp&rank=1.

98. Zehender M, Kasper W, Kauder E, et al. Right ventricular infarction as an independent predictor of prognosis after acute inferior myocardial infarction. N Engl J Med 1993;328:981–8.

99. Serrano Junior CV, Ramires JA, Cesar LA, et al. Prognostic significance of right ventricular dysfunction in patients with acute inferior myocardial infarction and right ventricular involvement. Clin Cardiol 1995;18:199–205.

100. Atiemo AD, Conte JV, Heldman AW. Resuscitation and recovery from acute right ventricular failure using a percutaneous right ventricular assist device. Catheter Cardiovasc Interv 2006;68:78–82.

101. Kapur NK, Paruchuri V, Korabathina R, et al. Effects of a percutaneous mechanical circulatory support device for medically refractory right ventricular failure. J Heart Lung Transplant 2011;30:1360–7.

102. Cheung A, Leprince P, Freed D. First clinical evaluation of a novel percutaneous right ventricular assist device: the Impella RP. J Am Coll Cardiol 2012;59:E872.

103. Liotta D, Hall CW, Henly WS, et al. Prolonged assisted circulation during and after cardiac or aortic surgery. Prolonged partial left ventricular bypass by means of intracorporeal circulation. Am J Cardiol 1963;12:399–405.

Left Ventricular Assist Device Management and Complications

Edo Y. Birati, MD, J. Eduardo Rame, MD, MPhil*

KEYWORDS

- Heart failure • Left ventricular assist device • Complications • Post-LVAD

KEY POINTS

- Mechanical assist devices have emerged as one of the main therapies of advanced heart failure.
- Patients on long-term LVAD support present unique challenges in the intensive care unit.
- Managing patients on mechanical circulatory support require basic understanding of the physiology and characteristics of the devices and awareness of its complications.

Heart failure (HF) is one of the most frequent medical diagnoses, with more than 650,000 new patients with HF diagnosed annually and more than 5 million persons in the United States currently suffering from HF.[1] HF is a very common cause for hospital admissions in the United States, with more than 37.5 million hospitalizations during the years 2001 to 2009.[2]

Patients with advanced HF suffer from severe circulatory compromise and require special care, including heart transplantation, mechanical assist device, inotropes, and hospice. These patients are very ill, suffering from significant HF symptoms during rest or mild exercise, and their prognosis without therapy is unfavorable, with life expectancy of less than 2 years.[3]

Heart transplantation remains the definitive therapy for advanced HF. However, because of the lack of organ supply and the substantial increase in the prevalence of HF, durable mechanical assist devices have emerged as one of the main therapies of advanced HF. Inotrope therapy can be given as an inpatient or outpatient therapy. Despite an improvement in symptoms, these drugs can foreshorten life.[4,5] Thus, inotropes should be given only as a bridge to definite advanced HF therapy (long-term mechanical support or transplantation), and only rarely as definite therapy for palliation.[3]

Division of Cardiovascular Medicine, University of Pennsylvania, Philadelphia, PA 19104, USA
* Corresponding author. Hospital of the University of Pennsylvania, 2 East Perelman Center for Advanced Medicine, 3400 Civic Center Boulevard, Philadelphia, PA 19104.
E-mail address: eduardo.rame@uphs.upenn.edu

Crit Care Clin 30 (2014) 607–627
http://dx.doi.org/10.1016/j.ccc.2014.04.001
0749-0704/14/$ – see front matter © 2014 Elsevier Inc. All rights reserved.

VENTRICULAR ASSIST DEVICES

A ventricular assist device (VAD) is a mechanical circulatory device that is used to partially or completely replace the function of a failing heart. The first-generation devices, the HeartMate I and Novacor, had pulsatile flow, trying to mimic the normal blood flow that the heart produces. These devices were shown to increase survival and quality of life of patients with end-stage HF compared with optimal medical therapy but had clear limitations. The primary limitation was the lack of durability noted across all the first-generation devices.[6] The pulsatile LVAD was approved in 1994 by the US Food and Drug Administration (FDA) as a bridge to heart transplantation and subsequently, in 2003 for those not eligible for transplantation as destination therapy (DT). The second-generation and third-generation devices, which are currently being used (mainly, HeartMate II and HeartWare), have continuous flow patterns, generating up to 10 L a minute. The HeartMate II trial[7] compared the treatment with continuous flow devices with the first-generation pulsatile flow devices. The results showed that continuous flow LVAD improved the primary end point of survival free from stroke and device failure at 2 years compared with a pulsatile device. In addition, patients with continuous flow devices had better survival rates after 2 years. The success of these devices is reflected in the number of implantations. Since FDA approval in 2006 of the first continuous flow device, more than 6000 implants have been reported in our national registry. Worldwide, more than an estimated 18,000 continuous flow devices have been implanted, and the number keeps increasing exponentially. Thus, the likelihood that the critical care physician will encounter one of these patients is becoming higher.

The physiologic basis and sequelae of circulatory support with a continuous flow device are not fully understood. As blood moves through the systemic circulation, the pulsatile flow in the aorta is progressively decreased, transforming into continuous flow at the level of the capillary (**Fig. 1**). This process suggests that a pattern of pulsatile flow may not be necessary for an end-organ to remain fully viable with adequate perfusion.[8] It is important for clinicians to recognize that left-sided continuous flow devices produce some pulsatility. This situation is because the flow of the device is influenced by the remnants of native left ventricular (LV) contractility, and all determinants that affect LV preload, such as right ventricular (RV) function and volume depletion, affect the pulsatility.

VADs may serve the RV (RVAD), LV (LVAD), or both (BiVAD). The LVAD configuration is the most common in the current era. Most devices are being developed and

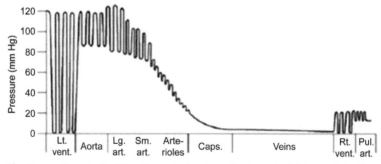

Fig. 1. The flow pattern in the blood vessels. Caps, capillaries; Lg art, large artery; Lt vent, left ventricle; Pul Art, pulmonary artery; Rt vent, right ventricle; Sm art, small artery. (*From* Sayer G, Naka Y, Jorde UP. Ventricular assist device therapy. Cardiovasc Ther 2009;27(2):142; with permission.)

manufactured for LV assist. No device has yet been approved for only RV assist. The inflow cannula of the device is placed in the apical part of the ventricle, allowing blood flow into the pump. The pump is attached to the outflow cannula, which is placed in the ascending aorta in patients with LVAD and in the pulmonary artery (PA) in patients with RVAD. The device is also connected through an electrical wire, called the percutaneous lead or driveline, to batteries located outside the body. **Fig. 2**A shows the HeartMate II (Thoratec, Pleasanton, CA), a second-generation axial continuous flow LVAD, and **Fig. 2**B shows the HeartWare device (HeartWare, Framingham, MA), a third-generation centrifugal flow device.

Surgical implantation is typically performed via a median sternotomy. Thus, access to the cardiac apex as well as the ascending aorta is gained. Differing device shapes and orientation have allowed for alternative surgical approaches, such as lateral thoracotomy and subcostal. The HeartMate II LVAD requires a pump pocket to be created below the diaphragm, whereas the HeartWare LVAD is fully contained within the pericardial space. Previous surgeries and adhesions make LVAD surgery more difficult, causing increased time on cardiopulmonary bypass and increasing the risk of bleeding. Plus, LVAD surgery creates more adhesions and increases the risk of subsequent surgeries such as LVAD exchange or heart transplantation.

Mechanical assist devices may be used as a bridge to transplantation (BTT), for candidates awaiting transplantation; as DT for patients who are ineligible for transplantation from various reasons (eg, age, severe diabetes); as a bridge to decision for patients that their suitability for transplantation is considered or additional

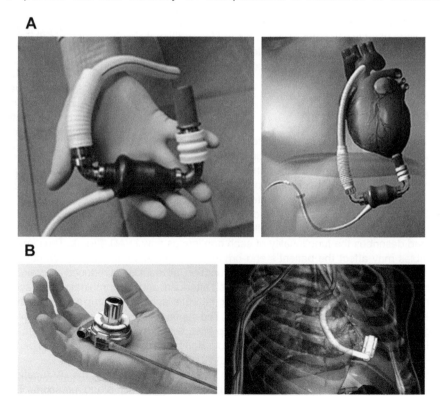

Fig. 2. (*A*) HeartMate 2 device. (*B*) HeartWare device. ([*A*] *Courtesy of* Thoratec, Pleasanton, CA; with permission; [*B*] Courtesy of HeartWare, Framingham, MA.)

therapeutic options need to be evaluated; and as a bridge to recovery among selected patients with an enhanced potential for reverse myocardial remodeling in chronic cardiomyopathy syndromes and acute cardiomyopathies (in the latter case, eg, patients with fulminant lymphocytic myocarditis, peripartum cardiomyopathy, and so forth).[3,9] INTERMACS (Interagency Registry of Mechanical Circulatory Support) is the formal US registry of patients treated with FDA-approved long-term mechanical assist devices. According to the fifth annual report of INTERMACS,[10] during 2012, 44% of mechanical assist device implants were designated as DT and only 21% as BTT. According to this registry, the survival of patients treated with continuous flow LVADs was 80% at 1 year and 70% at 2 years. The survival of patients treated with LVAD as DT or BTT is similar, and after adjusting other variables, the difference in predicted 1-year survival between the groups is approximately 5%.[10]

The INTERMACS clinical profiles allow further classification and risk stratification of patients with New York Heart Association (NYHA) class III to IV symptoms and provides more information on the disease severity and prognosis.[3,11] Patients with INTERMACS profile 1 to 3 are being treated with some form of temporary mechanical or inotropic support. Patients who are profile 3 are clinically stable on inotropes, whereas patients with profile 1 suffer from hypotension and critical organ hypoperfusion on escalating inotropic support and by definition require some form of temporary circulatory support within hours for preservation of end-organ function. Patients with profile 4 to 7 are not inotrope dependent.[3,11] Patients with INTERMACS profiles 1 and 2 have postimplantation mortality that is 44% higher than patients with INTERMACS profile 3 or 4.[12] **Table 1** provides detail on the INTERMACS clinical profiles. The importance of correct classification of the patient in cardiogenic shock cannot be stressed enough to identify when the immediate need for additional circulatory support (INTERMACS I) is present **Box 1**, and **Table 2** summarizes the current indication for all mechanical assist devices, as published by the American Heart Association and European Society of Cardiology.

BASIC VAD MANAGEMENT

Pulsatile devices depend on adequate preload, a fixed stroke volume, and rate to determine pump flow. In contrast, continuous flow pumps depend on a pressure difference across the pump to determine the pump flow. The pressure differential or head pressure is the systemic blood pressure – LV pressure. The pump flow is also determined by the LVAD speed in revolutions per minute (RPM), which is the only parameter on an LVAD that can be adjusted. The combination of head pressure plus LVAD speed determines flow and can be shown on a plot called the pressure-flow (HQ) curve, which is unique for and describes the functionality of each continuous flow LVAD (**Fig. 3**). Thus, many variables may affect the patient's end-organ perfusion, such as dehydration caused by overdiuresis, bleeding, and right RV dysfunction, all resulting in reduced LV preload; uncontrolled hypertension results in increased afterload, and the combination of these 2 elements can result in a significant pressure differential across the pump and a reduction of the pump flow, resulting in hypoperfusion. The continuous pumps also have the ability to generate negative pressures at the pump inlet, which may result in septal shift, LV collapse, and RV dysfunction, also leading to a significant decrease in end-organ perfusion in patients who are dependent on the LVAD for circulatory support.

It is essential to repeatedly estimate the effective volume status, the RV function, valvular regurgitation, and accurately estimate the systemic blood pressure. The pump speed must be adequate in relation to these variables. The pump speed effectively determines the degree of LV mechanical unloading, and this in turn affects RV

Table 1
INTERMACS clinical profiles

Level	Description	Hemodynamic Status	Time Frame for Intervention
1	Critical cardiogenic shock, crash and burn	Persistent hypotension despite rapidly escalating inotropic support and intra-aortic balloon pump, and critical organ hypoperfusion	Within hours
2	Progressive decline on inotropic support, sliding on inotropes	Intravenous inotropic support with acceptable values of blood pressure and continuing deterioration in nutrition, renal function, or fluid retention	Within days
3	Stable but inotrope dependent, dependent stability	Stability reached with mild to moderate doses of inotropes but showing failure to wean from them because of hypotension, worsening symptoms, or progressive renal dysfunction	Elective over weeks to months
4	Resting symptoms, frequent flyer	Possible weaning of inotropes but experiencing recurrent relapses, usually fluid retention	Elective over weeks to months
5	Exertion intolerant, housebound	Severe limited tolerance for activity, comfortable at rest with some volume overload and often with some renal dysfunction	Variable urgency, dependent on nutrition and organ function
6	Exertion limited, walking wounded	Less severe limited tolerance for activity and lack of volume overload, fatigue easily	Variable urgency, dependent on nutrition and organ function
7	Advanced NYHA III symptoms, placeholder	Patient without current or recent unstable fluid balance, NYHA class II or III	Not currently indicated

From Peura JL, Colvin-Adams M, Francis GS, et al, American Heart Association Heart Failure and Transplantation Committee of the Council on Clinical Cardiology, Council on Cardiopulmonary, Critical Care, Perioperative and Resuscitation, Council on Cardiovascular Disease in the Young, Council on Cardiovascular Nursing, Council on Cardiovascular Radiology and Intervention, and Council on Cardiovascular Surgery and Anesthesia. Recommendations for the use of mechanical circulatory support: device strategies and patient selection: a scientific statement from the American Heart Association. Circulation 2012;126(22):2657; with permission.

function and the degree of mitral and aortic regurgitation, which in turn affects the systemic blood pressure and perfusion of the patient. In this regard, blood pressure optimization is crucial, not only to optimize cardiac support and pump performance but also to reduce the stroke rate (ischemic and hemorrhagic). Mean arterial blood pressure (MAP) should be maintained between 70 and 80 mm Hg and should not exceed 90 mm Hg.[11] In the case of the HeartWare HVAD, an intrapericardial centrifugal pump, the recommended target for systemic blood pressure should not exceed 85 mm Hg.

Box 1
Recommendations for mechanical circulatory support (MCS)

1. MCS for BTT indication should be considered for transplant-eligible patients with end-stage HF who are failing optimal medical, surgical, or device therapies and at high risk of dying before receiving a heart transplantation (class I; level of evidence B).

2. Implantation of MCS in patients before the development of advanced HF (ie, hyponatremia, hypotension, renal dysfunction, and recurrent hospitalizations) is associated with better outcomes. Therefore, early referral of advanced patients with HF is reasonable (class IIa; level of evidence B).

3. MCS with a durable, implantable device for permanent therapy or DT is beneficial for patients with advanced HF, high 1-year mortality resulting from HF, and the absence of other life-limiting organ dysfunction; who are failing medical, surgical, or device therapies; and who are ineligible for heart transplantation (class I; level of evidence B).

From Peura JL, Colvin-Adams M, Francis GS, et al, American Heart Association Heart Failure and Transplantation Committee of the Council on Clinical Cardiology, Council on Cardiopulmonary, Critical Care, Perioperative and Resuscitation, Council on Cardiovascular Disease in the Young; Council on Cardiovascular Nursing, Council on Cardiovascular Radiology and Intervention, and Council on Cardiovascular Surgery and Anesthesia. Recommendations for the use of mechanical circulatory support: device strategies and patient selection: a scientific statement from the American Heart Association. Circulation 2012;126(22):2661; with permission.

Because there is variability in the ability to palpate a pulse, measurement of blood pressure is difficult. Early in the postoperative period, there is often some pulsatility because of the inotropes and pressors often used. With much controversy about blood pressure techniques, direct arterial line measurement remains the standard to obtaining an MAP. A Doppler occlusion pressure obtained at the brachial artery correlates reasonably well with central arterial monitoring. An automatic or manual auscultated blood pressure often underestimates the MAP. Further, because

---

Table 2
Recommendations for surgical implantation of LVADs in patients with systolic HF

Recommendations	Class[a]	Level[b]
An LVAD or BiVAD is recommended in selected patients with end-stage HF despite optimal pharmacologic and device treatment and who are otherwise suitable for heart transplantation, to improve symptoms and reduce the risk of HF hospitalization for worsening HF and to reduce the risk of premature death while awaiting transplantation	I	B
An LVAD should be considered in highly selected patients who have end-stage HF despite optimal pharmacologic and device therapy and who are not suitable for heart transplantation, but are expected to survive >1 y with good functional status, to improve symptoms, and reduce the risk of HF hospitalization and of premature death	IIa	B

[a] Class of recommendation.
[b] Level of evidence.
From McMurray JJ, Adamopoulos S, Anker SD, et al, ESC Committee for Practice Guidelines. ESC Guidelines for the diagnosis and treatment of acute and chronic heart failure 2012: The Task Force for the Diagnosis and Treatment of Acute and Chronic Heart Failure 2012 of the European Society of Cardiology. Developed in collaboration with the Heart Failure Association (HFA) of the ESC. Eur Heart J 2012;33(14):1787–847, 835 [Erratum in Eur Heart J 2013;34(2):158]; with permission.

HeartWare centrifugal LVAD
1800 – 4000 RPM curves

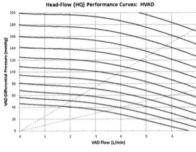

HeartMate II axial LVAD
6000-15,000 RPM curves

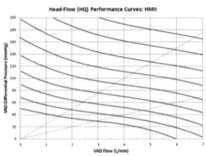

Fig. 3. The pressure-flow (HQ) curve.

pulsatility is variable, pulse oximetry can be unreliable also. Unbelievable values should be confirmed by arterial blood gas measurement.

PA catheters are frequently used in the postoperative period, because the patient with an LVAD is generally moved from the operating room with the PA catheter in place. They can be used early to assess the appropriateness of the LVAD speed settings with rapidly changing volume status and weaning inotropes and pressors from the surgery. Further, changes in preload and afterload can occur with awakening from anesthesia, extubation from the ventilator, and upright posture. For these rapid changes early after LVAD surgery, a PA catheter to assess filling pressures and cardiac output is generally useful along with the MAP and LVAD parameters. PA catheters are also useful in diagnosing subsequent hemodynamic complications with the patient with an ongoing LVAD or LVAD parameter abnormalities.

Echocardiography remains another valuable diagnostic tool. It is not often needed immediately perioperatively. However, in very ill patients with rapidly changing hemodynamics, continuous transesophageal echocardiography monitoring with a disposable probe has been used. Echocardiography is useful in troubleshooting a variety of parameter abnormalities, new symptoms, new alarms, or evaluating for myocardial and valvular function in patients with an ongoing LVAD. There is a ramp protocol (speed increased over discrete and short time intervals) with echocardiogram that can show the dynamic response of the myocardium, VAD, or valves to escalating LVAD speeds. There is a growing literature that shows that LVAD occlusion can be diagnosed with LVAD ramp protocol echocardiograms.

The International Society of Heart and Lung Transplantation (ISHLT) guidelines for early postoperative management[13] incorporate each of these assessments in the intensive care unit management of these patients to diagnose and treat problems (**Figs. 4 and 5, Table 3**).

INTERPRETING THE LVAD PARAMETERS

Each type of assist device has several parameters that can be informative in monitoring the patient and in identifying certain complications of the devices, such as VAD thrombosis, obstruction, suction events, hydration, and valvular insufficiency. Here, we focus on the most frequently used assist devices, HeartMate II and HeartWare HVAD.

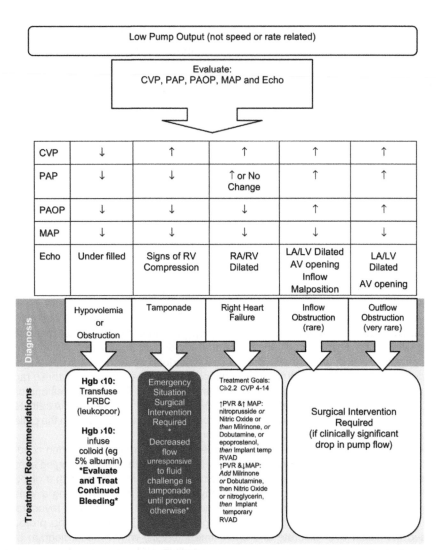

Fig. 4. Treatment algorithm for low pump output. AV, arteriovenous; CI, cardiac index; CVP, central venous pressure; Hgb, hemoglobin; LA, left atrium; PAOP, pulmonary artery occlusion pressure; PAP, pulmonary artery pressure; PRBC, packed red blood cells; PVR, peripheral vascular resistance; RA, right atrium. (*From* Feldman D, Pamboukian SV, Teuteberg JJ, et al, International Society for Heart and Lung Transplantation. The 2013 International Society for Heart and Lung Transplantation Guidelines for mechanical circulatory support: executive summary. J Heart Lung Transplant 2013;32(2):167; with permission.)

PARAMETERS OF HEARTMATE II

The device parameters include speed, power, pulsatility index (PI), and flow. Power and pump speed (RPM) are the only direct measurement of the device, and both the flow and the PIs are estimated values determined from power and pump speed.

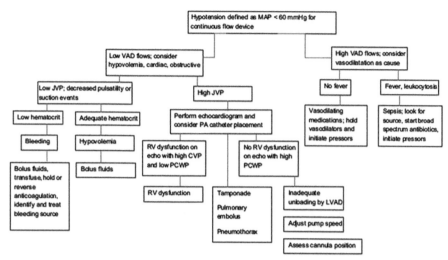

Fig. 5. Algorithm for assessment of hypotension after implant. CVP, central venous pressure; JVP, jugular venous pressure; PCWP, pulmonary capillary wedge pressure. (*From* Feldman D, Pamboukian SV, Teuteberg JJ, et al. International Society for Heart and Lung Transplantation. The 2013 International Society for Heart and Lung Transplantation Guidelines for mechanical circulatory support: executive summary. J Heart Lung Transplant 2013;32(2):170; with permission.)

Table 3
Treatment recommendations for early postoperative hemodynamic management

Cardiac Index (L/min/m²)	MAP (mm Hg)	LV Ejection	Primary Recommendation	Alternative
<2.2	<65	No	Epinephrine Vasopressin Norepinephrine	Dopamine
		Yes	Increase pump speed	Volume for low central venous pressure
	>65	No	Dobutamine	Milrinone
		Yes	Increase pump speed	
	>90	No	Milrinone	Sodium nitroprusside
		Yes	Sodium nitroprusside Nitroglycerin Hydralazine	Milrinone Nicardipine
>2.2	<65	No	Norepinephrine	Vasopressin
		Yes	Norepinephrine	Vasopressin
	>65 and <90	No	No intervention	
		Yes	No intervention	
	>90	No	Sodium nitroprusside Nitroglycerin Hydralazine	Milrinone Nicardipine
		Yes	Sodium nitroprusside	Nicardipine

From Feldman D, Pamboukian SV, Teuteberg JJ, et al, International Society for Heart and Lung Transplantation. The 2013 International Society for Heart and Lung Transplantation Guidelines for mechanical circulatory support: executive summary. J Heart Lung Transplant 2013;32(2): 166; with permission.

PI

The PI is the magnitude of change in flow through the VAD during the cardiac cycle associated with heart rate and contractility over a 15-second interval. The PI value is inversely related to the amount of assistance provided by the pump with unloading of the LV. The PI is directly proportional to the strength of contraction of the LV. Low PI may indicate a decrease in circulating blood volume or an obstruction associated with thrombosis.

Pump Speed

Pump speed is a direct measurement of the speed of the pump. According to the manufacturer, pump speed should be between 8600 and 9800 RPM. The optimal speed should be determined by hemodynamic and echocardiographic measurements. The optimal speed is achieved when the cardiac index and LV size are within normal range and there is no rightward or leftward shift of the septum. Suction events precipitate decrease in speed to the lower speed limit.

Power

Power is a direct measure of current and voltage applied to the motor. An increase in pump speed results in an increase in pump power, and a decrease in pump speed results in a decrease in the power. A decrease in the power occurs with flow obstruction that does not contact with the pump rotor, whereas flow obstruction secondary to thrombus in contact with the rotor can result in increased power. Gradual increase in the power may also indicate thrombosis formation on the rotor.

Flow

Flow is an approximation of the blood flow through the LVAD estimated from pump speed and power. Flow estimation should be used for trending changes rather than as an absolute measurement of flow. Abnormal power increase can result in overestimation of flow.[11]

PARAMETERS OF HEARTWARE HVAD

The HeartWare HVAD device estimates the blood flow rate using the characteristics (electrical current, RPM) and blood viscosity. Viscosity is calculated from the patient's hematocrit level, and the patient's updated hematocrit level should be entered in to the monitor to receive the flow estimation.

Flow

Flow is given in liters per minute and is an approximation of blood flow through the LVAD. The flow is determined by the speed of the impeller as well as by the pressure differential across the pump. This flow is more accurate in a centrifugal pump because of its physical characteristics.

Speed

Speed is a direct measure of the LVAD rotor speed measured in RPM. Along with the hematocrit level, it is another parameter that can be input. The recommended pump speed is between 2400 and 3200 RPM. Like in the HeartMate II device, the optimal speed of the pump should be determined by hemodynamic and echocardiographic measurements, ensuring that the interventricular septum does not shift toward the RV or the LV.[14] If the pump speed is too low, the device may not generate enough forward pressure, and a retrograde flow (flow from the aorta back through the device and into the LV) occurs.

Power

Power is a direct measure of current and voltage applied to the motor to maintain the set speed. It is similar to the power consumption in the HeartMate II described earlier.

Pulsatility

Although PI is not calculated for the HeartWare HVAD, the HVAD does have a pulse flow profile through the VAD, which can be imaged in real time and provide information on the flow variation (high pulsatility, low pulsatility) over time. Again, factors that affect the pulsatility (flow variability) include the volume status, degree of RV dysfunction, the presence of arrhythmias, and the intrinsic contractile state of the LV. A centrifugal pump tends to have larger swings in pulsatility and flow during the cardiac cycle than an axial flow pump.

VAD COMPLICATIONS
LVAD Thrombosis

VAD thrombosis is one of the most devastating complications of LVAD, previously described to occur in 2% of the patients treated with VAD as BTT[15] and 4% of patients treated as DT.[7] This prevalence is likely substantially higher, with an increasing number of cases in the last 2 years.[16]

By definition, VAD thrombosis is the development of a blood clot in one of the components of the VAD, including the inflow cannula, outflow cannula, and the rotor/propeller. Several risk factors have been linked to the formation of VAD thrombosis, including patient-associated, pump-related, and management-related factors. Patient-related factors include noncompliance to anticoagulation therapy, inherited hypercoagulable state, atrial fibrillation, or infection. Pump-related factors include pump heating and inflow cannula malposition. Management-related factors include subtherapeutic international normalized ratio (INR), absence of adequate antiplatelet therapy, inflow cannula malposition, or low pump flow.[17]

The clinical presentation can vary from very mild and nonspecific symptoms to HF decompensation or cardiogenic shock. Some patients may present with tea-colored urine, as a result of the severe hemolysis. Sustained LVAD power increase can be the first clue for thrombosis formation, and mandates further evaluation. Laboratory tests are essential for this diagnosis and consist of measurements of hemolysis, such as increased lactate dehydrogenase (LDH) levels (>3 times the upper limit of normal) and plasma free hemoglobin levels (>40 mg/dL).[17] Some investigators advocate the routine imaging with plain radiograph to exclude malposition of the inflow cannula and chest computed tomography (CT) angiogram to diagnose inflow cannula malposition or outflow obstruction.[17] Echocardiography has an important role and can show dilated ventricle, severe mitral regurgitation, and frequent aortic valve opening. The echocardiographic ramp study is specific and sensitive test for the diagnosis of VAD thrombosis with flow obstruction when used in conjunction with LDH levels. This test consists of serial echocardiogram recording of LV end-diastolic diameter (LVEDD) with increasing LVAD speed. In LVAD thrombosis, the LVEDD fails to decrease in response to increasing LVAD speed.[18] **Fig. 6** shows the algorithm for the diagnosis and management of pump thrombus.

Patients with suspected VAD thrombosis should be admitted to the intensive care unit because of the suboptimal performance of the LVAD, their congestive HF

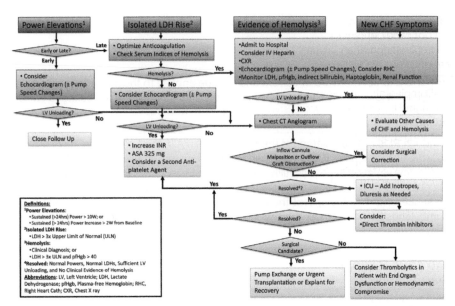

Fig. 6. Diagnosis and management of VAD thrombosis. (*From* Goldstein DJ, John R, Salerno C, et al. Algorithm for the diagnosis and management of suspected pump thrombus. J Heart Lung Transplant 2013;32(7):668; with permission.)

symptoms, and the possibility of rapid progression. Treatment of their HF may require diuresis and inotropic support depending on its severity. Administration of intravenous heparin is recommended in most cases, unless contraindicated. In some cases, treatment with heparin and supportive care may result in resolution of findings (power spikes, hemolysis, and HF signs and symptoms). These patients should be further followed, with consideration of increasing the aspirin dosage to 325 mg/d, increasing the INR target level to 2.5, or adding second antiplatelet therapy. Clopidogrel and dipyridamole have been used as a second agent. Intravenous direct thrombin inhibitors and glycoprotein IIb/IIIa inhibitors have also been sporadically tried for LVAD pump thrombosis in the hospital. No good trial has defined efficacy of these agents for pump thrombosis. If patient symptoms and hemolysis persist, the recommended therapy is dependent on the LVAD type: in patients with a HeartWare HVAD, tissue plasminogen activator trial is recommended before LVAD pump exchange, whereas direct surgical pump exchange is usually warranted in HeartMate II devices. If the patient's condition does not allow surgical intervention, only the option of aggressive antithrombotic therapy is left. Suitable patients should be considered for heart transplantation.[17] LVAD pump thrombosis is a reason to be moved into high-priority transplant waiting status, because of the increased mortality associated with this complication.

Right HF

RV failure is a common problem occurring early after LVAD implantation, occurring in 20% to 50% of patients in the current era of mechanical assist device support.[19] Patients suffer significant morbidity and mortality after LVAD implant if the RV is unable to pump sufficient blood and adequately fill the left heart.[11,20,21] Before LVAD implantation, it is essential to evaluate the RV function for adequate function by imaging and hemodynamics. Patients suffering from severe, chronic RV dysfunction that is not reversed by pulmonary venous decongestion or unloading of the pulmonary impedance with inodilator therapy such as milrinone should be considered high risk and not candidates for LVAD implantation.[11]

If implantation of an LVAD achieves adequate LV unloading and reduction in mitral regurgitation, an expected improvement in RV function occurs. This improvement recouples RV function to a lower pulmonary impedance. In a subset of patients, LVAD implantation may challenge the functional reserve of the RV and can result in severe right HF, with cardiogenic shock and multisystem organ failure. The physiology behind the RV improving from the LVAD implantation is based on the following premise. The LVAD should decrease the left ventricular end-diastolic pressure (LVEDP), followed by a decrease in left pulmonary capillary wedge pressure and the pulmonary vascular resistance (PVR), thus decreasing the afterload of the RV. However, the increase in the RV preload during and after the implantation surgery together with the decrease in the LV size and LVEDPs may result in significant leftward septal shift. An abnormal RV geometry ensues, adversely affecting RV function. A high speed setting can further flatten the LV, shift the septum, and worsen the RV function. Thus, high RPMs should be avoided in these patients. Large volume shifts in the early postoperative period may also cause changes in RV geometry. It is crucial to perform an echocardiogram during the first days after the implantation to assess ventricular geometry. With any hemodynamic deterioration on LVAD support, immediately after implant or late, an echocardiogram should be repeated to assess the RV function. Potentially, pump speed can be adjusted. Transthoracic echocardiography is adequate, because the RV is an anterior structure and imaged best through the chest wall.

Any atrial and ventricular arrhythmias should be treated promptly; their tachycardic effect on RV function can be substantial. Hemodynamic measurements with a PA catheter may assist in adjusting treatment in the first few days after implantation. Increased right atrial pressure (>15 mm Hg) may necessitate treatment with furosemide, ultrafiltration, or renal replacement therapy, or decreasing the LVAD flow. In patients with low right atrial pressure (<10 mm Hg), intravenous saline may be needed to improve hemodynamics and organ perfusion.[19] Significant RV dysfunction with or without increased PVR should be treated with milrinone or dobutamine early after the LVAD implantation to improve RV perfusion and function. For those with increased PVR (>3 Wood units), pulmonary vasodilator therapy such as phosphodiesterase type 5 inhibition, nitric oxide therapy, or Flolan should be used and dosed to the desired effect of adequate RV function.[5,9] In patients with RV dysfunction and low systemic vascular resistance (<800 dyn/s/cm⁵) it is essential to add inotropic support and a vasopressor agent, to increase the transmyocardial perfusion of the RV (MAP – central venous pressure).[22]

Up to 15% of patients with early post-LVAD right HF require RVAD implantation. These patients are in severe refractory right HF with end-organ renal or hepatic dysfunction with or without cardiogenic shock. These patients should be taken to the operating room for RVAD support as soon as possible.[22] They have mortality as high as 50% to 70%. Several studies have reported improved survival in the group of patients who were supported with an RVAD early as opposed to late with refractory right HF and cardiogenic shock despite maximal pharmacologic therapy.[23]

Active Bleeding

Bleeding is the most frequent adverse event associated with LVAD, accounting for 9% of the total mortality associated with LVADs.[24] Postoperative bleeding can be observed after LVAD implantation, but the high incidence of both surgical and nonsurgical bleeding among patients with LVAD is unique. It is believed to involve complex pathophysiologic mechanisms and is not fully understood.[24] The theory involves the development of acquired von Willebrand syndrome, secondary to polymer deformation by the rotating impeller of the LVAD, leading to deficiency of the von Willebrand factors.

The second-generation and third-generation continuous flow LVADs led to an increase in the nonsurgical gastrointestinal (GI) bleeding incidence, secondary to formation to arteriovenous malformations. It has been hypothesized that the reduced pulse pressure (or pulsatility) induced by continuous flow LVADs results in hypoperfusion of the GI mucosa and neovascularization with friable vessels prone to bleeding.[24] It is reasonable in patients with previous episodes of GI bleeding to reduce the LVAD flow to increase the PI and prevent further bleeding. The mechanism described earlier and the fact that all patients with LVAD are treated with both anticoagulation and antiplatelet therapies increase the incidence of significant bleeding.

The hemodynamic consequences of significant bleeding can be fatal, because the LVAD is dependent on the preload of the LV. Every change in the effective systemic volume may result in suck-down effect (collapse of the LV walls), with clinical deterioration (**Fig. 7**). Patients with RV dysfunction are sensitive to significant bleeding because of their dependence on RV preload and coronary perfusion. Acute bleeding should promote a thorough investigation, volume repletion with close hemodynamic monitoring, and echocardiography if needed to assess ventricular function.

Diagnosis of GI bleeding in patients with LVAD should include upper and lower endoscopy. However, because the source of bleeding is often the small bowel, video capsule endoscopy is often warranted.[25] Initial management of patients with suspected significant bleeding, including GI bleeding, should include discontinuation of the antiplatelet and anticoagulation therapy.[25] the need to reverse the anticoagulation using fresh frozen plasma should be considered, although this may result in increased risk of LVAD thrombosis formation.

The treatment of GI bleeding in patients with LVAD includes endoscopic guided therapy with or without intravenous proton pump inhibitor therapy (**Fig. 8**).

In refractory bleeding, some advocate treatment with octreotide infusion[26] or desmopressin acetate.[27] Anticoagulation treatment should be restarted once the bleeding stops and hemoglobin levels stabilize. As detailed earlier, some patients may benefit from decreasing the RPM, with resultant increase in pulsatility. This maneuver should be performed under the direct vision of echocardiogram and hemodynamic monitoring, from simple blood pressure monitoring to PA catheter monitoring in selected individuals.

Sepsis

One-third of the patients treated with LVAD suffer from systemic infection.[28] This burden is likely to increase with the use of LVAD as long-term DT.[28] According to

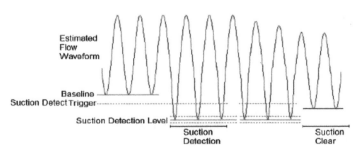

Fig. 7. HeartWare HVAD wave form during suction event. (*Courtesy of* Thoratec, Pleasanton, CA; with permission.)

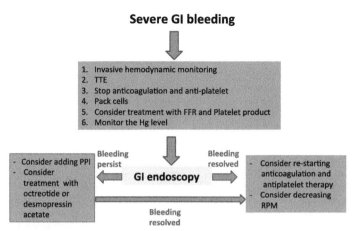

Severe GI bleeding

1. Invasive hemodynamic monitoring
2. TTE
3. Stop anticoagulation and anti-platelet
4. Pack cells
5. Consider treatment with FFR and Platelet product
6. Monitor the Hg level

- Consider adding PPI
- Consider treatment with octreotide or desmopressin acetate

Bleeding persist

GI endoscopy

Bleeding resolved

- Consider re-starting anticoagulation and antiplatelet therapy
- Consider decreasing RPM

Bleeding resolved

Fig. 8. Severe GI bleeding. (*Data from* Suarez J, Patel CB, Felker GM, et al. Mechanisms of bleeding and approach to patients with axial-flow left ventricular assist devices [review]. Circ Heart Fail 2011;4(6):781.)

the ISHLT data,[29] 87% of LVAD infections are bacterial, with the remainder being mostly fungal. In patients with VAD with bacteremia and sepsis, the prognosis becomes poor, even with transplantation. Standard sepsis treatments with antibiotics and pressors should be used in an attempt to reverse the sepsis before an overwhelming systemic inflammatory response syndrome process ensues.

The ISHLT Infectious Diseases Working Group[30] defined 3 subgroups of infection: (1) VAD-specific infections related to the device hardware, occurring only in patients with VAD (this includes pump and cannula infections, pocket infections, and driveline infections); (2) VAD-related infections can occur also in patients who do not have VAD (however, they require special consideration in respect to diagnosis and clinical management, eg, infective endocarditis, mediastinitis); (3) non-VAD infections are infections that are unlikely to relate to the VAD therapy.

The ISHLT Infectious Diseases Working Group[30] redefined the criteria for the diagnosis of pump and cannula infections based on the modified Duke criteria. A patient must have at least one of the microbiologic, pathologic, echocardiographic, or clinical criteria to achieve a firm diagnosis. **Boxes 2** and **3** show the diagnostic criteria for pump and cannula infections.

Pocket infections are another important source of infection. These infections occur in the body space that was created to hold the pump, usually within the abdominal wall or close to the pericardium and the diaphragm.[30]

Percutaneous driveline infections are the most prevalent infections in patients with VAD and may reflect the presence of a deeper infection of the device hardware (pump, cannula) or the pocket space. Patients with suspected diagnosis of percutaneous driveline infections should be further defined according to the depth of the infection (superficial vs deep infection) and to the certainty of the diagnosis (proven, probable, and possible infection).[30] CT and ultrasonography (US) imaging are mandated in most patients to show fluid collection around the drivelines, cannula, and pump.

The clinical presentation of patients with VAD infections may be nonspecific, with symptoms such as lethargy, fatigue, or anorexia, or classic presentation with fever and severe shock. A driveline or pump pocket infection can often be seen externally, with localized erythema, warmth, and purulence. Often, there is tenderness locally. A fever and increased white blood count can be seen. One needs a high index of

---

Box 2
Definition of terms used for the diagnosis of VAD-specific pump or cannula

Major Clinical Criteria

- If the VAD is not removed, then an indistinguishable organism (genus, species, and antimicrobial susceptibility pattern) recovered from 2 or more peripheral blood cultures taken greater than 12 hours apart with no other focus of infection or
  All of 3 or most of 4 or more separate positive blood cultures (with the first and last sample drawn at least 1 hour apart) with no other focus of infection

- When 2 or more positive blood cultures are taken from the CVC and peripherally at the same time, and defined by criteria in **Box 3** as either BSI-VAD-related or presumed VAD-related

- Echocardiogram positive for VAD-related IE (TEE recommended for patients with prosthetic valves, rated at least possible IE by clinical criteria, or complicated IE [paravalvular abscess] and in any patient in whom VAD-related infection is suspected and TTE is nondiagnostic; TTE as first test in other patients) defined as follows: intracardiac mass suspected to be vegetation adjacent to or in the outflow cannula, or in an area of turbulent flow such as regurgitant jets, or consistent with a vegetation on implanted material, or abscess, or new partial dehiscence of outflow cannula.

Minor Clinical Criteria

- Fever 38°C or higher

- Vascular phenomena, major arterial emboli, septic pulmonary infarcts, mycotic aneurysm, intracerebral or visceral, conjunctival hemorrhage, and Janeway lesions

- Immunologic phenomena: glomerulonephritis. Osler nodes, Roth spot

- Microbiological evidence: positive blood culture that does not meet criteria as noted above (excluding single positive culture for coagulase-negative staphylococci excluding *Staphylococcus lugdunensis*)

Abbreviations: BSI, blood stream infection; CVC, central venous cannula; IE, infective endocarditis; TEE, transesophageal echocardiogram; TTE, transthoracic echocardiogram.
From Hannan MM, Husain S, Mattner F, et al, International Society for Heart and Lung Transplantation. Working formulation for the standardization of definitions of infections in patients using ventricular assist devices. J Heart Lung Transplant 2011;30(4):379; with permission.

---

suspicion for infection and should respond promptly. Echocardiography (transthoracic and transesophageal), US, and CT have become first line in imaging of a patient with VAD suspected of infection. For an infection external to the LVAD, US can often show a fluid collection, as can a noncontrast CT scan. For an infection internal to the LVAD, there is no good modality to image inside the pump itself. Thus, echocardiography may identify associated cardiac valve infections but may identify only flow characteristics of blood entering and exiting the LVAD. It is crucial to consult an infectious disease expert and start broad-spectrum antibiotic coverage as soon as infection is suspected. Driveline infections should be treated with antimicrobial therapy tailored to *Staphylococcus* and *Pseudomonas* species.[31] In many cases, medical therapy cannot eradicate the infection, and surgical intervention, with possible device explantation, is warranted. The driveline of the LVAD cannot be disconnected from the LVAD. Thus, any driveline removal must be accompanied by a full exchange of the LVAD pump itself. Localized surgical debridement can be performed around the LVAD components. Definitive therapy is removal of the LVAD, thus often requiring heart transplantation. Transplantation has not been shown to be adversely affected by a localized LVAD infection. Infection of an LVAD is 1 reason that patients awaiting heart

Box 3
Definitions of VAD-specific pump infections or cannula infection

Proven

- Microbiology: Isolation of indistinguishable organism (genus, species, antimicrobial susceptibility pattern) at explanation or intraoperatively from

  o 2 or more positive internal aspect culture samples from pump or cannula or

  o 1 positive peripheral blood culture and 1 positive culture from VAD internal aspect aspirate or endovascular brushings, (internal aspect refers to the inner lumen of the cannula) or

  o In the case of coagulase-negative staphylococci excluding *Staphylococcus lugdunensis*, 2 or more positive sets of peripheral blood cultures and a positive internal aspect culture of pump or cannula

- Histologic features of infection from heart tissue samples from around the VAD pump or cannula at explantation or intraoperatively

- Clinical criteria (see **Box 2**)

  o 2 major criteria

Probable

- 1 major criterion and 3 minor criteria or

- 4 minor criteria

Possible

- 1 major and 1 minor or

- 3 minor

Rejected

- Firm alternative diagnosis explaining the clinical findings

- Resolution of evidence of pump or cannula infection with antibiotic therapy for up to 4 days or

- No pathologic evidence of pump or cannula infection at surgery or autopsy with antibiotic therapy for up to 4 days or

- Does not meet criteria for possible pump or cannula infection

From Hannan MM, Husain S, Mattner F, et al, International Society for Heart and Lung Transplantation. Working formulation for the standardization of definitions of infections in patients using ventricular assist devices. J Heart Lung Transplant 2011;30(4):379; with permission.

transplant can move to a higher priority status. Sustained antimicrobial therapy is often needed at least until the time of LVAD explantation.

Aortic insufficiency

Aortic regurgitation is common among patients with LVAD, with the prevalence increasing with the duration of LVAD support. LVAD flow causes higher transvalvular pressures across the aortic valve, with decrease in the LV pressures and increase in the aortic pressures, especially during diastole. This situation may lead to regurgitation, which creates a vicious cycle that reduces the effectiveness of the LVAD function. As a result, the patient may suffer from HF symptoms as well as from hemolysis. All preimplant patients should undergo valvular function evaluation routinely, and those with moderate to severe aortic regurgitation should be considered for aortic valve repair if possible or replacement with a biological valve prosthesis.

Noncardiac surgery in patients with LVAD

Performing noncardiac surgery on a patient with LVAD can be challenging. With the increased use of mechanical assist devices and the improved survival, the need to perform these surgeries is increasing and will continue to increase. Only small studies have been published on this topic. All data support that noncardiac operations can be performed safely on patients with LVAD.[32–36] Because of the anticoagulation and antiplatelet therapy, these patients are at higher risk for bleeding. There is no consensus regarding the discontinuation of anticoagulation before the operation. Previous studies had shown that the risk of LVAD thrombosis is extremely low on preoperative discontinuation of anticoagulation. However, because the risk of LVAD thrombosis is increasing, we recommend that the decision should be individualized for each patient according to the risk of bleeding associated with surgery and previous history of suspected or confirmed LVAD thrombosis.

It is crucial to obtain continuous hemodynamic measurements throughout the operation and treat any change in MAP appropriately. The patients may require temporary inotropic support of RV function, and in patients with known RV dysfunction or right HF, it may be appropriate to use inotropic support preoperatively and postoperatively. All patients should be accompanied by an experienced LVAD coordinator, who is familiar with the device management and alerts.

VENTRICULAR ARRHYTHMIAS

Ventricular arrhythmias (ventricular tachycardia and fibrillation) are common, affecting 30% of patients treated with long-term LVAD support.[37] The arrhythmias tend to occur early after device implantation and are 10 times more likely to occur in the first month.[38] Several risk factors are correlated with the occurrence of ventricular arrhythmias in patients with LVAD; the most prominent factor is a history of ventricular arrhythmias before LVAD support.[37]

Although ventricular arrhythmias can be well tolerated in patients with LVAD, their occurrence can be associated with significant adverse outcome, including increased mortality.[39]

Two mechanisms are unique for patients with VAD, and understanding them may result in successful treatment. The first is suction event, which occurs as a result of a decrease in the LV preload (dehydration secondary to overdiuresis or bleeding, RV dysfunction) or as a result of an increased pump speed. All these factors can result in negative pressure at the inflow cannula, leading to a suction event, in which 1 or more of the ventricular walls become closer to the inflow cannula, causing mechanical stimulation of arrhythmia, tissue injury, and reduced inflow to the pump.[37,40,41] The second mechanism involves malposition of the inflow cannula, resulting in similar mechanical stimulation of arrhythmias and even VAD thrombosis. This condition may require surgical repositioning of the cannula.[42]

Although limited data support their use in patients with LVAD, antiarrhythmic drugs (eg, amiodarone, lidocaine) are commonly used in the treatment of ventricular arrhythmias. Further, reversible causes of arrhythmias include rehydration in cases of excessive diuresis or adjusting the pump speed for right HF.[37] Clinicians must also be vigilant for signs of VAD thrombosis (hemolysis, power surges), because ventricular arrhythmias may be the presenting symptom of VAD thrombosis. In cases of recurrence of ventricular arrhythmias, it is reasonable to proceed with ventricular tachycardia ablation.

SUMMARY

Patients on long-term LVAD support present unique challenges in the intensive care unit. It is crucial to always know the status of end-organ perfusion, and this may require invasive hemodynamic monitoring with a systemic arterial and PA catheter. Depending on the indication for LVAD support (bridge to decision or cardiac transplantation vs DT), it is also important to readdress goals of care with the patient (if possible) and their family after major events have occurred that challenge the survival of the patient.

REFERENCES

1. Yancy CW, Jessup M, Bozkurt B, et al. 2013 ACCF/AHA guideline for the management of heart failure: a report of the American College of Cardiology Foundation/American Heart Association Task Force on Practice Guidelines. Circulation 2013;128(16):e240–327.
2. Blecker S, Paul M, Taksler G, et al. Heart failure–associated hospitalizations in the United States. J Am Coll Cardiol 2013;61(12):1259–67.
3. Peura JL, Colvin-Adams M, Francis GS, et al. Recommendations for the use of mechanical circulatory support: device strategies and patient selection: a scientific statement from the American Heart Association. Circulation 2012;126(22):2648–67.
4. Hershberger RE, Nauman D, Walker TL, et al. Care processes and clinical outcomes of continuous outpatient support with inotropes (COSI) in patients with refractory endstage heart failure. J Card Fail 2003;9:180–7.
5. Gorodeski EZ, Chu EC, Reese JR, et al. Starling prognosis on chronic dobutamine or milrinone infusions for stage D heart failure. Circ Heart Fail 2009;2:320–4.
6. Rose EA, Gelijns AC, Moskowitz AJ, et al. Long-term use of a left ventricular assist device for end-stage heart failure. N Engl J Med 2001;345(20):1435–43.
7. Slaughter MS, Rogers JG, Milano CA, et al. Advanced heart failure treated with continuous-flow left ventricular assist device. N Engl J Med 2009;361(23):2241–51.
8. Sayer G, Naka Y, Jorde UP. Ventricular assist device therapy. Cardiovasc Ther 2009;27(2):140–50.
9. McMurray JJ, Adamopoulos S, Anker SD, et al. ESC guidelines for the diagnosis and treatment of acute and chronic heart failure 2012: The task force for the diagnosis and treatment of acute and chronic heart failure 2012 of the European Society of Cardiology. Developed in collaboration with the Heart Failure Association. Eur J Heart Fail 2013;15(3):361–2.
10. Kirklin JK, Naftel DC, Kormos RL, et al. Fifth INTERMACS annual report: risk factor analysis from more than 6,000 mechanical circulatory support patients. J Heart Lung Transplant 2013;32(2):141–56.
11. Slaughter MS, Pagani FD, Rogers JG, et al. Clinical management of continuous-flow left ventricular assist devices in advanced heart failure. J Heart Lung Transplant 2010;29(Suppl 4):S1–39.
12. Alba AC, Rao V, Ivanov J, et al. Usefulness of the INTERMACS scale to predict outcomes after mechanical assist device implantation. J Heart Lung Transplant 2009;28(8):827–33.
13. Feldman D, Pamboukian SV, Teuteberg JJ, et al. The 2013 International Society for Heart and Lung Transplantation Guidelines for mechanical circulatory support: executive summary. J Heart Lung Transplant 2013;32(2):157–87.

14. HeartWare instructions. Available at: http://www.heartware.com/sites/default/files/uploads/resources/ifu00001_rev17_hvasinstructionsforuse_us.pdf.

15. Miller LW, Pagani FD, Russell SD, et al. Use of a continuous-flow device in patients awaiting heart transplantation. N Engl J Med 2007;357:885–96.

16. Starling RC, Moazami N, Silvestry SC, et al. Unexpected abrupt increase in left ventricular assist device thrombosis. N Engl J Med 2014;370(1):33–40.

17. Goldstein DJ, John R, Salerno C, et al. Algorithm for the diagnosis and management of suspected pump thrombus. J Heart Lung Transplant 2013;32(7):667–70.

18. Uriel N, Morrison KA, Garan AR, et al. Development of a novel echocardiography ramp test for speed optimization and diagnosis of device thrombosis in continuous-flow left ventricular assist devices: the Columbia ramp study. J Am Coll Cardiol 2012;60(18):1764–75.

19. Meineri M, Van Rensburg AE, Vegas A. Right ventricular failure after LVAD implantation: prevention and treatment. Best Pract Res Clin Anaesthesiol 2012;26(2):217–29.

20. Lazar JF, Swartz MF, Schiralli MP, et al. Survival after left ventricular assist device with and without temporary right ventricular support. Ann Thorac Surg 2013;96(6):2155–9 pii:S0003-4975(13) 01543-9.

21. Kormos RL, Teuteberg JJ, Pagani FD, et al. Right ventricular failure in patients with the HeartMateII continuous-flow left ventricular assist device: incidence, risk factors, and effect on outcomes. J Thorac Cardiovasc Surg 2010;139:1316–24.

22. MacGowan GA, Schueler S. Right heart failure after left ventricular assist device implantation: early and late. Curr Opin Cardiol 2012;27(3):296–300.

23. Patlolla B, Beygui R, Haddad F. Right-ventricular failure following left ventricle assist device implantation. Curr Opin Cardiol 2013;28:223–33.

24. Kirklin JK, Naftel DC, Kormos RL, et al. Third INTERMACS Annual Report: the evolution of destination therapy in the United States. J Heart Lung Transplant 2011;30:115–23.

25. Demirozu ZT, Radovancevic R, Hochman LF, et al. Arteriovenous malformation and gastrointestinal bleeding in patients with the HeartMate II left ventricular assist device. J Heart Lung Transplant 2011;30(8):849–53.

26. Aggarwal A, Pant R, Kumar S, et al. Incidence and management of gastrointestinal bleeding with continuous flow assist devices. Ann Thorac Surg 2012;93(5):1534–40.

27. Meyer AL, Malehsa D, Bara C, et al. Acquired von Willebrand syndrome in patients with an axial flow left ventricular assist device. Circ Heart Fail 2010;3(6):675–81.

28. Adzic A, Patel SR, Maybaum S. Impact of adverse events on ventricular assist device outcomes. Curr Heart Fail Rep 2013;10(1):89–100.

29. Holman WL, Pae WE, Teutenberg JJ, et al. INTERMACS: interval analysis of registry data. J Am Coll Surg 2009;208(5):755–61.

30. Hannan MM, Husain S, Mattner F, et al, International Society for Heart and Lung Transplantation. Working formulation for the standardization of definitions of infections in patients using ventricular assist devices. J Heart Lung Transplant 2011;30(4):375–84.

31. Topkara VK, Kondareddy S, Malik F, et al. Infectious complications in patients with left ventricular assist device: cause and outcomes in the continuous-flow era. Ann Thorac Surg 2010;90(4):1270–7.

32. Goldstein DJ, Mullis SL, Delphin ES, et al. Noncardiac surgery in long-term implantable left ventricular assist-device recipients. Ann Surg 1995;222:203–7.

33. Morgan JA, Paone G, Nemeh HW, et al. Non-cardiac surgery in patients on long-term left ventricular assist device support. J Heart Lung Transplant 2012;31(7): 757–63.
34. Schmid C, Wilhelm M, Dietl KH, et al. Noncardiac surgery in patients with left ventricular assist devices. Surgery 2001;129:440–4.
35. Votapka TV, Pennington DG, McBride LR, et al. Noncardiac operations in patients supported with mechanical circulatory support devices. J Am Coll Surg 1994; 179:318–20.
36. Eckhauser AE, Melvin WV, Sharp KW. Management of general surgical problems in patients with left ventricular assist devices. Am Surg 2006;72:158–61.
37. Pedrotty DM, Rame JE, Margulies KB. Management of ventricular arrhythmias in patients with ventricular assist devices. Curr Opin Cardiol 2013;28(3):360–8.
38. Kühne M, Sakumura M, Reich SS, et al. Simultaneous use of implantable cardioverter-defibrillators and left ventricular assist devices in patients with severe heart failure. Am J Cardiol 2010;105(3):378–82.
39. Brenyo A, Rao M, Koneru S, et al. Risk of mortality for ventricular arrhythmia in ambulatory LVAD patients. J Cardiovasc Electrophysiol 2012;23(5):515–20.
40. Gregory SD, Timms D, Gaddum NR, et al. In vitro evaluation of a compliant inflow cannula reservoir to reduce suction events with extracorporeal rotary ventricular assist device support. Artif Organs 2011;35(8):765–72.
41. Vollkron M, Voitl P, Ta J, et al. Suction events during left ventricular support and ventricular arrhythmias. J Heart Lung Transplant 2007;26(8):819–25.
42. Milano CA, Simeone AA, Blue LJ, et al. Presentation and management of left ventricular assist device inflow cannula malposition. J Heart Lung Transplant 2011; 30:838–40.

Post–Heart Transplant Complications

Edo Y. Birati, MD, J. Eduardo Rame, MD, MPhil*

KEYWORDS

• Heart transplant • Complications • Immunosuppression • Rejection

KEY POINTS

- Managing patients after heart transplantation is challenging.
- After heart transplantation, patients have unique clinical complications (associated with the immunosuppressive therapy and cardiac allograft rejection) together with atypical clinical presentations for infection and systemic inflammatory response syndrome.
- High vigilance, early diagnosis, and appropriate intervention for allograft-related and non–allograft-related syndromes with significant morbidity and mortality are the keys to long-term survival of patients after transplantation.

INTRODUCTION

Heart transplantation remains the only definitive therapy for advanced heart failure. Approximately 2000 heart transplantations are performed annually in the United States.[1] The survival rates have improved with the use of new immunosuppressive drugs, with median survival of approximately 11 years.[1]

Soon after the transplantation, all patients should receive 3 classes of immunosuppressive drugs: glucocorticoids, calcineurin inhibitors (cyclosporine, tacrolimus), and antiproliferative agents (azathioprine, mycophenolate mofetil).[2] Glucocorticoids are gradually weaned 6 months after the transplantation. It is beyond the scope of this article to discuss the detailed mechanism and side effects of the immunosuppressive drugs.

INDICATIONS FOR HEART TRANSPLANTATION

Heart transplantation is recommended in various cardiac diseases. The most important indication is end-stage heart failure. These patients are American Heart Association stage D, New York Heart Association class III or IV with objective evidence of impaired functional capacity (peak oxygen consumption <14 mL/kg/min) despite optimal medical therapy.[1]

Division of Cardiology, Perelman School of Medicine, University of Pennsylvania, Philadelphia, PA 19104, USA
* Corresponding author. Hospital of the University of Pennsylvania, 2 East Perelman Center for Advanced Medicine, 3400 Civic Center Boulevard, Philadelphia, PA 19104.
E-mail address: eduardo.rame@uphs.upenn.edu

Crit Care Clin 30 (2014) 629–637
http://dx.doi.org/10.1016/j.ccc.2014.03.005
0749-0704/14/$ – see front matter © 2014 Elsevier Inc. All rights reserved.

Infrequent medical conditions requiring cardiac transplantation include (1) recurrent life-threatening ventricular arrhythmias, despite medical therapy and electrophysio-logic interventions; (2) intractable angina despite maximal medical therapy and not amenable to revascularization; (3) primary cardiac tumors; (4) severe hypertrophic or restrictive cardiomyopathy.[1]

Current contraindications for heart transplantation include (1) severe irreversible pulmonary hypertension (pulmonary artery systemic pressure >60 mm Hg, mean transpulmonary gradient >15 mm Hg, and/or peripheral vascular resistance [PVR] >5 Wood units on maximal vasodilator therapy. When these patients are trans-plantable, they usually have right ventricle allograft failure); (2) significant peripheral vascular disease; (3) severe diabetes mellitus with end-organ damage; (4) severe irre-versible hepatic, renal, or pulmonary disease (unless dual-organ transplantation is planed); (5) active infection; (6) ongoing tobacco use; (7) high or low body mass index (>30 or <20); (8) age (in most centers the age limit is 70 years, although some centers use alternative listing for elderly patients).[1]

GRAFT REJECTION

Graft rejection can be classified according to its acuity (hyperacute, acute, and chronic rejection) and to the mechanism of the rejection (cell-mediated rejection vs antibody-mediated rejection). Hyperacute rejection is mediated by preexisting anti-bodies to allogenic antigens and occurs within minutes to hours after the transplanta-tion, causing rapid occlusion of graft vasculature with rapid graft failure. It rarely occurs with the current blood and human leukocyte antigen (HLA) typing techniques. Acute rejection can be subdivided into cell-mediated and humoral-mediated rejection. Acute cellular rejection may occur in the first week to several years after the transplan-tation. The inflammatory response of cell-mediated rejection consists mainly of T-cell lymphocytes.[3–5] To date, there are no sensitive serologic markers for acute rejection and myocardial biopsy remains the gold standard for this diagnosis.[3] In most institu-tions myocardial biopsies are done on a regular basis at least during the first year after the transplantation. It is essential to perform the biopsy on a routine basis regardless of symptoms, because patients can be asymptomatic during the rejection. Low compliance with immunosuppressive drugs remains the major risk factor for the occurrence of acute rejection. Humoral-mediated (or antibody-mediated) rejection consists mainly of antibodies directed against the donor HLA, and may occur during the first days to years after the implantation.[3,4] Chronic rejection may occur months to years after the implantation. It causes an irreversible graft dysfunction.[6]

As stated earlier, the diagnosis of acute cellular rejection is based on the biopsy re-sults. Thus, endomyocardial biopsy should be performed as early as possible in any clinical suspicion of rejection. Every biopsy is graded according to the revised nomen-clature of the International Society for Heart and Lung Transplantation (ISHLT)[5]:

- Grade 0: no rejection
- Grade 1 R, mild: interstitial and/or perivascular infiltrate with up to 1 focus of my-ocyte damage
- Grade 2 R, moderate: 2 or more foci of infiltrate with associated myocyte damage
- Grade 3 R, severe: diffuse infiltrate with multifocal myocyte damage, with or without edema, hemorrhage, or vasculitis[5]

All patients with acute cellular or antibody rejection should be admitted and undergo basic evaluation, including echocardiogram and blood tests. Those who have acute heart failure or hemodynamic compromise should be admitted to the intensive care unit and undergo right heart catheterization. Treatment with inotropes, pressors, diuretics and antiarrhythmic medications should be considered, according to the clinical presentation. The initial therapy for antibody-mediated rejection includes high-dose intravenous (IV) corticosteroid (CS) with plasmapheresis and/or low dose of IV immunoglobulin. Rituximab can be added to reduce the risk of recurrent rejection.[7]

Acute symptomatic cellular rejection should be treated with high-dose IV CS, regardless of ISHLT biopsy grade. According to the ISHLT guidelines, antithymocyte antibodies should be added in cases of hemodynamic compromise or if there is no clinical improvement within 12 to 24 hours of IV CS administration.[7]

Cardiac allograft vasculopathy (AV), likely a manifestation of chronic rejection, is characterized by intimal thickening and fibrosis, leading to luminal narrowing or occlusion of the coronary arteries and graft ischemia.[6,8] Based on the ISHLT registry, AV occurs in 8% of the patients during the first year after the transplantation and in 32% of the patients after 5 years.[9] AV correlates with persistent inflammation and a higher degree of HLA mismatch. Although AV is predominately a secondary immunologic reaction, the classic cardiovascular risk factors, such as hypertension, diabetes mellitus, and hyperlipidemia, may enhance local inflammation and exacerbate the coronary narrowing.[8]

Diagnosis of AV is limited not only by the lack of ischemic symptoms in the denervated allograft but also by the underestimation of the extent of the disease during routine coronary angiography.[10] In one study, the positive predictive power of coronary angiography was only 44%.[11] Intravascular ultrasonography (IVUS) is the most sensitive tool and is regarded as the gold standard for the diagnosis of AV.[8] Thus, some institutions advocate performance of IVUS routinely 1 month and 12 months after the transplantation to identify high-risk patients for future cardiovascular events. However, coronary angiography remains the standard for the diagnosis of cardiac AV in most transplant centers.[8] Some transplant centers screen their patients for AV using noninvasive tests. Dobutamine stress echocardiography is frequently used to screen the patients. It has sensitivity of 80% compared with coronary angiography[12] and specificity of 88% compared with IVUS.[13] Myocardial single-photon emission computed tomography (SPECT) has a high negative predictive value and seems to be well suited to screening for significant AV.[14] Multidetector computed tomography with has a sensitivity and specificity of 86% and 99%, respectively[15]; however, this modality is not optimal for patients after transplantation, because these patients have higher resting heart rates, which may impair the imaging quality.[8] In addition, the use of contrast media and radiation increase the risk for worsening renal insufficiency and cancer, respectively, and thus this modality is not frequently used in most transplant centers.[8]

In order to prevent AV, some prophylactic regimens have been advocated, including statin therapy, which reduces the progression of the AV and improves survival after heart transplant[16]: angiotensin-converting enzyme (ACE) inhibitors, which improve allograft microvascular endothelial dysfunction, endothelin activation, and have been associated with plaque regression[17,18]; and calcium channel blockers, which seem to slow the progression of AV.[19] Some immunosuppressive drugs, such as sirolimus, have been associated with slower development of AV[20]; some correlate with certain infections, such as cytomegalovirus (CMV) infection and AV.[21] Ganciclovir treatment seems to reduce the progression of AV,[22] whereas lack of aggressive CMV prophylaxis is correlated with greater lumen loss.[23]

Revascularization procedures for AV do not affect the long-term survival, and may be used only to alleviate symptoms. Most centers perform percutaneous coronary intervention in patients who have symptoms and abnormal physiologic stress tests.[8]

Bypass grafting is associated with a high mortality, and is rarely used. Retransplantation is the only definitive treatment of AV.[24]

EARLY POSTOPERATIVE CARE OF PATIENTS AFTER HEART TRANSPLANTATION

During the early postoperative period, the allograft usually requires active hemodynamic management, and this period requires a focus on the maintenance of hemodynamic stability as the allograft restores its normal cardiac function. All patients should be monitored with continuous electrocardiographic recording and continuous measurements of the arterial pressure, central venous pressure or right atrial pressure, cardiac output, urinary output, and oxygen saturation. It is essential to perform either a transthoracic or transesophageal echocardiogram early in the postoperative period in order assess heart allograft function, particularly in the setting of acute hemodynamic instability or clinical suspicion of rejection, right ventricle failure, or tamponade.[7]

ESTIMATION OF FLUID STATUS

The fluid status should be estimated based on clinical findings (for example, jugular venous pressure, extremities edema) as well as on the fluid input and output. Many patients require a high dosage of diuretics after transplantation to overcome diuretic resistance. Patients with volume overload who are resistant to diuretics should be treated with ultrafiltration or renal replacement therapies. It is essential to solve this volume overload because it may cause graft right ventricular (RV) dysfunction.[7]

LEFT VENTRICULAR AND RV FUNCTION

It is essential to evaluate the left ventricular (LV) and RV function. LV systolic dysfunction may suggest poor heart quality or early rejection (hyperacute) and mandate further evaluation and treatment. LV diastolic dysfunction may occur, secondary to prolonged ischemic time and donor LV hypertrophy.[7] RV dysfunction may occur secondary to high PVR, severe volume overload, decrease in preload (for example, overdiuresis, severe bleeding), poor preservation of the graft, and significant donor/recipient size mismatch.[25] Most patients can be managed conservatively, using mainly inotropic therapy and diuretics. However, some patients may need additional support, such as intra-aortic balloon pump and left or right mechanical assist devices.

HEART RATE

Heart rate after heart transplantation usually ranges from 90 to 110 beats per minute. The rapid heart rate is secondary to parasympathetic denervation during the transplant procedure. Patients may have relative bradycardia secondary to preprocedural sinus node injury or before treatment with amiodarone, requiring treatment with isoproterenol or theophylline and may mandate cardiac pacing.[7] In cases of significant undersizing of the donor heart, the heart rate should be even higher in order to allow adequate end-organ perfusion, because the stroke volumes of small hearts are smaller.[26] Heart rate early after transplantation remains a significant driver of cardiac output because of the early diastolic stiffness of transplanted hearts.

PRIMARY GRAFT FAILURE AND RV DYSFUNCTION

Graft failure is associated with increased short-term and long-term mortality. Primary graft failure is defined as the presence of severe mechanical dysfunction, requiring 2 inotropic agents or mechanical circulatory support, without anatomic or immunologic causes (ie, it is not the result of rejection).[7,27] Isolated RV failure is more common than biventricular failure and is one of the most serious complications of heart transplantation. Patients with isolated RV failure have high right atrial pressures (>20 mm Hg) with low pulmonary capillary wedge pressure (<10 mm Hg) and low cardiac output and arterial pressures.[7,28] It is essential to screen patients' PVR and transpulmonary gradients before listing them for transplantation and to monitor these pressures on a regular basis while waiting for transplantation in order to prevent this complication. Isolated LV failure is rare after heart transplantation, and should prompt investigation for coronary disease in the donor heart.[7]

The goal of therapy in graft failure is to reduce the RV afterload and preload while maintaining adequate RV preload. The blood pressures should be closely monitored in order to allow end-organ perfusion as well as RV coronary perfusion. Patients are usually treated with an inotropic agent (milrinone or a combination of dopamine and dobutamine) in addition to a vasodilatory agent, such as nitroprusside or nitroglycerine.[29] Prostaglandins and inhaled NO reduce the PVR with less systemic effect on blood pressures, allowing treatment in patients with borderline systemic blood pressures.[7,30] Sildenafil, a phosphodiesterase type 5 inhibitor, may be used as a treatment of RV dysfunction after transplantation.

Refractory patients should be treated with mechanical circulatory support (MCS). The ISHLT guidelines recommend that an intra-aortic balloon pump (IABP) should be used as the first option after pharmacologic therapy because it is the least invasive form of MCS.[7] Extracorporeal membrane oxygenation and ventricular assist devices (either right, left, or biventricular assist devices) should be used next in refractory cases. Although the rule should be that these MCS devices should be used for the shortest possible time because of the immunosuppression therapy and the risks of infection, when a ventricular assist device is implanted, weaning attempts should be made not sooner than 48 hours after the implantation.

Isolated RV failure may result in LV failure secondary to inadequate LV filling (decreased LV preload). These patients should be treated with IABP in addition to inotropes to allow a decrease in the LV afterload in addition to improvement in the RV perfusion.[7]

VALVULAR DYSFUNCTION

The most common valvular abnormality is tricuspid regurgitation (TR), occurring in 19% to 84% of patients, depending on the definition of significant regurgitation.[31] In the early stages after transplantation, most TR is functional and is mostly secondary to geometric distortion of the AV annular ring, and preservation of atrial and tricuspid annulus geometry may prevent the development of TR.[31] The ISHLT guidelines recommend that patients who are identified after surgery as having moderate to severe TR should have a repeat echocardiogram in the first 24 hours after the transplantation.[7] Most patients can be managed conservatively, mainly with diuretics, and only rarely do they require surgical intervention.[7]

The second common valvular abnormality is mitral regurgitation (MR), occurring in the perioperative period in more than 50% of all patients receiving transplants.[32] MR is usually mild, does not cause symptoms, and does not require treatment.[7]

SYSTEMIC VASODILATATION

Soon after the transplantation, some patients develop hypotension secondary to systemic vasodilatation. The exact cause for this vasodilatation is not clear and it may reflect a systemic inflammatory response syndrome secondary to cytokine release during the cardiopulmonary bypass (CPB). It may also reflect a deficiency in vasopressin or the preoperative use of vasodilating agents, such as ACE inhibitors.[7] Clinicians should always suspect the occurrence of sepsis in these patients, and perform a thorough investigation when appropriate.

Treatment varies according to the severity and responsiveness of the vasodilatation. Mild vasodilatation may be a response to single alpha-adrenergic agent, whereas more refractory and profound hypotension may require multiple vasoconstrictors. Low-dose arginine vasopressin[33] and methylene blue[34] have been used in severe refractory cases.

BLEEDING

Bleeding after heart transplantation can be subdivided into bleeding associated with the surgery and bleeding not associated with the surgery. Nonsurgical bleeding occurs secondary to coagulopathy that results from the CPB. CPB can cause coagulopathy for various reasons, mainly because of a decrease in both coagulation factors and platelets and activation of fibrinolysis. Inflammatory cascade may further promote the abnormal hemostasis. In addition, anticoagulation with IV heparin is routinely used before initiation of CPB, as well as hypothermia therapy, which is commonly used in many centers as part of the CPB procedure. Both anticoagulation and hypothermia may further exacerbate the abnormal hemostasis.

In order to decrease the risk of bleeding, patients treated with warfarin should have their International Normalized Ratio reversed before the transplantation, using vitamin K, fresh frozen plasma, prothrombin complex concentrates, or recombinant active factor VII (the last 2 of these therapies are not approved in the United States and are used only in Europe).[7]

Pharmacologic therapies for bleeding include aprotinin, tranexamic acid, and epsilon-aminocaproic acid. The last 2 agents are currently not approved by the US Food and Drug Administration. Aprotinin, a serine proteases inhibitor, decreased bleeding among patients after heart transplantation.[35] However, it may cause an increased risk of renal failure, myocardial infarction, heart failure, and stroke.[36] Tranexamic acid and epsilon-aminocaproic acid have antifibrinolytic activity, with tranexamic acid being 10 times more potent than epsilon-aminocaproic acid.[37] Unlike aprotinin, tranexamic acid and epsilon-aminocaproic acid do not cause cardiovascular and cerebral side effects.[37]

Prophylactic use of platelet transfusion and fresh frozen plasma is generally not recommended.[38] According to the guidelines, platelet transfusion should be given when there is bleeding with excessive blood loss and usually in cases in which the platelet count is less than 50,000/μL.[7]

SEPSIS

Infection remains a major complication among patients after transplantation, causing approximately 20% of the deaths within the first year after the transplantation as well as being a major cause of morbidity and mortality during the rest of the patient's life.[3]

Before transplantation, all patients must be vaccinated against pneumococcal and influenza infections. Soon after the procedure, prophylactic therapy against Pneumocystis carinii, Herpes simplex virus, and oral candidiasis should be started in all patients, and CMV-seropositive donors/seronegative recipients must be treated with valganciclovir as well.

During the first month after transplantation, most infections are nosocomial, related to the catheters, surgical procedure, and mechanical ventilation. Because these patients are immunosuppressed, various infections, including protozoal, fungal, bacterial, and viral, may occur, with mortality being the highest with fungal infections. Viral infection, especially CMV, may enhance immunosuppression, causing a vicious cycle that may result in secondary infection.[3]

The clinical presentation of sepsis may vary among patients after transplantation, from mild or atypical symptoms to severe refractory shock. Thus, a high level of vigilance is warranted in order to diagnose and treat these patients in the early stages of the infection. Therapy includes broad-spectrum antibiotics, with or without antiviral and antifungal agents, as the clinical suspicions mandate. In addition, clinicians should consider decreasing the immunosuppressive therapy in accordance with the severity of the infection. Many patients are treated with steroids for many months to years after the transplantation. These patients should be treated with stress-dosage steroids during the acute infectious episode.

In conclusion, managing patients after heart transplantation is challenging. These patients have unique clinical complications (associated with the immunosuppressive therapy and cardiac allograft rejection) together with atypical clinical presentations for infection and systemic inflammatory response syndrome. High vigilance, early diagnosis, and appropriate intervention for allograft-related and non–allograft-related syndromes with significant morbidity and mortality are the keys to the long-term survival of patients after transplantation.

REFERENCES

1. United Health Group. Transplant review guidelines. 2013.
2. Lindenfeld J, Miller GG, Shakar SF, et al. Drug therapy in the heart transplant recipient: part II: immunosuppressive drugs. Circulation 2004;110(25):3858–65.
3. Acker MA, Jessup M. Surgical management of heart failure. In: Bonow RO, Mann DL, Zipes DP, et al, editors. Braunwald's heart disease: a textbook of cardiovascular medicine. 9th edition. St. Louis (MO): Elsevier Saunders; 2012. p. 601–16.
4. Singh N, Pirsch J, Samaniego M. Antibody-mediated rejection: treatment alternatives and outcomes. Transplant Rev (Orlando) 2009;23(1):34–46.
5. Stewart S, Winters GL, Fishbein MC, et al. Revision of the 1990 working formulation for the standardization of nomenclature in the diagnosis of heart rejection. J Heart Lung Transplant 2005;24(11):1710–20.
6. Jessup M, Brozena S. State-of-the-art strategies for immunosuppression. Curr Opin Organ Transplant 2007;12:536.
7. Costanzo MR, Dipchand A, Starling R, et al. The International Society of Heart and Lung Transplantation guidelines for the care of heart transplant recipients. J Heart Lung Transplant 2010;29(8):914–56.
8. Schmauss D, Weis M. Cardiac allograft vasculopathy: recent developments. Circulation 2008;117(16):2131–41.
9. Taylor DO, Edwards LB, Boucek MM, et al. Registry of the International Society for Heart and Lung Transplantation: twenty-third official adult heart transplantation report: 2006. J Heart Lung Transplant 2006;25:869–79.
10. Weis M, von Scheidt W. Coronary artery disease in the transplanted heart. Annu Rev Med 2000;51:81–100.
11. Stork S, Behr TM, Birk M, et al. Assessment of cardiac allograft vasculopathy late after heart transplantation: when is coronary angiography necessary? J Heart Lung Transplant 2006;25:1103–8.
12. Ciliberto GR, Massa D, Mangiavacchi M, et al. High-dose dipyridamole echocardiography test in coronary artery disease after heart transplantation. Eur Heart J 1993;14:48–52.

13. Spes CH, Mudra H, Schnaack S, et al. Dobutamine stress echocardiography for noninvasive diagnosis of cardiac allograft vasculopathy a comparison with angiography and intravascular ultrasound. Am J Cardiol 1996;78:168–74.
14. Carlsen J, Toft JC, Mortensen SA, et al. Myocardial perfusion scintigraphy as a screening method for significant coronary artery stenosis in cardiac transplant recipients. J Heart Lung Transplant 2000;19:873–8.
15. Sigurdsson G, Carrascosa P, Yamani MH, et al. Detection of transplant coronary artery disease using multidetector computed tomography with adaptative multisegment reconstruction. J Am Coll Cardiol 2006;48:772–8.
16. Wenke K, Meiser B, Thiery J, et al. Simvastatin initiated early after heart transplantation: 8-year prospective experience. Circulation 2003;107:93–7.
17. Steinhauff S, Pehlivanli S, Bakovic-Alt R, et al. Beneficial effects of quinaprilat on coronary vasomotor function, endothelial oxidative stress, and endothelin activation after human heart transplantation. Transplantation 2004;77:1859–65.
18. Bae JH, Rihal CS, Edwards BS, et al. Association of angiotensin-converting enzyme inhibitors and serum lipids with plaque regression in cardiac allograft vasculopathy. Transplantation 2006;82:1108–11.
19. Schroeder JS, Gao SZ, Alderman EL, et al. A preliminary study of diltiazem in the prevention of coronary artery disease in heart-transplant recipients. N Engl J Med 1993;328:164–70.
20. Mancini D, Pinney S, Burkhoff D, et al. Use of rapamycin slows progression of cardiac transplantation vasculopathy. Circulation 2003;108:48–53.
21. Streblow DN, Orloff SL, Nelson JA. Acceleration of allograft failure by cytomegalovirus. Curr Opin Immunol 2007;19:577–82.
22. Valantine HA. Cardiac allograft vasculopathy: central role of endothelial injury leading to transplant "atheroma." Transplantation 2003;76:891–9.
23. Fearon WF, Potena L, Hirohata A, et al. Changes in coronary arterial dimensions early after cardiac transplantation. Transplantation 2007;83:700–5.
24. Musci M, Loebe M, Wellnhofer E, et al. Coronary angioplasty, bypass surgery, and retransplantation in cardiac transplant patients with graft coronary disease. Thorac Cardiovasc Surg 1998;46:268–74.
25. Leeman M, Van CM, Vachiery JL, et al. Determinants of right ventricular failure after heart transplantation. Acta Cardiol 1996;51(5):441–9.
26. Sethi GK, Lanauze P, Rosado LJ, et al. Clinical significance of weight difference between donor and recipient in heart transplantation. J Thorac Cardiovasc Surg 1993;106(3):444–8.
27. Segovia J, Pulpon LA, Sanmartin M, et al. Primary graft failure in heart transplantation: a multivariate analysis. Transplant Proc 1998;30(5):1932.
28. Marasco SF, Esmore DS, Negri J, et al. Early institution of mechanical support improves outcomes in primary cardiac allograft failure. J Heart Lung Transplant 2005;24(12):2037–42.
29. Stobierska-Dzierzek B, Awad H, Michler RE. The evolving management of acute right-sided heart failure in cardiac transplant recipients. J Am Coll Cardiol 2001; 38(4):923–31.
30. Kieler-Jensen N, Lundin S, Ricksten SE. Vasodilator therapy after heart transplantation: effects of inhaled nitric oxide and intravenous prostacyclin, prostaglandin E1, and sodium nitroprusside. J Heart Lung Transplant 1995;14(3): 436–43.
31. Wong RC, Abrahams Z, Hanna M, et al. Tricuspid regurgitation after cardiac transplantation: an old problem revisited. J Heart Lung Transplant 2008;27(3): 247–52.

32. Rees AP, Milani RV, Lavie CJ, et al. Valvular regurgitation and right-sided cardiac pressures in heart transplant recipients by complete Doppler and color flow evaluation. Chest 1993;104(1):82–7.
33. Argenziano M, Choudhri AF, Oz MC, et al. A prospective randomized trial of arginine vasopressin in the treatment of vasodilatory shock after left ventricular assist device placement. Circulation 1997;96(Suppl 9). II-286-90.
34. Leyh RG, Kofidis T, Struber M, et al. Methylene blue: the drug of choice for catecholamine-refractory vasoplegia after cardiopulmonary bypass? J Thorac Cardiovasc Surg 2003;125(6):1426–31.
35. Prendergast TW, Furukawa S, Beyer AJ III, et al. Defining the role of aprotinin in heart transplantation. Ann Thorac Surg 1996;62(3):670–4.
36. Mangano DT, Tudor IC, Dietzel C. The risk associated with aprotinin in cardiac surgery. N Engl J Med 2006;354(4):353–65.
37. Karkouti K, Beattie WS, Dattilo KM, et al. A propensity score case-control comparison of aprotinin and tranexamic acid in high-transfusion-risk cardiac surgery. Transfusion 2006;46(3):327–38.
38. Fremes SE, Wong BI, Lee E, et al. Metaanalysis of prophylactic drug treatment in the prevention of postoperative bleeding. Ann Thorac Surg 1994;58(6):1580–8.

Index

Note: Page numbers of article titles are in **boldface** type.

Crit Care Clin 30 (2014) 639–655
http://dx.doi.org/10.1016/S0749-0704(14)00042-6
0749-0704/14/$ – see front matter © 2014 Elsevier Inc. All rights reserved.

criticalcare.theclinics.com

648 Index

Moving?

Make sure your subscription moves with you!

To notify us of your new address, find your **Clinics Account Number** (located on your mailing label above your name), and contact customer service at:

Email: journalscustomerservice-usa@elsevier.com

800-654-2452 (subscribers in the U.S. & Canada)
314-447-8871 (subscribers outside of the U.S. & Canada)

Fax number: 314-447-8029

Elsevier Health Sciences Division
Subscription Customer Service
3251 Riverport Lane
Maryland Heights, MO 63043

*To ensure uninterrupted delivery of your subscription, please notify us at least 4 weeks in advance of move.

Printed and bound by CPI Group (UK) Ltd, Croydon, CR0 4YY

03/10/2024

01040491-0012